BIOLOGY AND TREATMENT OF COLORECTAL CANCER METASTASIS

DEVELOPMENTS IN ONCOLOGY

F.J. Cleton and J.W.I.M. Simons, eds.: Genetic Origins of Tumour Cells. 90-247-2272-1.
J. Aisner and P. Chang, eds.: Cancer Treatment and Research. 90-247-2358-2.
B.W. Ongerboer de Visser, D.A. Bosch and W.M.H. van Woerkom-Eykenboom, eds.: Neuro-oncology: Clinical and Experimental Aspects. 90-247-2421-X.
K. Hellmann, P. Hilgard and S. Eccles, eds.: Metastasis: Clinical and Experimental Aspects. 90-247-2424-4.
H.F. Seigler, ed.: Clinical Management of Melanoma. 90-247-2584-4.
P. Correa and W. Haenszel, eds.: Epidemiology of Cancer of the Digestive Tract. 90-247-2601-8.
L.A. Liotta and I.R. Hart, eds.: Tumour Invasion and Metastasis. 90-247-2611-5.
J. Banoczy, ed.: Oral Leukoplakia. 90-247-2655-7.
C. Tijssen, M. Halprin and L. Endtz, eds.: Familial Brain Tumours. 90-247-2691-3.
F.M. Muggia, C.W. Young and S.K. Carter, eds.: Anthracycline Antibiotics in Cancer. 90-247-2711-1.
B.W. Hancock, ed.: Assessment of Tumour Response. 90-247-2712-X.
D.E. Peterson, ed.: Oral Complications of Cancer Chemotherapy. 0-89838-563-6.
R. Mastrangelo, D.G. Poplack and R. Riccardi, eds.: Central Nervous System Leukemia. Prevention and Treatment. 0-89838-570-9.
A. Polliack, ed.: Human Leukemias. Cytochemical and Ultrastructural Techniques in Diagnosis and Research. 0-89838-585-7.
W. Davis, C. Maltoni and S. Tanneberger, eds.: The Control of Tumor Growth and its Biological Bases. 0-89838-603-9.
A.P.M. Heintz, C. Th. Griffiths and J.B. Trimbos, eds.: Surgery in Gynecological Oncology. 0-89838-604-7.
M.P. Hacker, E.B. Double and I. Krakoff, eds.: Platinum Coordination Complexes in Cancer Chemotherapy. 0-89838-619-5.
M.J. van Zwieten. The Rat as Animal Model in Breast Cancer Research: A Histopathological Study of Radiation- and Hormone-Induced Rat Mammary Tumors. 0-89838-624-1.
B. Lowenberg and A. Hogenbeck, eds.: Minimal Residual Disease in Acute Leukemia. 0-89838-630-6.
I. van der Waal and G.B. Snow, eds.: Oral Oncology. 0-89838-631-4.
B.W. Hancock and A.M. Ward, eds.: Immunological Aspects of Cancer. 0-89838-664-0.
K.V. Honn and B.F. Sloane, eds.: Hemostatic Mechanisms and Metastasis. 0-89838-667-5.
K.R. Harrap, W. Davis and A.N. Calvert, eds.: Cancer Chemotherapy and Selective Drug Development. 0-89838-673-X.
V.D. Velde, J.H. Cornelis and P.H. Sugarbaker, eds.: Liver Metastasis. 0-89838-648-5.
D.J. Ruiter, K. Welvaart and S. Ferrone, eds.: Cutaneous Melanoma and Precursor Lesions. 0-89838-689-6.
S.B. Howell, ed.: Intra-Arterial and Intracavitary Cancer Chemotherapy. 0-89838-691-8.
D.L. Kisner and J.F. Smyth, eds.: Interferon Alpha-2: Pre-Clinical and Clinical Evaluation. 0-89838-701-9.
P. Furmanski, J.C. Hager and M.A. Rich, eds.: RNA Tumor Viruses, Oncogenes, Human Cancer and Aids: On the Frontiers of Understanding. 0-89838-703-5.
J.E. Talmadge, I.J. Fidler and R.K. Oldham: Screening for Biological Response Modifiers: Methods and Rationale. 0-89838-712-4.
J.C. Bottino, R.W. Opfell and F.M. Muggia, eds.: Liver Cancer. 0-89838-713-2.
P.K. Pattengale, R.J. Lukes and C.R. Taylor, eds.: Lymphoproliferative Diseases: Pathogenesis, Diagnosis, Therapy. 0-89838-725-6.
F. Cavalli, G. Bonadonna and M. Rozencweig, eds.: Malignant Lymphomas and Hodgkin's Disease. 0-89838-727-2.
L. Baker, F. Valeriote and V. Ratanatharathorn, eds.: Biology and Therapy of Acute Leukemia. 0-89838-728-0.
J. Russo, ed.: Immunocytochemistry in Tumor Diagnosis. 0-89838-737-X.
R.L. Ceriani, ed.: Monoclonal Antibodies and Breast Cancer. 0-89838-739-6.
D.E. Peterson, G.E. Elias and S.T. Sonis, eds.: Head and Neck Management of the Cancer Patient. 0-89838-747-7.
D.M. Green: Diagnosis and management of Malignant Solid Tumors in Infants and Children. 0-89838-750-7.
K.A. Foon and A.C. Morgan, Jr., eds.: Monoclonal Antibody Therapy of Human Cancer. 0-89838-754-X.
J.G. McVie, et al, eds., Clinical and Experimental Pathology of Lung Cancer. 0-89838-764-7.
K.V. Honn, W.E. Powers and B.F. Sloane, eds.: Mechanisms of Cancer Metastasis. 0-89838-765-5.
K. Lapis, L.A. Liotta and A.S. Rabson, eds.: Biochemistry and Molecular Genetics of Cancer Metastasis. 0-89838-785-X.

BIOLOGY AND TREATMENT OF COLORECTAL CANCER METASTASIS

Proceedings of the
National Large Bowel Cancer Project
1984 Conference on Biology and Treatment of
Colorectal Cancer Metastasis
Houston, Texas — September 13–15, 1984

edited by

Anthony J. Mastromarino
The University of Texas System Cancer Center
M. D. Anderson Hospital and Tumor Institute
Texas Medical Center
Houston, Texas

Martinus Nijhoff Publishing
a member of the Kluwer Academic Publishers Group
Boston/Dordrecht/Lancaster

Distributors for North America:
Kluwer Academic Publishers
190 Old Derby Street
Hingham, Massachusetts 02043, USA

Distributors for the UK and Ireland:
Kluwer Academic Publishers
MTP Press Limited
Falcon House, Queen Square
Lancaster LA1 1RN, UNITED KINGDOM

Distributors for all other countries:
Kluwer Academic Publishers Group
Distribution Centre
Post Office Box 322
3300 AH Dordrecht, THE NETHERLANDS

Library of Congress Cataloging-in-Publication Data

National Large Bowel Cancer Project Conference on
   Biology and Treatment of Colorectal Cancer
   Metastasis (1984 : Houston, Tex.)
   Biology and treatment of colorectal cancer
metastasis.

   (Developments in oncology)
   Includes bibliographies and index.
   1. Colon (Anatomy)—Cancer—Congresses. 2. Rectum—
Cancer—Congresses. 3. Metastasis—Congresses.
4. Liver—Cancer—Congresses. I. Mastromarino,
Anthony J. II. National Large Bowel Cancer Project
(U.S.) III. Title. IV. Series. [DNLM: 1. Colonic
Neoplasms—congresses. 2. Neoplasm Metastasis—
congresses. 3. Rectal Neoplasms—congresses.
W1 DE998N / WI 520 N2775b]
RC280.C6N38   1984   616.99 '4347   85–29747
ISBN-13:978-1-4612-9417-7   e-ISBN-13:978-1-4613-2301-3
DOI: 10.1007/978-1-4613-2301-3

The proceedings of the final National Large Bowel Cancer Project workshop are dedicated to all the individuals, including the many grantees of the project, who contributed to its success, with special remembrance of the contributions of Dr. Murray M. Copeland. Throughout the history of the National Large Bowel Cancer Project, the primary goal of all the research conducted was understanding the biology of colorectal cancer, its early detection, and more efficacious therapy for improved patient care and management. This volume is written with the hope that research knowledge derived with support from the National Large Bowel Cancer Project will be of benefit to all the patients diagnosed with colorectal cancer.

CONTENTS

CONTRIBUTING AUTHORS   xi

PREFACE   xv

ACKNOWLEDGMENTS   xxi

I. The Biology of Colorectal Cancer Metastasis

1. Natural History of Liver Metastasis and Resective Treat-
    ment
    Martin A. Adson   3

2. The Use of Nude Mice to Ascertain the Malignant Capacity
    of Human Colon Cancer
    Ian R. Hart   23

3. The Cotton-Top Tamarin as an Animal Model of Colorectal
    Cancer Metastasis
    Neal K. Clapp, Clarence C. Lushbaugh, Gretchen L. Humason,
    Barbara L. Gangaware, and Marsha A. Henke   31

4. Clinicopathologic Studies on Mechanisms of Metastasis
    in Man and Other Vertebrates
    David Tarin   41

5. Metastatic Colorectal Carcinoma: Pathobiologic Subsets
    Lewis A. Johnson   53

6. The Use of Lectins in Biochemical Studies on Colorectal
    Carcinoma Metastasis
    Tatsuro Irimura, David M. Ota, Karen R. Cleary, and Garth L.
    Nicolson   57

II. Controversies in the Management of Patients with Colorectal Cancer Metastasis

7. Quality of Life: A Cerebral Affair
    Frank Adams and Theresa Adams   75

8. Quality of Life and Cost Effectiveness Issues in the
    Management of Patients with Hepatic Metastases from
    Colorectal Cancer
    Paul H. Sugarbaker, Martin A. Adson, Ivan Barofsky, Edward M.
    Copeland III, Sallie Martin Foley, Kevin S. Hughes, Frank E. Jones,
    M. Margaret Kemeny, Bernard Levin, Philip D. Schneider,
    Marshall Urist, and Paul V. Woolloy, III   83

III. The Prevention and Local Treatment of Colorectal Metastasis

9. Regional Infusion Chemotherapy for Colorectal Hepatic
    Metastases
    John M. Daly and Nancy Kemeny   101

10. Local Surgical Treatment of Hepatic Metastases from Colorectal Carcinoma: Survival Times and Sites of Recurrence
    Nicholas J. Petrelli, Lemuel Herrera, and Arnold Mittelman   117

11. Endoscopic Laser Surgery for Colonic Neoplasia
    John H. Bowers, Randall W. Burt, and John A. Dixon   129

12. Pharmacokinetics of Hepatic Arterial Chemotherapy
    William D. Ensminger and John W. Gyves   137

13. Adjuvant Radiation Therapy for Colorectal Cancer
    Tyvin A. Rich   145

14. Hepatic Resection for Colorectal Carcinoma Metastases: Present Status and Future Prospects
    Kevin S. Hughes, David A. August, Reyer T. Ottow, and Paul H. Sugarbaker   159

15. New Diagnostic Techniques in Hepatic Mass Detection
    Michael E. Bernardino   179

16. Predictive Assays of Clinical Response for Primary and Metastatic Colorectal Cancer
    Daniel D. Von Hoff   187

17. Radiolabeled Antibodies for Gastrointestinal Malignancies
    Stanley E. Order   197

IV. Criteria of Response

18. Problems with Response Criteria
    Philip T. Lavin   211

19. Accuracy of Diagnostic Techniques with Follow-Up and Evaluation of Disease Recurrence
    Michael E. Bernardino   225

20. The Evaluation of Serial Marker Measurements for Monitoring Patients at Risk of Recurrent Cancer: Application to Colorectal Cancer
    Mitchell H. Gail   235

21. Prognostic Factors for Liver Metastases from Colorectal Cancer
    Daniel G. Haller   253

V. Analysis of Failure

22. Clinical Patterns of Failure After Resection of Colon and Rectum Carcinoma Metastases to the Liver
    Glenn D. Steele, Jr.   267

23.   Drug Resistance in Colon Cancer
      Gregory A. Curt and Bruce A. Chabner   281

24.   Biology of Colon Cancer Resistance to Treatment
      Paul V. Woolley, III, Daniel D. Von Hoff, Gregg W. Kyle,
      Shailendra Kumar, Robert A. Nagourney, Thu-Trang P. Luc,
      and Kenneth L. Mossman   295

25.   Circumvention of Neoplastic Heterogeneity by System-
      ically Activated Macrophages
      Isaiah J. Fidler, J. Milburn Jessup, Eugenie S. Kleinerman,
      William E. Fogler, and Amitabha Mazumder   311

INDEX   323

CONTRIBUTING AUTHORS

Frank Adams, M.D., FRCP(C)
Department of Internal Medicine
The University of Texas System
  Cancer Center
M. D. Anderson Hospital and Tumor
  Institute
6723 Bertner Avenue
Houston, Texas 77030

Theresa Adams, B.A.
Department of Chemotherapy Research
The University of Texas System
  Cancer Center
M. D. Anderson Hospital and Tumor
  Institute
6723 Bertner Avenue
Houston, Texas 77030

Martin A. Adson, M.D.
Mayo Medical School
200 First Street, S.W.
Rochester, Minnesota 55905

David A. August, M.D.
Surgery Branch
Division of Cancer Treatment
National Cancer Institute
Bethesda, Maryland 20892

Ivan Barofsky, Ph.D.
Institute of Social Oncology
Silver Spring, Maryland 20904

Michael E. Bernardino, M.D.
Department of Radiology
Emory University School of Medicine
1365 Clifton Road, N.E.
Atlanta, Georgia 30322

John H. Bowers, M.D.
Department of Surgery
University of Utah School of Medicine
4E504 Medical Center
Salt Lake City, Utah 84132

Randall W. Burt, M.D.
Department of Internal Medicine
University of Utah School of Medicine
4E504 Medical Center
Salt Lake City, Utah 84132

Bruce A. Chabner, M.D.
Division of Cancer Treatment
National Cancer Institute
Building 31, Room 3A52
Bethesda, Maryland 20892

Neal K. Clapp, D.V.M., Ph.D.
Marmoset Research Program
Oak Ridge Associated Universities
Medical and Health Sciences Division
P.O. Box 117
Oak Ridge, Tennessee 37831-0117

Karen R. Cleary, M.D.
Department of Pathology
The University of Texas System
  Cancer Center
M. D. Anderson Hospital and Tumor
  Institute
6723 Bertner Avenue
Houston, Texas 77030

Edward M. Copeland III, M.D.
Department of Surgery
University of Florida College of
  Medicine
Box J 286
J. Hillis Miller Health Center
Gainesville, Florida 32610

Gregory A. Curt, M.D.
Division of Cancer Treatment
National Cancer Institute
Building 31, Room 3A52
Bethesda, Maryland 20892

John M. Daly, M.D.
Department of Surgery
Memorial Sloan-Kettering Cancer Center
1275 York Avenue
New York, New York 10021

John A. Dixon, M.D.
Department of Surgery
University of Utah School of Medicine
4E504 Medical Center
Salt Lake City, Utah 84132

William D. Ensminger, Ph.D., M.D.
Department of Internal Medicine and
 Pharmacology
Upjohn Center for Clinical Pharmacology
The University of Michigan Medical
 School
3709 Upjohn Center
Ann Arbor, Michigan 48109

Isaiah J. Fidler, D.V.M., Ph.D.
Department of Cell Biology
The University of Texas System
 Cancer Center
M. D. Anderson Hospital and Tumor
 Institute
6723 Bertner Avenue
Houston, Texas 77030

William E. Fogler, Ph.D.
Department of Cell Biology
The University of Texas System
 Cancer Center
M. D. Anderson Hospital and Tumor
 Institute
6723 Bertner Avenue
Houston, Texas 77030

Sallie Martin Foley, M.S.W.
Dept. of Ambulatory Care Social Work
The University of Michigan
Upjohn Center for Clinical Pharmacology
W4642 Clinical Research Center
Ann Arbor, Michigan 48109

Mitchell H. Gail, M.D., Ph.D.
Biometry Branch
Division of Cancer Prevention and
 Control
National Cancer Institute
Landow Building, Room 3C37
Bethesda, Maryland 20892

Barbara L. Gangaware, B.S.
Oak Ridge Associated Universities
P.O. Box 117
Oak Ridge, Tennessee 37831-0117

John W. Gyves, M.D.
Dept. of Internal Medicine and
 Pharmacology
Upjohn Center for Clinical Pharmacology
University of Michigan Medical School
3709 Upjohn Center
Ann Arbor, Michigan 48109

Daniel G. Haller, M.D.
Department of Medicine
Hospital of the University of
 Pennsylvania
3400 Spruce Street
Philadelphia, Pennsylvania 19104

Ian R. Hart, D.V.M., Ph.D.
Biology of Metastasis Laboratory
Imperial Cancer Research Fund
 Laboratories
P.O. Box 123
Lincoln's Inn Field
London, England WC2A 3PX
United Kingdom

Marsha A. Henke, M.S.
Oak Ridge Associated Universities
P.O. Box 117
Oak Ridge, Tennessee 37831-0117

Lemuel Herrera, M.D.
Department of Surgical Oncology
New York State Department of Health
Roswell Park Memorial Institute
666 Elm Street
Buffalo, New York 14263

Kevin S. Hughes, M.D.
Surgery Branch
Division of Cancer Treatment
National Cancer Institute
Bethesda, Maryland 20892

Gretchen L. Humason, M.S.
Oak Ridge Associated Universities
P.O. Box 117
Oak Ridge, Tennessee 37831-0117

Tatsuro Irimura, Ph.D.
Department of Tumor Biology
The University of Texas System
 Cancer Center
M. D. Anderson Hospital and Tumor
 Institute
6723 Bertner Avenue
Houston, Texas 77030

J. Milburn Jessup, M.D.
Department of Surgery
The University of Texas System
  Cancer Center
M. D. Anderson Hospital and Tumor
  Institute
6723 Bertner Avenue
Houston, Texas 77030

Lewis A. Johnson, M.D.
Department of Pathology
Roger Williams General Hospital
825 Chalkstone Avenue
Providence, Rhode Island 02908

Frank E. Jones, M.D.
Department of Surgery
Medical College of Wisconsin
8700 W. Wisconsin Avenue
Milwaukee, Wisconsin 53226

Margaret Kemeny, M.D.
Dept. of General and Oncology Surgery
City of Hope Hospital
1500 E. Duarte Road
Duarte, California 91010

Nancy Kemeny, M.D.
Memorial Sloan-Kettering Cancer Center
1275 York Avenue
New York, New York 10021

Eugenie S. Kleinerman, M.D.
Department of Cell Biology
The University of Texas System
  Cancer Center
M. D. Anderson Hospital and Tumor
  Institute
6723 Bertner Avenue
Houston, Texas 77030

Gregg W. Kyle, M.S.
Division of Medical Oncology
Georgetown University Medical Center
800 Reservoir Road, N.W.
Washington, D.C. 20007

Shailendra Kumar, M.S.
Division of Medical Oncology
Georgetown University Medical Center
800 Reservoir Road, N.W.
Washington, D.C. 20007

Philip T. Lavin, Ph.D.
Consulting Statisticians, Inc.
A Crowntek Company
20 William Street
Wellesley Hills, Massachusetts 02181

Bernard Levin, M.D.
Division of Medicine
The University of Texas System
  Cancer Center
M. D. Anderson Hospital and Tumor
  Institute
6723 Bertner Avenue
Houston, Texas 77030

Thu-Trang P. Luc, B.A.
Division of Medical Oncology
Georgetown University Medical Center
800 Reservoir Road, N.W.
Washington, D.C. 20007

Clarence C. Lushbaugh, Ph.D., M.D.
Medical and Health Sciences Division
Oak Ridge Associated Universities
P.O. Box 117
Oak Ridge, Tennessee 37831-0117

Amitabha Mazumder, M.D.
Department of Medicine
Baylor College of Medicine
1 Baylor Plaza
Houston, Texas 77030

Arnold Mittelman, M.D.
Department of Surgical Oncology
New York State Department of Health
Roswell Park Memorial Institute
666 Elm Street
Buffalo, New York 14263

Kenneth L. Mossman, Ph.D.
Division of Medical Oncology
Georgetown University Medical Center
800 Reservoir Road, N.W.
Washington, D.C. 20007

Robert A. Nagourney, M.D.
Division of Medical Oncology
Georgetown University Medical Center
800 Reservoir Road, N.W.
Washington, D.C. 20007

Garth L. Nicolson, Ph.D.
Department of Tumor Biology
The University of Texas System
  Cancer Center
M. D. Anderson Hospital and Tumor
  Institute
6723 Bertner Avenue
Houston, Texas 77030

Stanley E. Order, M.D., Sc.D.
Department of Radiation Oncology
Johns Hopkins Hospital
600 N. Wolfe Street
Baltimore, Maryland 21205

David M. Ota, M.D.
Division of Surgery
The University of Texas System
  Cancer Center
M. D. Anderson Hospital and Tumor
  Institute
6723 Bertner Avenue
Houston, Texas 77030

Reyer T. Ottow, M.D.
Surgery Branch
Division of Cancer Treatment
National Cancer Institute
Bethesda, Maryland 20892

Nicholas J. Petrelli, M.D.
Department of Surgical Oncology
New York State Department of Health
Roswell Park Memorial Institute
666 Elm Street
Buffalo, New York 14263

Tyvin A. Rich, M.D.
Department of Radiotherapy
The University of Texas System
  Cancer Center
M. D. Anderson Hospital and Tumor
  Institute
6723 Bertner Avenue
Houston, Texas 77030

Philip D. Schneider, M.D., Ph.D.
Department of Surgery
University of California, Davis
4301 X Street
Sacramento, California 95817

Glenn D. Steele, Jr., M.D., Ph.D.
Department of Surgery
New England Deaconess Hospital
110 Francis Street
Boston, Massachusetts 02115

Paul H. Sugarbaker, M.D.
Surgery Branch
Division of Cancer Treatment
National Cancer Institute
Building 10, Room 2B07
Bethesda, Maryland 20892

David Tarin, D.M., M.R.C.Path
Nuffield Department of Pathology
University of Oxford
John Radcliffe Hospital
Headington, Oxford
0X3 9DU England

Marshall Urist, M.D.
Department of Surgery
University of Alabama at Birmingham
320 Kracke Building
Birmingham, Alabama 35294

Daniel Von Hoff, M.D.
Department of Medicine
The University of Texas Health Science
  Center at San Antonio
7703 Floyd Curl Drive
San Antonio, Texas 78284

Paul V. Woolley, III, M.D.
Division of Medical Oncology
Georgetown University Medical Center
800 Reservoir Road, N.W.
Washington, D.C. 20007

xiv

PREFACE

The theme of the current workshop was identified several years ago and was considered by the working group of the National Large Bowel Cancer Project to be an appropriate workshop topic. Although the subject was important then, it was not possible to conduct such a workshop at that time. In the interim, not only did the problems associated with colorectal metastasis still exist, but new insights on the biology and treatment of colorectal cancer metastasis emerged, making the workshop topic especially important and relevant. With input from an expert Planning Committee, a unique program was designed to provide an opportunity for information exchange between basic scientists and clinical investigators.

The published proceedings reflect the organization of the workshop which consisted of five sections:

Section I.   The Biology of Colorectal Cancer Metastasis co-chaired by Drs. J. Isaiah Fidler and George Poste
Section II.   Controversies in the Management of Patients with Colorectal Cancer Metastasis co-chaired by Drs. Edward M. Copeland, III and Frank Adams
Section III.   The Prevention and Local Treatment of Colorectal Metastasis co-chaired by Drs. Nicholas Petrelli and Paul V. Woolley, III
Section IV.   Criteria of Response co-chaired by Drs. Philip T. Lavin and Bernard Levin
Section V.   Analysis of Failure co-chaired by Drs. Glenn D. Steele, Jr. and John Marsh

The chapters examine relevant questions related to the clinical management of patients with hepatic metastases from colorectal cancer and the important, but less well-defined issue, their quality of life; the better design and evaluation of clinical trials; and the biologic phenomenon associated with metastasis. In so doing, questions were posed and potential approaches were suggested for examining problems and analyzing results.

Of the 138,000 new cases of colorectal cancer in the United States in 1985, an estimated 60,000 will die and the five-year survival, which is related to the stage of disease at diagnosis, is only 44%. Although primary prevention and early detection are desirable goals, the fact is that too many patients present with more advanced disease at diagnosis. The prognosis for those patients presenting with distant metastasis at diagnosis or with recurrent metastatic disease is not good. The chapters of this volume examine an important clinical problem and the advances being made in the clinic as well as the problems, complexities, and approaches associated with studying colorectal cancer metastasis experimentally. Despite these complexities, experimental strategies are emerging which may result in progress for the more effective therapy of this disease.

The first six chapters (Section I) examine the natural history of hepatic metastases in colorectal cancer in a retrospective study of patients with biopsy-proven, hepatic metastases that were not resected, a variety of models of metastases using three different species (the nude mouse, the marmoset, and man), careful histological and cytological differentiation and classification of colon tumors as prognostic factors, and the inherent biological properties of colorectal cancer metastases. Collectively, these chapters address a formidable problem facing clinicians and laboratory investigators, namely, tumor cell heterogeneity. Looking at the natural history of this disease process as well as using model systems and biochemical approaches, attempts are made to define what it is that endows particular colon tumor cells with the ability to metastasize selectively and at what stage in tumor progression these metastatic colon tumor cells emerge. The variety of approaches offer new avenues of practical and experimental significance.

Chapters 7 and 8 (Section II) address the complex issue involving controversies in the management of patients with colorectal cancer metastases. The focus of this section is on the issues affecting quality of life. Two themes emerged. The first is the need to develop and incorporate quality of life parameters by which to assess various treatments in clinical trials, and the second is an adequate neuropsychiatric assessment of patients with cancer with special emphasis on brain-behavior relations in oncology. Clearly, doing something simply for the sake of doing something may not always be wise. In selecting treatment options, patients should be evaluated thoroughly, spoken with compassionately, listened to, and involved in choosing the most therapeutically-effective and cost-effective approach.

The third section focuses on approaches to the prevention and treatment of colorectal metastases. Taken together, these nine chapters review recent data from studies using a variety of procedures that may offer better therapeutic response or assist in selecting more effective therapeutic approaches for patients with hepatic metastases from colorectal cancer. One such study compared the response rates and survival data for patients treated with systemic infusion versus intra-arterial infusion therapy. Not unsurprisingly, many patients on systemic infusion developed liver disease while patients on intrahepatic therapy had extrahepatic disease progression without liver progression. This suggests the possibility of combining these two approaches to optimize control, and to maximize response rate and duration of response to hepatic and extrahepatic disease. Two studies describe the selective advantage of hepatic resection for metastases from colorectal carcinoma in carefully selected subsets of patients. These two studies call attention to the relative safety of hepatic resection as a surgical procedure, the tendency for recurrence in extrahepatic sites, the need to include matched, untreated controls in study designs, and the obvious need for more effective therapeutic agents.

The potential role of laser surgery in the palliative treatment of patients with colorectal cancer is described. Efforts to achieve selective therapy using pharmacokinetic data as a rationale for prolonged regional infusion are also presented. The advantages of adjuvant radiotherapy for colorectal cancer is reviewed, including approaches to minimize the irradiation of underlying organs and tissues during radiotherapy for colon cancer. Two important questions are raised relative to the use of radiotherapy for patients with rectal cancer. The first relates to the optimal dose of preoperative radiotherapy and the second to the selection criteria used in selecting rectal cancer patients to be treated with radiotherapy.

This section concludes with chapters reviewing newer, sophisticated diagnostic and staging techniques for imaging the liver, the current role of the clonogenic assay of colon tumors in predicting clinical response and in selecting therapeutic regimens, and the use of radiolabelled antibodies for diagnosis and therapy of colorectal cancer metastases. Despite advancing diagnostic technologies, at present computerized tomographic scans remain the modality of choice for diagnosis and follow-up of patients with hepatic metastases from colorectal cancer. Optimization of this modality is possible using delayed iodine imaging. Although the clonogenic assay is reproducible, methodological inadequacies, including poor tumor growth and low plating efficiency exist. At present this approach represents an experimental research tool only and currently has no place in the clinical management of patients with colorectal cancer. However, new approaches are being evaluated to improve the assay so that it may be predictive of clinical response. Finally, a balanced appraisal of the methodologies, limitations, and potential applicability of using radiolabelled antibodies for diagnosis and therapy is presented. At present, this approach is still experimental.

A recurring theme throughout the workshop was the lack of adequate definition of terms, many of which are fundamental to interpreting and comparing data reported in the literature. Thus, the fourth section adresses the topic of criteria of response. The first of the four chapters in this section presents an overview of the concerns and questions of more than theoretical interest relative to response criteria, including deficiencies and defining categories of response. Four models and several methods of measuring antitumor activity, each with specific application to the design and analysis of clinical trial data are described. The use of such models permits significant sample size reduction in the design of clinical studies. Technological advances in detecting and measuring disease recurrence add to the problem of defining response and are addressed in the second chapter of this section. The serial measurement of tumor markers constitutes another complementary approach in evaluating patient response to therapy and recurrence. The adaptation of the time-dependent covariant model to solve some of the statistical problems associated with the analysis of marker data is presented as an approach to assess elevated relative risk of recurrence. Data are presented suggesting that monitoring a marker alone, such as CEA, may be as good or better than clinical monitoring. Not only is this provocative, but it would result in cost reduction and greatly reduced inconvenience to patients. With the availability of marker measurements at regular time intervals, one can choose from a variety of statistical techniques to estimate absolute risk of recurrence.

The final chapter of Section IV presents a literature review of prognostic factors for liver metastases from colorectal cancer. The need to appreciate and report data on prognostic variables in evaluating clinical trials is emphasized.

The last section consists of an analysis of failure in the treatment of patients with hepatic metastases from colorectal cancer. It is essential to identify problems before devising solutions. Critical analysis of failures in other diseases has led to successful treatment strategies. For example, the recognition that recurrence in advanced Hodgkin's disease following chemotherapy-induced complete remission has led to the successful use of radiotherapy to those areas of previous macroscopic disease following chemotherapy. In this section, not only are the clinical patterns of failure reviewed, but the biology of treatment failure in colorectal cancer relative to drug resistance and tumor heterogeneity is also reviewed. The clinical patterns of failure clearly point out that there are different subsets of patients who reflect the biologic heterogeneity of colon tumors and their metastases. Of particular note is the observation that patients with surgically resectable, isolated hepatic metastases represent a biologically selected subset with good prognoses. It is important to note that the concept of pleiotropic drug resistance involving a number of mechanisms is applicable to the resistance noted in colon carcinomas. This is evident in the general refractoriness of colon tumors to different classes of therapeutic agents. However, this knowledge provides a biochemical rationale for the development of future strategies aimed at overcoming drug resistance in colon tumors. The theme of biological resistance of colon carcinoma to treatment is reiterated. Empirical testing of agents is not a productive approach, rather assays ought to be targeted using a spectrum of appropriate models. Clearly, the data presented suggest that the resistance of colon tumor cells is inherent and represents a multifactorial phenomenon. Despite these generally pessimistic results, the final presentation suggests some optimism for the treatment of heterogeneous cancer metastases by systemic activation of macrophages. This technique is enhanced by activating the macrophages using immunomodulators encapsulated in liposomes to achieve sustained release. Although preliminary data are encouraging, the limitations of such treatment for disseminated metastatic disease are obvious and relate both to the availabily of macrophages and the tumor burden.

While definitive answers to very complex and perplexing problems may not be presented, important questions are identified and important new approaches and directions for research initiatives in the area of metastases are identified. The chapters provide an update of the state-of-the-art treatment of colorectal cancer metastases without necessarily providing a consensus as there is some disagreement in certain areas of patient management. Nevertheless, the presentations should provide a better understanding of the patterns and mechanisms of colon tumor spread, both experimentally and in the natural history of the disease. In addition, the chapters evaluate the biologic and biochemical reasons for colon tumor resistance, better define criteria of response to therapy, and hopefully will stimulate new research approaches and define important and relevant clinical questions requiring additional laboratory investigation. The latter will best be achieved through complementary interaction of basic scientists of varying disciplines with clinical investigators. Finally, for progress to be made in this area, it is suggested that a national registry for surgical treatment of hepatic metastases be established to accumulate data from hepatic resections. These data could be derived from both retrospective and prospective studies, and would be useful in designing future studies and in evaluating the most effective therapy of hepatic metastases and the best treatment of extrahepatic disease. It is hoped that the contents of this volume will be of benefit in providing improved management of patients with hepatic metastases from colorectal cancer.

Throughout the proceedings basic science concepts have been integrated with clinically relevant questions and studies. In this way, the proceedings should be of interest, not only to clinicians treating patients with hepatic metastases from colorectal cancer, but also to laboratory investigators of diverse disciplines interested in elucidating the biology of the metastatic process. In fact, many of the concepts and approaches presented in these proceedings have more widespread applicability to sites other than large bowel cancer.

Anthony J. Mastromarino

ACKNOWLEDGMENTS

This volume, The Biology and Treatment of Colorectal Cancer Metastasis, represents the contributions of many individuals. The workshop itself, held at the Stouffer's Greenway Plaza Hotel, Houston, September 13-15, 1984, was the last of 18 multidisciplinary workshops sponsored by the National Large Bowel Cancer Project during its 12-year administration at the University of Texas System Cancer Center, M. D. Anderson Hospital and Tumor Institute, Houston, Texas. From 1972 to 1984 the headquarters of the National Large Bowel Cancer Project was supported by grant R26 CA14140 from the National Cancer Institute (NCI). During that time the National Large Bowel Cancer Project received encouragement and support from the administration of The University of Texas System Cancer Center, M. D. Anderson Hospital and Tumor Institute, especially from Dr. R. Lee Clark, Dr. Robert C. Hickey, and Dr. Charles A. LeMaistre, and was under the capable direction of Dr. Murray M. Copeland (1972-1982), Dr. Edward M. Copeland III (1982-1983), and Dr. Richard G. Martin (1983-1984). During this period, each project director was complemented by a scientific support staff which included Drs. Rulon W. Rawson, William Spears, Birger Jansson, Marvin M. Romsdahl, Michael G. Brattain and myself, a working group of outstanding, dedicated consultants and advisors from numerous institutions, and an office staff of highly skilled and technically competent individuals. In addition, the National Large Bowel Cancer Project enjoyed the constant support and assistance of the Organ Systems Program Branch at the NCI, especially from Dr. Andrew Chiarodo and Dr. Vincent Cairoli, Program Director for the National Large Bowel Cancer Project. Since I am so indebted to all of the above individuals, I wish this volume to be a tribute to all those who made the National Large Bowel Cancer Project the success that it was.

As with the proceedings of any workshop its success is predicated on the contributions of many. This conference was no different. As chairman of the conference and editor of the proceedings, I am especially indebted to those who served on the Planning Committee. Their suggestions resulted in an integrated program of basic scientists and clinical investigators, the identification of key topics to be discussed, and the selection of an outstanding program faculty. I am also gratefully indebted to those who served as Session Chairpersons, and of course, to all the speakers and workshop discussants and participants for their active role in the workshop and for their contributions to the proceedings. This workshop and its published proceedings have fulfilled one of the important objectives of the National Large Bowel Cancer Project, that is, information transfer between clinical investigators and basic scientists from diverse disciplines.

From my perspective as editor, the most important components in the completion of this project were the relentless dedication of my executive secretary, Ms. Deborah Maloney, and the cooperation and expertise provided by the staff of the Department of Scientific Publications. Those persons, specifically, Ms. Carol Kakalec, editor, and her assistant Kathleen Robertson as well as Ms. Dorothy Kisling and Ms. Mary Deiss, were invaluable in editing and assisting Ms. Maloney in entering the manuscripts on the word processor for camera-ready copy. The product speaks for itself and attests to their competence and dedication to detail. The success of the workshop is attributable to their collective efforts, skillful planning, and organizational capabilities.

Anthony J. Mastromarino

Program Planning Committee Members:

Michael Bernardino, M.D.
Emory University School
  of Medicine
Atlanta, Georgia

Michael G. Brattain, Ph.D.
Baylor College of Medicine
Houston, Texas

Edward M. Copeland, III, M.D.
University of Florida
  College of Medicine
J. Hillis Miller Health Center
Gainesville, Florida

Isaiah J. Fidler, D.V.M., Ph.D.
The University of Texas System
  Cancer Center
M. D. Anderson Hospital and
  Tumor Institute
Houston, Texas

Young S. Kim, M.D.
University of California
Veterans Administration Hospital
San Francisco, California

Daniel L. Kisner, M.D.
The University of Texas Health
  Science Center- San Antonio
San Antonio, Texas

Philip T. Lavin, Ph.D.
Consulting Statisticians, Inc.
A Crowntek Company
Wellesley Hills, Massachusetts

Anthony J. Mastromarino, Ph.D.
The University of Texas System
  Cancer Center
M. D. Anderson Hospital and
  Tumor Institute
Houston, Texas

Alka Palekar, M.D.
Shady Side Hospital
Pittsburgh, Pennsylvania

Glenn D. Steele, Jr., M.D., Ph.D.
New England Deaconess Hospital
Boston, Massachusetts

Paul Sugarbaker, M.D.
Surgery Branch
National Cancer Institute
Bethesda, Maryland

SECTION I.

THE BIOLOGY OF COLORECTAL CANCER METASTASIS

1

NATURAL HISTORY OF LIVER METASTASIS AND RESECTIVE TREATMENT

Martin A. Adson

SUMMARY

Five-year survival after resection of hepatic metastases from colorectal cancer is 25%. Although resection palliates the disease in some patients who do not live that long, 50% of patients so treated are not helped at all. Until ignorance of a cancer's real stage is resolved by improved techniques, the evaluation and choice of therapy can be based only upon knowledge of the natural history of untreated metastases and determinants of prognosis derived from treated patients. Analysis of the survival rates of 252 patients who had biopsy-proven, unresected hepatic metastases that were the only evidence of residual disease shows the extent to which natural history, rather than resection, may determine length of survival. It also indicates the need for critical analysis of two- and three-year survival rates reported after any therapy. Study of 141 patients who had hepatic metastases resected shows that the stage of the primary lesion, being female, and the absence of extrahepatic metastases are significant determinants of favorable prognosis after resection of hepatic metastases.

INTRODUCTION

The natural history of untreated cancer is the standard against which the value of any therapy should be measured, but nowadays it seldom is. Historically, medicine, "the youngest science," has involved the study of the natural history of disease because once that was about all that could be studied. The good physician who was totally in want of useful therapy had studied natural history of disease in a scientific way and could make an accurate diagnosis and predict a reliable prognosis. There is much good literature to give evidence of the science of that art.

However, as Lewis Thomas has observed (1), the recorded history of the reported benefits of therapeutic efforts ". . . based on nothing more than pure whim--make horrifying reading today". The learned authors who recount the benefits of bleeding, cupping, purging, use of leeches, immersion of patients in water that was either too hot or too cold, or administration of botanical extracts were convincing in their day, but now we see that physicians were trying to take credit for what nature could have done alone.

Therapeutic efforts, then as well as now, are evidence of caring of two sorts, not only the physician's concern for the patient, but also concern for self. I am not criticizing this dual obligation that has so much to do with human motivation when these two concerns are so inseparable, so long as physicians put the patients' needs above their own. Physicians really cannot serve others without some need to serve themselves. Also, when both the doctor and the patient must contend with so much that is bad, it is natural for physicians either to want to make things better or, failing that, to try to make things look better to and for themselves. However, we know that these goals must be tempered for proper balance, if the patient is to get a fair share of caring and concern. In the twelfth century, Maimonides saw this need for balance and stated in his code, "May the love of my art actuate me at all times, may neither avarice nor miserliness nor thirst for glory or a great reputation engage my mind; for as enemies of truth and philanthropy, they could easily deceive me and make me forget my lofty aim of doing good to thy children" (2).

Against this background, it is interesting to look at what is going on today. The remarkable impact of true science upon medical and surgical therapy in general is less evident in oncology. Bacteria have given into science more easily than have cancer cells, but still ". . . the endless list of botanical extracts cooked up and mixed together under the influence of pure whim . . ." (1) have been replaced by growing lists of their botanical descendants that have been scientifically discovered and even surgical progress has been scientific, in a way. Therefore, it is hard to understand why the introduction of science into the therapy of cancer has been accompanied by some neglect of the scientific method for use in the evaluation of results. The concept of natural history is so simple that lately it has been ignored, and the science of statistics, if misused, may become an enemy of truth.

Some of this disparity within oncologic science has to do with the bias of investigative therapists who are inclined to make things look better than they are. But, it has more to do with the problem of observation--the difficulty of measuring what the cancer is doing and what is happening to the host. If the mechanism of disease--a cancer's birth, growth, and spread--could be observed clinically from day to day or if the results of most therapy for cancer were obviously successful, there would be no need to study the natural history of cancer today. But, for now, there is still a need to know more about the natural history of hepatic metastases from large bowel cancer to help us with our choice of therapy and with our evaluation of results.

4

STUDY OF NATURAL HISTORY OF CANCER TODAY

"Natural history can be studied best in prospective randomized therapeutic trials. However, most clinicians are unwilling to give uneven effort, and those who recognize the needs and niceties of science have trouble recruiting patients for study that involves a choice of having nothing done. Therefore, it is difficult to study natural history today when so little is left to nature" (3).

The natural history of untreated large bowel cancer has been studied in a general way (4-23), but only two of many reports (22-23) have taken into account the presence of uncontrolled primary or regional growth, the extent of hepatic involvement, or the presence or absence of extrahepatic metastases. Thus, longevity and quality of life of these studied patients was determined by many factors (a variety of sites of growth and spread) that obscured the natural history of hepatic metastases alone.

It is easy to recognize what we need to know about hepatic metastasis, in order to assess its effect on longevity and the quality of life. The hard part is knowing how to find out because we cannot see enough of what goes on between a cancer's beginning and the patient's end. What can be seen at the beginning is evident to cellular biologists who can study tumor models, but cannot see our patients well, and, looking backward, the anatomic pathologist can tell us what happened just before the end, but not when it happened. Thus, neither of these views can tell us when the clinician might have altered the natural history of the disease by use of treatments now at hand.

The view from either end is discouraging to surgeons or to other therapists who try to deal with regional disease. I have never seen a cancer start to grow, but understand that most cancers can shed into the blood stream after only 20 doublings, when a tumor is so small (1 mm) that the clinician has no way to know that it is even there. This means that the capacity to metastasize precedes clinical detectability by many months or even years (24).

Data from studies conducted at autopsy are equally disheartening. Pickren (25) found that of 733 patients who had large bowel cancer and died, 383 (52%) also had hepatic metastases. Only 12% had solitary liver lesions, and some, or maybe most, of these patients had extrahepatic metastases as well. Thus, there is good evidence to show that most often cancer has the head start on the surgeon, and that in the end, most large bowel cancers have gone to more places than the surgeon can remove.

This potential for wide systemic spread observed at the beginning, and the successful dissemination that is so often evident at the end should discourage surgeons and other focal therapists (medical oncologists and radiation therapists) from their efforts to deal with local or regional disease. However, these observations show nothing

5

of what goes on in between the beginning and the end, and there is some evidence to show that the metastatic process is erratic and unreliable in a way that might allow focal therapists to alter the advance of malignant disease.

Looking again at the threat, a cancer's capacity to shed precedes detectability, and usually, many, many cells are shed into the liver, which is a sieve made up of fertile soil from which metastases can metastasize again. However, this opportunity for success is not always realized. It is hard to put the metastatic process in order when so much disorder can be seen and when so much of what can be seen looks like whimsy. This is because many shed cancer cells cannot thrive in other sites; most cells that are shed singly die in the blood stream. Aggregates of cancer cells must achieve neovascularity and survive host defenses, and even then, cellular proliferation involves growth factors and cell loss. Thus, successful distant growth requires a selective subpopulation of cancer cells.

This accounts for the fact that about 50% of patients who die from large bowel cancer do not have hepatic metastases, and also explains some other observations that indicate that the ablation of some hepatic metastases by clinicians might alter the natural history of this disease.

It is true that most postmortem studies show a predominance of multiple hepatic metastases. However, such multiplicity may come about in two different ways. I used to envision only showers of cells given off from the primary lesion to both hepatic lobes, but lately have seen something that was always there--multiple unilobular hepatic metastases of unequal size (big lesions with small satellites)--and have wondered where the smaller ones might have come from. Good observations of this phenomena are wanting because the word "multiple" has so many discouraging implications that most observers have not tried to look beyond it. However, Willis, a gifted pathologist and thoughtful observer who must be a surgeon at heart, has studied multiplicity of hepatic metastases more carefully than others have. He believes ". . . that embolism to the liver from the primary source is responsible for few (or only one) hepatic metastases seen at autopsy; and that the great majority of hepatic growths are local intrahepatic descendants, generations removed from the pioneer metastasis" (26).

We already know that solitary hepatic metastases are discouragingly uncommon, but mutiple unilobar metastases that are resectable may be more common than we have been led to think they are. Moreover, the fact remains that some or many bilateral hepatic metastases may get from one side to the other over a span of time different from which the surgeon and the patient might consider to be relevant.

However, this good news for regional therapists (who hope that better systemic therapy soon will prevail) must be tempered by the frequency with which metastases are

6

found outside the liver during postmortem examinations. These observations indicate that in the end, given enough time, most cancers will spread and grow beyond the scope of regional therapy. However, such studies do not show what was happening at one time somewhere between the beginning and the end when hepatic metastases might have been the only sites of tumor that remained to grow. Reported incidences of "liver only" metastases seems to be determined, in part, by what has gone on before. Postmortem studies of patients who had primary lesions that could not be treated well have cancer nearly everywhere (25), but Willis (26), whose autopsy observations were based in large part upon patients whose primary tumors were removed, found that 11 (19%) of 59 necropsy cases of large bowel cancer had only hepatic metastases.

NATURAL HISTORY EVIDENT IN THERAPEUTIC FAILURE

From this oblique view of the natural history of the disease, we might infer that hepatic metastasis may, at least for that time during the life history of a cancer's growth and the patient's death, be the independent sole determinant of prognosis. If that is so, it could be a reasonable target for regional therapy at some point. In fact, there is other evidence that shows that this is true. Twenty-five percent of patients who have had hepatic metastases surgically removed live five years or more (27). I bring this up only to show what might be learned of natural history from this unnatural view--from analysis of treated patients. Today's treatment of hepatic metastasis benefits so few patients that we can learn as much or more from our therapeutic failures as we can from our successes. This involves a different way of looking at the benefits of resecting hepatic metastases, but it is an easy thing to do.

To identify determinants of prognosis for comparison with natural history, we have recently studied all of our clinic patients (n=141) who had hepatic metastases removed between 1948 and 1982 (27). We found that location and grade of the primary tumor and time of removal of the metastasis (that is whether they were synchronous or metachronous) were not significant. Size of lesions and extent of resections related only to operative mortality.

Also, we found, contrary to an earlier observation (23), that survival of patients who had multiple liver metastases resected did not differ from those who had apparent solitary lesions taken out. The nearly identical survival curves of patients who had multiple lesions and those who had solitary lesions resected are shown on Figure 1. The overall survival curve is mostly hidden by the other two curves.

7

COMPARATIVE SURVIVAL

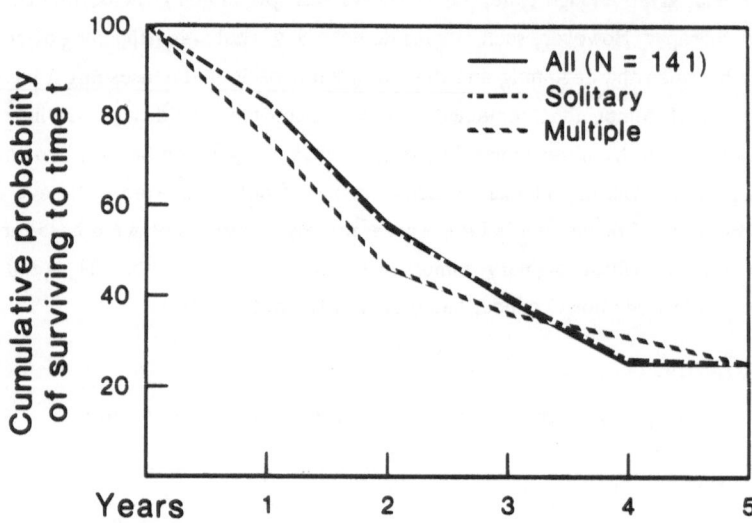

FIGURE 1.   Survival curves for patients who underwent resection of multiple (n=37) or solitary (n=104) lesions.

This finding requires some pondering because it seems to contradict a reasonable armchair view of the metastatic process. It is reasonable to suppose that multiplicity of metastases in the liver would most often be associated with dissemination of many other cells outside the liver that should compromise survival. This is true for small metastases, but we found that patients who had multiple lesions, larger than 4 cm, removed lived longer than did patients who had smaller multiple lesions resected (Table 1).

This finding must have something to do with separate generations of bloodborne metastases and with time, the time required for them to have grown so large. It may be that the time it takes for those metastases to become so large also offers time for tiny metastases to become large enough to be seen.

It is exciting for a surgeon to observe something that an anatomic pathologist has seen in another way. The conclusion of Willis that ". . . the great majority of hepatic growths are likely local intrahepatic descendants, generations removed from the pioneer metastasis . . ." (26) should excite anyone who is trying to work with the tools that we have at hand.

Three other determinants of prognosis were identified in our study of patients who had hepatic metastases resected. The first had to do with gender. Being female has some advantage that has borderline statistical significance. (P=.054)

8

Table 1. Relationship of Size and Multiplicity of Hepatic Metastases to Survival Rate*

	Small Lesions				Large Lesions			
	Synchronous		Metachronous		Synchronous		Metachronous	
	1	>1	1	>1	1	>1	1	>1
Survival, yr	(n=27)	(n=2)	(n=24)	(n=16)	(n=4)	(n=1)	(n=43)	(n=18)
3	37	50	56	21	25	0	30	50
5	26	50	33	0	0	0	18	37
10	11	0	22	0	0	0	18	0

* Values expressed are percentage of patients who survived. Small lesions were less than 4 cm, and large lesions, 4 cm or larger. 1 indicates solitary lesions, and >1, multiple lesions.

Two other determinants of prognosis have significance, the stage of the primary lesion and the influence of the extrahepatic metastases that were found and removed when hepatic lesions were resected.

Figures 2 and 3 show what can be achieved by surgical resection. However, it is easy to look at these data the other way around to show what can be learned from failure.

Figure 2 shows that patients who had more extensive disease involvement of the lymph nodes that were removed at the primary operation did not do as well as others who had minimal lymph node involvement when hepatic metastases were removed. This simply shows that the invisible extrahepatic metastases that accompany more extensive local growth are more likely to determine the patients' outcome than are hepatic metastases that can be removed.

COMPARATIVE SURVIVAL

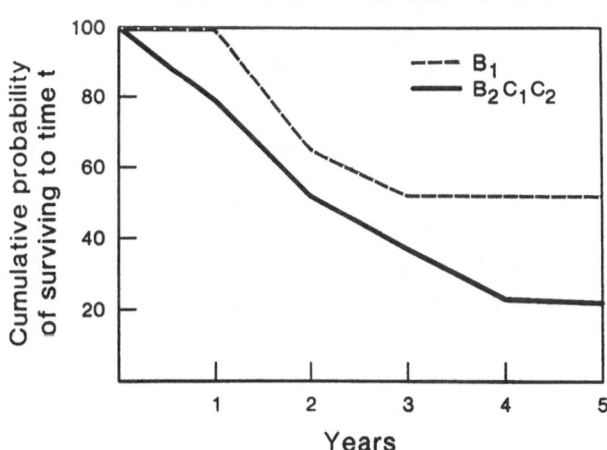

FIGURE 2. Survival curves for patients after resection of hepatic metastases from Dukes' stage BI (dashed line) (n=16) or B2/C1/C2 (solid line) (n=125) primary lesions.

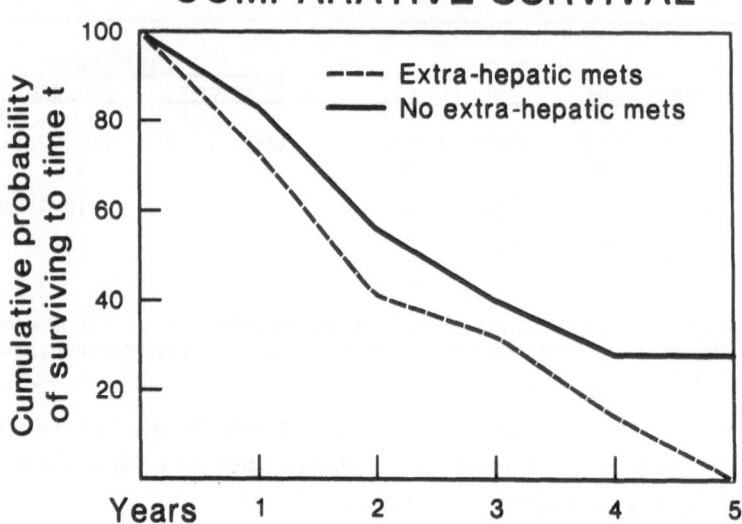

COMPARATIVE SURVIVAL

FIGURE 3. Survival curves for patients after resection of hepatic metastases with (dashed line) (n=25) or without (solid line) (n=116) extrahepatic metastases.

This phenomena can be seen more clearly as one compares, in Figure 3, the survival of patients who had visible extrahepatic metastases when their liver metastases were removed with the survival of patients who had no evident extrahepatic spread.

It may seem unfair to look at the natural history of the disease by studying treated patients, but this study of the counterparts of success confirms what we have suspected all along--it is not what we have seen and taken out that kills the patient, but what was unseen and left in to grow. The studies of prognostic factors reported by Lahr et al. (8) and by Goslin and others (29) generally confirm that view.

THE NATURAL HISTORY OF UNRESECTED HEPATIC METASTASES

We studied 252 patients who had unresected hepatic metastases for use as historical controls (3). This study of natural history is retrospective for reasons that have been explained and may be faulted by problems in interpretation of some operative reports. However, if there is bias in selection of our sample, it involves inclusion of some patients who may have had extrahepatic residua that unfavorably influenced survival. Nevertheless, study of this sample does give perspective to therapeutic efforts for selecting therapy and for assessing results.

10

The operative reports of 466 patients seen at Mayo between 1943 and 1976 were reviewed. All had biopsy-proven hepatic metastases found when their primary colorectal cancers were resected. In order to identify a group of patients whose hepatic metastases were likely the major determinant of their survival, we excluded 214 patients whose survival was obviously threatened in other ways.

Most of the exclusions shown on Table 2 are those patients who died in the hospital soon after operation and those who either had their liver lesions resected or had residual tumor elsewhere that would have compromised survival. The remaining 252 patients can be seen as historical controls for patients who have had hepatic metastases resected or treated in other ways because our process of exclusion for this study was the same method that we use clinically to select patients for resection of their hepatic metastases.

Thirty-nine lesions were solitary and 31 were multiple, but confined to portions of the liver that could be resected by lobectomy or right-sided trisegmentectomy. One hundred eighty-two patients had widespread bilateral unresectable metastases. Thus, 70 lesions (28%) were resectable, but were, for reasons determined by the individual surgeons, not resected.

Table 2. Biopsy-proven Hepatic Metastases Found When Primary Colorectal Cancers Were Resected (466 Patients: 1943-1976)

To study the natural history of hepatic metastases, we excluded 214 patients who:

Died within 30 days	13
Had liver metastases resected	56
Had residual extrahepatic spread	98
Had residual primary tumor	19
Had jaundice, ascites, or another primary cancer	19
Had insufficient data for our study	9

The basic analysis of survival rates calculated from our retrospective study is shown on Figure 4. Patients who have hepatic metastases that were left in to grow and who have no other detectable tumor residua live longer than we have been led to think they would. This is because most other studies of survival rates of patients who had untreated hepatic metastases have included many patients who had untreated or untreatable extrahepatic metastases as well (4-21). The extent of hepatic involvement is

11

a definite determinant of longevity that is statistically significant. Median survival rates of patients who had unresected solitary and multiple unilobar lesions are 21 and 15 months, respectively and more than 20% of patients who had unresected solitary liver lesions lived three years or more. These survival rates are similar to those reported by Wanebo et al. (21), Wilson and Adson (22), and Wood et al. (23) in their observations of selected patients.

The observations shown on Figure 4 may be enough to know. However, we were moved by curiosity to look at our data in some other ways. These analyses are statistically soft owing to small sample size, lack of prospective randomization, and subjective judgements involved in our selection of patients for comparative analysis. Nevertheless, the observations shown in Figures 2 to 7 are clinically interesting and deserving of thoughtful analysis.

EXTENT OF HEPATIC METASTASES

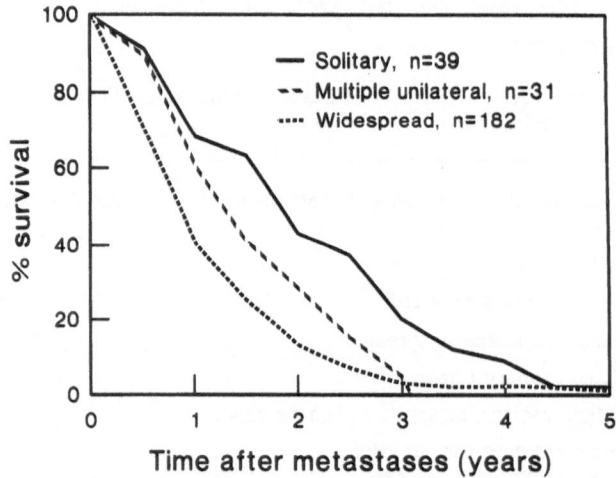

FIGURE 4. Survival rates of patients who had unresected hepatic metastases without evidence of other residual disease, classified with respect to extent and site of hepatic involvement. Three-year survival rates: solitary lesions 21%; multiple unilateral 6%; and widespread 4%. Five-year survival rates: 3%, 0%, and 2%, respectively.

The observation (Figure 5) that will excite most oncologists is the apparent difference between the survival of patients who had adjuvant chemotherapy (about half of the total sample) for unresected hepatic lesions and those who did not. The effects of the therapeutic intrusion must be admitted. However, this comparison is neither

12

statistically nor clinically significant because patients were given chemotherapeutic agents selectively, most often long after operative evaluation and only then when their hepatic disease became clinically measurable (before good imaging techniques were available), or became locally, not systemically symptomatic. Figure 5 shows that about 10% of patients who had a solitary metastasis and were not given antitumor drugs died just a few months after operation. If these patients, who were infirm and therefore were not offered chemotherapy, are discounted, the survival curves are much the same. This figure is reproduced only to show how little is left to nature and cannot be used to show that drugs that have unproved value had benefit for our studied patients (30).

HEPATIC METASTASES -- NOT RESECTED

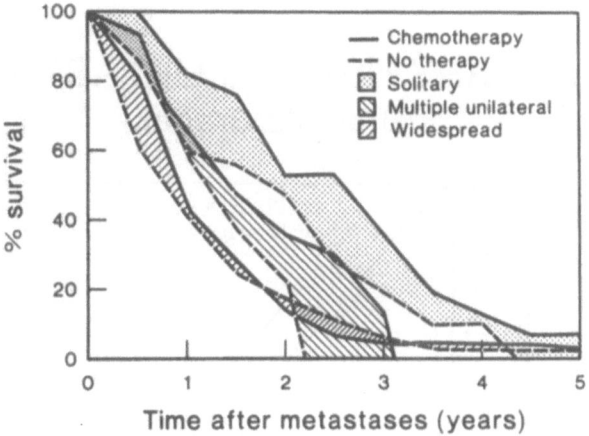

FIGURE 5. Survival rates of patients who had unresected hepatic metastases of varied extent who were and were not treated with chemotherapeutic agents.

Figures 6-8 show the influence of the stage and grade of the primary colorectal lesion upon survival, which seems to make a difference when hepatic involvement is minimal or less advanced. However, these factors have negligible influence when extensive hepatic spread and growth predominate.

13

SOLITARY HEPATIC METASTASES

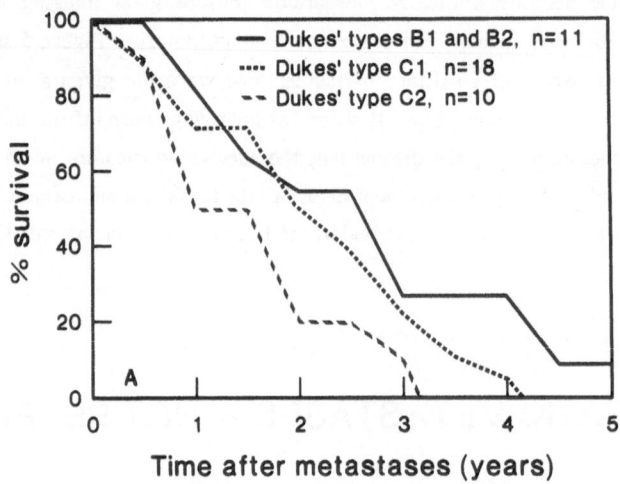

SOLITARY HEPATIC METASTASES
(Broder's Grades)

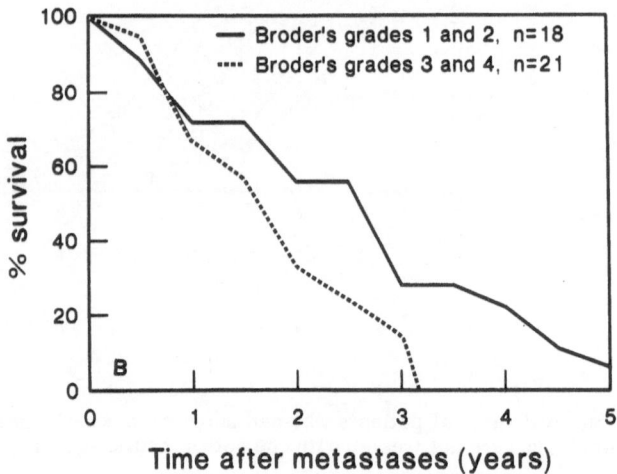

FIGURE 6A & B. The influence of stage (A) and grade (B) of the primary tumor upon survival of patients who had unresected solitary hepatic metastases without evidence of other residual disease.

14

MULTIPLE UNILATERAL HEPATIC METASTASES

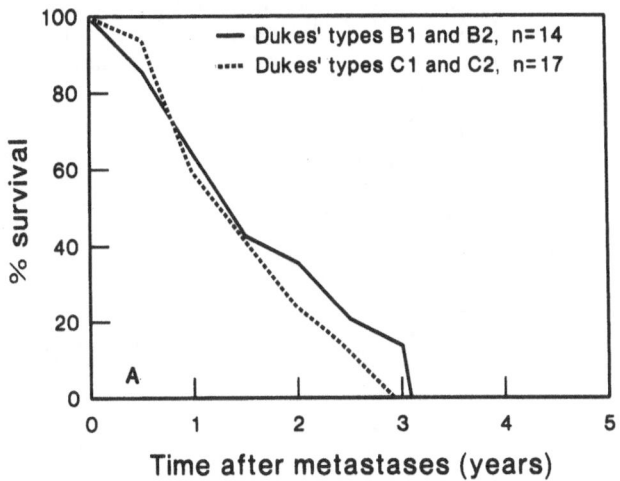

MULTIPLE UNILATERAL HEPATIC METASTASES

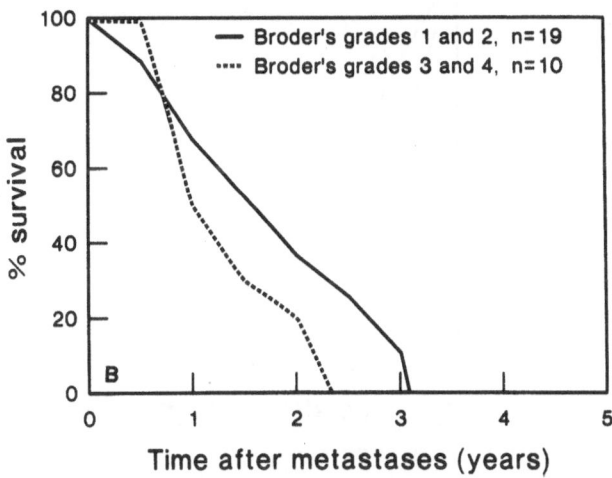

FIGURE 7A & B. The influence of stage (A) and grade (B) of the primary tumor upon survival of patients who had unresected multiple unilobar liver lesions without evidence of other residual disease.

WIDESPREAD HEPATIC METASTASES

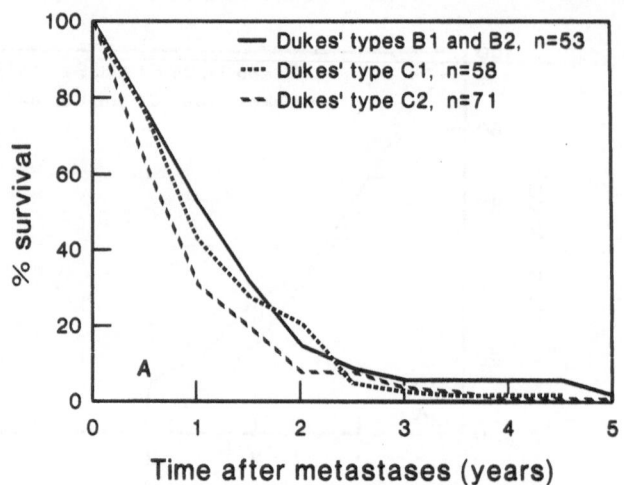

WIDESPREAD HEPATIC METASTASES

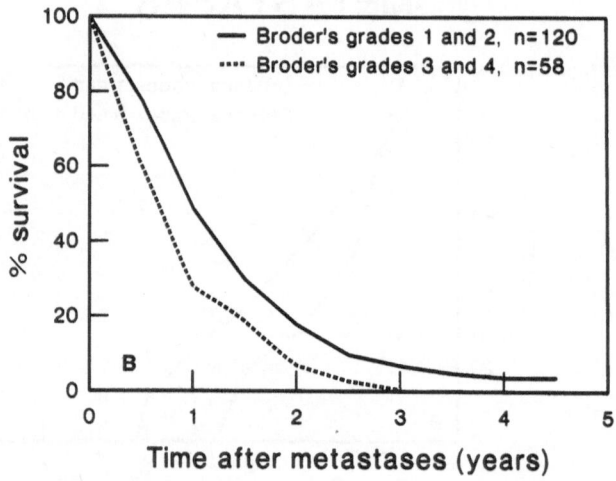

FIGURE 8A & B. The influence of stage (A) and grade (B) of the primary tumor upon survival of patients who had unresectable widespread bilobar hepatic metastases without evidence of other residual disease.

Figures 9A and B show that survival related to lung metastases that coexist with lesions in the liver is similarly related to the predominant extent of hepatic growth of cancer. Considered in another way, these curves show the consequence of disseminated growth and, in a way, indicate that something might be gained by use of focal or regional therapy.

SOLITARY HEPATIC METASTASES

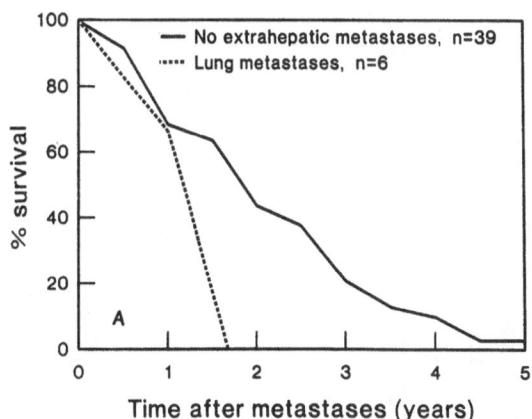

WIDESPREAD HEPATIC METASTASES

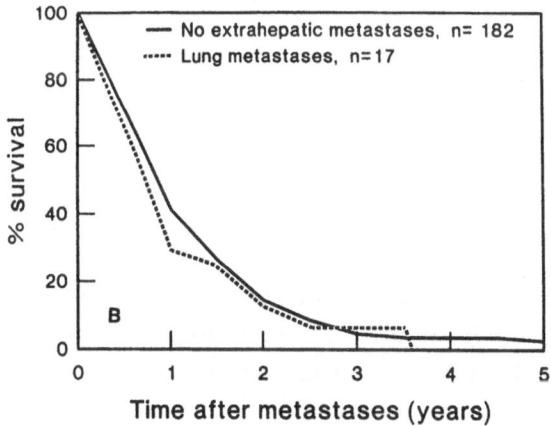

FIGURE 9A & B. A comparison of the influence of extrahepatic (lung) metastases upon survival of patients who had (A) unresected solitary and (B) widespread hepatic metastases without evidence of other residual disease.

These many observations support the view that the natural history of a cancer's growth and spread is a major determinant of survival. We must compare our therapeutic efforts critically with what nature can do alone, evaluate our treatments objectively, and not take credit for what might have happened anyway.

EXTENT OF HEPATIC METASTASES

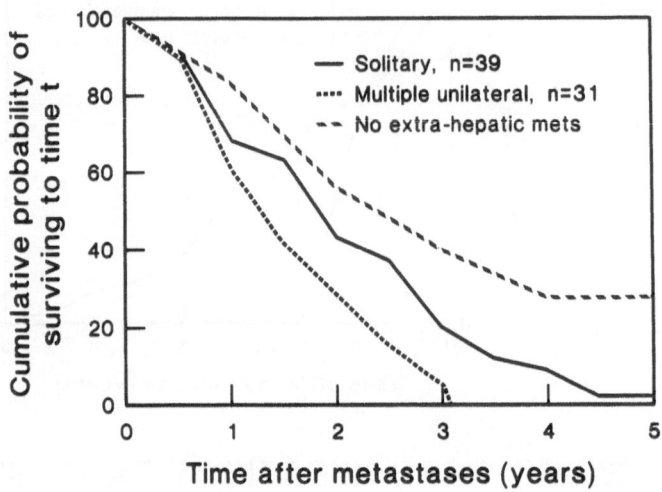

FIGURE 10. The top line is the survival curve of 116 patients who had solitary and multiple hepatic metastases resected when there was no evidence of residual primary tumor or of extrahepatic metastases, compared with patients who had unresected solitary (n=39) and multiple, unilateral hepatic (n=31) metastases.

DISCUSSION

These gross correlations of prognosis with the primary tumor's stage have some use clinically for selecting patients who might be helped by resection of their liver lesions. However, these observations do not help us to determine the value of treatment for most of the patients who are treated.

Figure 10, which compares survival rates of patients treated surgically and those not, shows us more than we can understand as we try to evaluate what we have done. The benefit given some patients is obvious, but it is clear that most patients that we try to help die early, not from what we have seen and taken out, but from unseen metastatic lesions that were left in to grow.

Comparison of these curves also shows that even though long-term survival rates are significantly affected by resection, (P=.0001), median survival rates (so grouped by nature in the middle of this graph) cannot be analyzed significantly. These observations of the role of natural history, however crude, should be considered by clinical practitioners who wish to publish prematurely and by academic statisticians who are unacquainted with disease.

Other things can be seen in our study. One has to do with the role of resection of hepatic metastases from colorectal cancer. What proportion of patients who have such lesions might be helped by resection of their liver lesions?

We have already seen that the 70 (28%) of 252 patients who had hepatic metastases that seemed to be the major determinant of their prognosis had either solitary or unilobar resectable lesions. Also, from our total sample of 466 patients, 56 patients had resectable lesions, which when added to the others, gives 27%. If one-fourth of these are truly helped by surgery, then only about 7% of patients who have hepatic metastases may benefit from surgical resection.

This leaves a predominance of patients who have widespread hepatic metastases and who will not benefit from resection. The natural history of these patients was also studied in our sample (Figure 1) and also should be studied and considered by those whose therapeutic efforts involve such lesions. Their therapeutic trials should either be randomized or compared critically with the natural history of disease.

When the inception, growth, and spread of cancer can be seen clinically in each patient and when biological manipulations can be used to kill all cancer cells, the natural history of cancer will have only historical interest. Then, this phenomena will be seen as the natural history of rational human thought and as evidence of man's capacity and need to rationalize. But, for now, there is need to know more about the natural history of hepatic metastases from large bowel cancer to help us with our choice of therapy and with evaluation of results.

References

1. Thomas L: The youngest science. New York, The Viking Press, 1983, pp 270.
2. Moses ben Maimon: Code for Physicians, 1135-1204 A.D.
3. Wagner JS, Adson MA, van Heerden JA, Adson MH, Ilstrup DM: The natural history of hepatic metastases from colorectal cancer. Ann Surg 199: 502-508, 1984.
4. Abrams MS, Lerner HJ: Survival of patients at Pennsylvania Hospital with hepatic metastases from carcinoma of the colon and rectum. Dis Colon Rectum 14: 431-434, 1971.

19

5. Bacon HE, Martin PV: The rationale of palliative resection for primary cancer of the colon complicated by liver and lung metastases. Dis Colon Rectum 7: 211-217, 1964.

6. Bengmark S, Hafstrom L: The natural history of primary and secondary malignant tumors of the liver. I. The prognosis for patients with hepatic metastases from colonic and rectal carcinoma by laparotomy. Cancer 23: 198-202, 1969.

7. Bengtsson G, Carlsson G, Hafstrom L, Per-Ebbe J: Natural history of patients with untreated liver metastases from colorectal cancer. Am J Surg 141: 586-589, 1981.

8. Cady B, Moncon DO, Swinton NW: Survival of patients after colonic resection from carcinoma with simultaneous liver metastases. Surg Gynecol Obstet 131: 697-700, 1970.

9. Flanagan J Jr., Foster JH: Hepatic resection for metastatic cancer. Am J Surg 113: 551-557, 1967.

10. Galante M, Dunphy JE, Fletcher WS: Cancer of the colon. Ann Surg 165: 732-744, 1967.

11. Jaffe BM, Donegan WL, Watson F: Factors influencing survival in patients with untreated hepatic metastases. Surg Gynecol Obstet 127: 1-11, 1968.

12. Lahey FH: Discussion. Ann Surg 121: 409-410, 1945.

13. Moolin J, Walker HSJ: Palliative resections in cancer of the colon and rectum. Cancer 2: 767-776, 1949.

14. Nielsen J, Balslev I, Jensen HE: Carcinoma of the colon with liver metastases. Acta Chir Scand 137: 463-465, 1971.

15. Oxley EM, Ellis H: Prognosis of carcinoma of the large bowel in the presence of liver metastases. Br J Surg 56: 149-152, 1969.

16. Pestana C, Reitemeier R, Moertel CG, Judd ES, Dockerty MB: The natural history of carcinoma of the colon and rectum. Am J Surg 108: 826-829, 1964.

17. Pettavel J, Morgenthaler F: Protracted arterial chemotherapy of liver tumors: An experience of 107 cases over a 12-year period. Prog Clin Cancer 7: 217-233, 1978.

18. Ransom HK: Carcinoma of the colon: A study of end results of surgical treatment. Arch Surg 64: 707-725, 1952.

19. Stearns MW Jr, Brinkley GJ: Palliative surgery for cancer of the rectum and colon. Cancer 7: 1016-1019, 1954.

20. Swinton NW, Samaan S, Rosenthal D: Cancer of the rectum and sigmoid. Surg Clin North Amer 47: 657-662, 1967.

21. Wanebo HJ, Semoglou C, Attiyeh F: Surgical management of patients with primary operable colorectal cancer and synchronous liver metastases. Am J Surg 135: 81-84, 1978.

22. Wilson SM, Adson MA: Surgical treatment of hepatic metastases from colorectal cancers. Arch Surg 111: 330-334, 1976.

23. Wood CB, Gillis CR, Blumgart LH: A retrospective study of the natural history of patients with liver metastases from colorectal cancer. Clin Oncol 2: 285-288, 1976.

24. Foster JH, Berman MM: Solid liver tumors. In: PA Ebert (ed), Major problems in clinical surgery, Vol. 22. WB Saunders, Philadelphia, 1977, pp 1-342.

25. Pickren JW, Tsukada Y, Lane WW: Liver metastasis: Analysis of autopsy data. In: L Weiss and HA Gilber (eds), Liver metastases. Boston, GK Hall, 1982, pp 2-18.

26. Willis J: Secondary tumours of the liver. In: RA Willis (ed), The spread of tumors in the human body. London, Butterworth & Co, 1973, pp 175-183.

27. Adson MA, van Heerden JA, Adson MH, Wagner JS, Ilstrup DM: Resection of hepatic metastases from colorectal cancer. Arch Surg 119: 647-651, 1984.

28. Lahr CJ, Seng-Jaw S, Cloud G, Smith J, Urist MM, Balch CM: A multifactorial analysis of prognostic factors in patients with liver metastases from colorectal carcinoma. J Clin Oncol 1: 720-726, 1983.

29. Goslin R, Steele G Jr, Zamcheck N, Mayer R, Macintyre J: Factors influencing survival in patients with hepatic metastases from adenocarcinoma of the colon or rectum. Dis Col Rectum 25: 749-754, 1982.
30. Moertel, CG: The liver. In: JF Holland and E Frei III (eds), Cancer medicine. Philadelphia, Lea and Febiger, 1973, pp 1541-1547.

2

THE USE OF NUDE MICE TO ASCERTAIN THE MALIGNANT CAPACITY OF HUMAN COLON CANCER

Ian R. Hart

SUMMARY

The metastatic behavior of 14 cell lines derived from 13 individual human tumor cell lines (six of which were colon carcinomas) have been assessed in athymic, nude mice. Many of these lines produced lung metastases after intravenous injection (experimental metastasis) and subcutaneous injection (spontaneous metastasis) into nude mice; however, the most dramatic expression of metastatic behavior was obtained after the injection of tumor cells into the spleens of recipient mice. With this route of cell inoculation, large tumor deposits frequently were found in the liver, the lungs, and the mesenteric and omental lymph nodes. Injection of human tumor lines into the spleens of athymic, nude mice appears to be a novel way of ascertaining the malignant capacity of neoplastic cells.

INTRODUCTION

Because tumor dissemination is an active process that occurs in a complex, responding host rather than within the relatively simple and benign two-dimensional constraints of the tissue-culture dish, there is an indispensable requirement for in vivo systems at some stage during any experimental studies on cancer metastasis (1). This requirement may be met by using fresh material isolated directly from patients within a short time of isolation, or it may be met by using autochthonous tumors from experimental animals; both of these possibilities are dealt with elsewhere in this volume. However, the transplantable tumor systems based upon inoculation with material derived from established tissue-culture lines provide the majority of experimental oncologists with their basic research systems. The advantages of these systems are associated with the simplicity of manipulation of the material, the ability to establish large and numerically significant experimental groups, and the degree of standardization that results from using pure populations of neoplastic cells free of contaminating host-cell infiltrates.

In recent years it has become common practice to graft human tumor material into immunologically compromised mice in the hope of studying its biology under the relatively natural circumstances of growth in a mammalian host. The existence of a wide range of tumor lines of human origin (2) has given rise to the possibility that the features that have made transplantable rodent tumors such attractive model systems can now be duplicated for the study of human neoplasms. Thus many investigators have used athymic, nude mice, which lack significant numbers of T-lymphocytes and are unable to reject grafts of foreign material, as vehicles for the propagation and expansion of human tumor lines (3-5). Tumor cells grown in nude mice have been shown to maintain their morphologic and biochemical identities to a remarkable degree (5,6). One characteristic that appears not to be fully conserved is that of malignancy (as opposed to tumorigenicity) defined as the ability to invade and metastasize; indeed, it frequently is stated that human tumors rarely metastasize in the nude mouse (7,8). Recently we have reported that this assumption (that nonmetastatic behavior is a general characteristic of all human tumor lines) may be invalid (9). Further, we have been able to show that relatively simple manipulations of either the recipient host or the injected tumor cells may facilitate and increase the observed incidence of human tumor spread in nude mice (9).

METASTATIC SPREAD OF HUMAN TUMOR CELL LINES IN NUDE MICE

The ability of a variety of human tumor lines to metastasize in nude mice was analyzed by injecting single-cell suspensions of these lines, harvested from plastic tissue-culture dishes and adjusted to similar concentrations, into young (3- to 6-week-old) athymic BALB/c nude mice using an intravenous (i.v.) or a subcutaneous (s.c.) route. The i.v. route of tumor-cell injection was used to assess what is termed "experimental" pulmonary metastasis. At a fixed time after i.v. injection (usually 6 to 8 weeks), the mice were killed and their lungs were removed, rinsed, and fixed in Bouin's solution to heighten the contrast between tumor nodules and normal lung parenchyma. Then the number of peripheral tumor nodules was counted under a dissecting microscope. The fixed lungs were subsequently sectioned and examined for the presence of microscopic tumor deposits.

So-called "spontaneous" metastasis was determined by examining animals in which the tumor cells had been injected subcutaneously. Tumors, located over the thorax or in a hind-foot pad, were allowed to grow until they were approximately 1 x 1 cm. They were then removed surgically. Mice were allowed to survive for a further 6 to 8 weeks, and then were killed and necropsied as described previously.

24

The individual tumor lines used in these studies are presented in Table 1. Initial studies utilized four malignant melanoma lines (A375-M was a more metastatic variant derived from the parental A375-P line by selection techniques) (10), two renal adenocarcinomas, two prostate carcinomas, and a single colon carcinoma line, HT-29. The behavior of the five additional lines derived from human colon carcinomas was assessed in subsequent experiments. Cell lines were obtained as acknowledged in our previous work (9) apart from the colon carcinoma lines Coll 5/3-112, LoVo, LS174T, SW48, and SW837, which were kindly supplied by Nigel Spurr (Imperial Cancer Research Fund, London).

Table 1. Human Tumor Lines Examined for Metastatic Capacity in BALB/c Nude Mice

Tumor Type	Cell Line
Malignant melanomas	A375-P
	A375-M
	DX-3
	SK-23
Prostate carcinomas	DU145
	PC3
Renal adenocarcinomas	769
	786-0
Colon carcinomas	HT-29
	Coll 5/3-112
	LoVo
	LS174T
	SW48
	SW837

Collated data from a number of initial experiments are presented in Table 2. It is apparent that while the metastatic capacities of the different cell lines vary widely, with the selected A375-M line exhibiting the most aggressive behavior, the general incidence of tumor spread is low, but not as rare as previous reports have suggested. From these results, it was determined that cultured human tumor cell lines could produce metastatic deposits in nude mice and that the application of selection techniques used with success in rodent tumor lines (11) could also be applied to at least some human tumor lines to produce variants with enhanced metastatic capacity (9,10).

Table 2. Experimental and Spontaneous Metastatic Capacity of Human Tumor Lines

Cell Line	Experimental Metastasis* Median No. (Range) of Pulmonary Nodules	Spontaneous Metastasis † No. of Mice with Metastasis/ No. of Mice Injected
A375-P	0 (0-3)	0/30
A375-M	69 (0-250)	28/30
DX-3	3 (0-68)	4/20
SK-23	0 (0-3)	ND ‡
DU-145	0	0/30
PC3-P	0	3/20
769	0	0/20
786-0	5 (0-55)	4/20
HT-29	0	7/10

*   Number of grossly evident tumor nodules determined with the aid of a dissecting microscope. Values, derived from at least 10 mice per group, represent one of two or more similar experiments.

†   Microscopically evident tumor foci. Data combined from subcutaneous sites over chest wall and in hind-foot pad.

‡   ND - Not done.

However, because it was apparent that the incidence of metastasis generally was low and that the size of secondary deposits produced after s.c. or i.v. injection was small, we sought to maximize the development of these metastatic lesions. A fibrous sheath or pseudocapsule frequently forms around human tumors xenografted into the nude mouse (12). This sheath may provide a strong anatomic barrier limiting invasion and spread, since injecting tumor cells within the peritoneum, where there is no restricting fibrous sheath, can produce widespread carcinomatosis and metastasis (13). Deposition of hybridoma cells in the spleens of recipient mice was reported recently to result in marked improvement in the growth of these tumors (14). In view of these two observations, it was decided to examine the behavior of human tumor cells injected into the spleens of nude mice. The spleen of a mouse under general anesthesia was exposed, received 5×10^5 viable cells in 0.05 ml volume by injection (with a 27-gauge needle) into the lateral spleen tip, and then was returned to the abdominal cavity. Six to eight weeks later, the animals were killed and autopsies were performed. Data in Table 3 show that injection into the spleen proved to be a way of producing widespread tumor development. Metastases frequently developed in several organs, including the mesenteric and omental lymph nodes (not reported in this table), but particularly striking in both number and size were the liver lesions. Thus, animals injected with A375-M, DX-3, PC3, 786-0, and HT-29 often had numerous, large neoplastic foci some greater than 5 mm in diameter, scattered throughout the liver parenchyma. Interestingly, the incidence of pulmonary tumor foci that developed after the injection of the prostate carcinoma PC3 and the colon carcinoma HT-29 lines was greater than that observed when direct i.v. injection in the tail vein was the route of inoculation. Of the nine tumor cell lines tested in this manner, four (A375-P, SK23, Dul45, and 769) failed to manifest any evidence of metastatic behavior. Thus, lines that may be described as metastatically indolent are not induced to change their behaviors when injected directly into the spleen. The behavior of the colon carcinoma line HT-29 suggested that intrasplenic tumor injection might be a suitable technique for evaluating the metastatic capacity of human colon tumors.

Table 3. Metastasis of Human Tumor Lines in Nude Mice Following Intrasplenic Injection of Tumor Cells

Cell Line	No. of Animals with Metastasis	
	Lung	Liver
A375-P	0/11	0/11
A375-M	0/15	8/15
DX-3	6/10	10/10
SK-23	0/15	0/15
DU145	3/10	0/10
PC3	16/20	20/20
769	1/10	0/10
786-0	6/10	4/10
HT-29	16/20	4/20

METASTATIC SPREAD OF HUMAN COLON CARCINOMA CELL LINES IN NUDE MICE

Groups of BALB/c mice were injected i.v. or intrasplenically with tumor cell suspensions obtained from colon carcinoma lines and subsequently were treated as already described. As shown in Table 4, none of these lines, when injected i.v., displayed any appreciable metastatic capacity. However, following injection into the spleen, both the LS174T and LoVo lines exhibited metastasis to the liver in many of the recipient mice (42% and 33% of animals, respectively). Again the large size of the metastatic deposits in the liver was perhaps more striking than the incidence of occurrence; in some mice bearing the LS174T line, greater than 50% of the liver was replaced by neoplastic tissue. Whether or not metastasis from the spleen occurred was independent of the in vivo growth rates of the various cell lines; although LS174T caused the fastest-growing tumors at the s.c. flank site (1 x 10^6 viable cells inoculated, mean tumor volume 0.69 mm^3 48 days after tumor injection) and the greatest number of mice bearing liver metastases, the LoVo line was much slower-growing than either the SW48 or SW837 lines (mean tumor volume 0.011 mm^3 versus 0.470 mm^3 or 0.205 mm^3 respectively, 48 days postinjection), but gave a higher incidence of metastasis from the spleen.

Table 4. Metastasis of Human Colon Carcinoma Cell Lines in Nude Mice

Cell Line	Experimental Metastasis Median No. (Range) of Lung Nodules	Metastasis from Spleen No. of Animals with Liver Nodules*
Coll 5/3-112	0	0/14
LoVo	0 (0-4)	4/13
LS174T	0 (0-4)	5/12
SW48	0	0/12
SW837	0 (0-1)	0/12

* Grossly evident tumor foci

DISCUSSION

The results presented here demonstrate that the metastatic spread of human tumors in nude mice is not an entirely uncommon event following i.v. or s.c. injection. However, intrasplenic injection of tumor cells allows the most dramatic overall expression of metastatic capacity (9). This observation has recently been confirmed in another laboratory (15) and suggests that this technique might prove a useful tool for experimental oncologists. Certainly, use of this route of tumor cell inoculation does not induce metastatic behavior in all lines tested; as suggested by Sharkey and Fogh (7), the intrinsic characteristics of the tumor line remain the major determinant in the regulation of metastatic spread. While the experiments reported here are somewhat preliminary in nature, they raise great possibilities for those interested in developing models of colon cancer metastasis and for the analysis of the underlying biology of this phenomenon. Can this route of cell injection be used to assay the malignant capacity of tumor material derived directly from patients? Since the metastatic behavior of the various cell lines appears to be due to intrinsic characteristics of the cells, is it possible to establish correlations between in vitro behavior and the degree of malignancy exhibited in this assay? We, and others, have already shown (8,10,16) that the application of in vivo or in vitro selection techniques, using passage through the nude mouse, can select out more malignant variant lines from starting heterogeneous populations. Will it prove possible to apply this protocol to human colon carcinoma lines to establish variants that produce metastasis in 100% of animals? If such variants are produced, will they supply us with relevant models for experimental therapy? It is to be hoped that the answers to these questions will be forthcoming in the near future. Certainly the development of model systems of human tumor metastasis based upon tumor spread in the athymic, nude mouse no longer looks as difficult as it appeared a few years ago.

ACKNOWLEDGMENTS

The author acknowledges the excellent technical assistance of Mavis Finch and Tony Carbonell.

References

1.   Hart IR: The role of animal models in the study of experimental metastasis. In: LA Liotta and IR Hart (eds), Tumor invasion and metastasis. Martinus Nijhoff, The Hague, 1982, pp 1-14.
2.   Fogh J, Fogh JM, Orfeo T: One hundred and twenty-seven cultured human tumor cell lines producing tumors in nude mice. J Natl Cancer Inst 59: 221-226, 1977.
3.   Fogh J, Orfeo T, Tiso J, Sharkey FE, Fogh JM, Daniels WP: Twenty-three new human tumor lines established in nude mice. Exp Cell Biol 48: 229-239, 1980.
4.   Kanazaki T, Hashimoto K, Bath DW: Heterotransplantation of human malignant melanoma cell lines in athymic nude mice. J Natl Cancer Inst 62: 1151-1153, 1979.
5.   Giovanella BC, Stehlin J, Williams LJ Jr: Heterotransplantation of human malignant tumors in "nude" thymusless mice. II. Malignant tumors induced by injection of cell cultures derived from solid tumors. J Natl Cancer Inst 52: 921-930, 1974.

6. Sordat B, Fritsche R, Mach JP, Carrel S, Ozzello L, Cerotini JC: Morphologic and functional evaluation of human solid tumors serially transplanted in nude mice. In: J Rygaard and CO Povlsen (eds), Proceedings of the First International Workshop on nude mice. Gustav-Fisher Verlag, Stuttgart, 1974, pp 269-277.

7. Sharkey FE, Fogh J: Metastasis of human tumors in athymic nude mice. Int J Cancer 24: 733-738, 1979.

8. Sordat BC, Ueyama Y, Fogh J: Metastasis of tumor xenografts in the nude mouse. In: J Fogh and BC Giovanella (eds), The nude mouse in experimental and clinical research, Vol 2. Academic Press, New York, 1982, pp 95-143.

9. Kozlowski JM, Fidler IJ, Campbell D, Xu Z-L, Kaighn ME, Hart IR: Metastatic behavior of human tumor cell lines grown in the nude mouse. Cancer Res 44: 3522-3529, 1984.

10. Kozlowski JM, Hart IR, Fidler IJ, Hanna N: A human melanoma line heterogeneous with respect to metastatic capacity in athymic nude mice. J Natl Cancer Inst 72: 913-917, 1984.

11. Fidler IJ: Selection of successive tumor lines for metastases. Nature 242: 148-149, 1973.

12. DeVore DO, Houches DP, Overjera AA, Dill GS, Hutson TB: Collagenase inhibitors retarding invasion of a human tumor in nude mice. Exp Cell Biol 48: 367-373, 1980.

13. Takahashi S, Konishi Y, Nakatoni K, Inui S, Kojima K, Shiratori T: Conversion of a poorly differentiated human adenocarcinoma to ascites form with invasion and metastasis in nude mice. J Natl Cancer Inst 60: 925-929, 1978.

14. Witte PL, Ber R: Improved efficiency of hybridoma ascites production by intrasplenic inoculation in mice. J Natl Cancer Inst 70: 575-577, 1983.

15. Vezeridis MP, Meinmer PA, Kajiji SM, Turner MD, Weimann MC, Calabresi P: Hepatic metastases of human tumor cell lines in nude mice (Abstract). Clin Res 32: 423, 1984.

16. Kerbel RS, Man MS, Dexter D: A model of human cancer metastasis: Extensive spontaneous and artificial metastasis of a human pigmented melanoma and derived variant sublines in nude mice. J Natl Cancer Inst 72: 93-108, 1984.

3

THE COTTON-TOP TAMARIN AS AN ANIMAL MODEL
OF COLORECTAL CANCER METASTASIS

Neal K. Clapp, Clarence C. Lushbaugh, Gretchen L. Humason,
Barbara L. Gangaware, and Marsha A. Henke

SUMMARY

The lack of satisfactory animal models for colorectal cancer has restricted the study of and significant progress in diagnosing and treating this very important human disease. High incidences of colon cancer in the cotton-top tamarin, Saguinus oedipus oedipus, mean that this animal is a potentially useful model for the study of causative agents and mechanistic and therapeutic aspects of this disease.

Age-dependent colonic carcinomas have been diagnosed in 35% of the tamarins that died after one year or more of colony-residence time. Colon cancer occurred in both sexes and in both feral and colony-born animals; all segments of the large bowel were affected. From January 1981 through July 1984, 70% (33/47) of the cotton-tops dying between 4 and 7 years of colony age had colonic cancer. Most tumors were diagnosed antemortem, diagnoses were followed by contrast radiography until the animal was moribund. The tumors metastasized early in the course of the disease (metastases have been found before the primary tumor was recognized grossly), first to the regional lymph nodes and eventually to the lungs, pancreas, and adrenals. No liver metastases have been found in the 81 cases diagnosed to date; the reason for the difference between the metastatic sites in tamarins and the common metastatic site of the liver in human colonic cancer is unknown. Colonic cancers in tamarins arise in the base of the crypts in flat (nonpolypoid) epithelium in the presence of chronic colitis, which can develop acute exacerbations with accompanying diarrhea and weight loss; this association resembles that between long-standing ulcerative colitis in humans and the carcinoma in situ that often develops subsequently. Not only can genetic and nutritional factors be manipulated in this animal model, but also experimental therapeutic protocols can be evaluated prior to human trials; such studies are not always feasible in humans. Investigations of immunologic, anatomic, and physiologic parameters as well as endoscopic biopsy examinations may help in understanding the causative agents, the development, and the metastatic characteristics of this disease and in identifying and developing diagnostic markers for colon cancer.

INTRODUCTION

Advances in diagnosing and treating human colorectal cancer have been made slowly, in part because of a lack of satisfactory animal models. Currently, increased numbers of tumors are being diagnosed in the right side of the colon in humans; these cancers are not only more difficult to diagnose than those on the left side, but are also more advanced in stage, frequently with extensive metastases. Most colorectal cancers metastasize relatively early in the course of the disease; the larger the number of lymph nodes involved, the poorer the prognosis. Early diagnosis prior to metastasis is essential for increased survival time, but often is not possible. Tumors chemically induced in rodents do not metastasize as frequently or as early as the spontaneous tumors observed in humans. Animal models of colon cancer are needed to study tumor diagnosis, tumor antigenicity, tumor biology, causative agents, metastatic potential, and therapeutic approaches.

TAMARIN COLON CANCER CHARACTERISTICS

Biology

High incidences of colonic cancer in the cotton-top tamarin, Saguinus oedipus oedipus, mean that this animal is a potentially useful model for the study of this important disease (1-3). Of cotton-tops that died after one year or more in the Oak Ridge Associated Universities (ORAU) colony between 1967 and 1984, 35% (79/225) had spontaneous colon cancer (2); in contrast, no colon cancer has been detected in several hundred necropsies of two other coexisting marmoset species, Saguinus fuscicollis illigeri and Callithrix jacchus (2,4). From January 1981 through July 1984, 70% (33/47) of deaths in cotton-tops between 4 and 7 years of colony age and 40% (6/15) 8 years or more of colony age were caused by colonic cancer (Table 1); in the end, the cause of death was usually intestinal obstruction. Colon carcinoma occurred in colony-born and imported S. o. oedipus of both sexes with a mean colony residence time of about 62 months (Table 2). All segments of the large bowel were affected; approximately 60% of the tumors involved the right side (from the cecum to the splenic flexure) (Table 3). Tamarin colon cancer was seen most often in young adults (3 to 7 years of colony age) (Figure 1) but also in older tamarins (up to 13 years of age); since 1980, only one cotton-top under 4 years of age has died with colon cancer. Colon cancer occurred as a single primary tumor or multiple primary tumors that metastasized readily, often before the primary was large enough to be diagnosed clinically (4). In certain affected families, more than

32

one generation have developed tumors. Detailed genealogical information has been
maintained on animals in the colony to provide information regarding hereditary
transmission.

Table 1. Frequency of Colonic Carcinomas in Recent S. o. oedipus Deaths

Year of Deaths	Colony Age No. Cancers/No. Deaths		
	1-3 Years	4-7 Years	$\geq$8 Years
1981	0/1	15/19	2/3
1982	0/0	8/13	2/5
1983	1/8	6/9	2/5
1984	0/1	4/6	0/2

Table 2. Mean Colony Ages at Death for S. o. oedipus with Colon Carcinoma

Origin	Males		Females	
	No. Animals	Mean Colony Age (Mos.)	No. Animals	Mean Colony Age (Mos.)
Imports	42	65	27	57
Colony-Born	3	59	9	68

Table 3. Location of Primary Carcinomas of the Large Bowel in S. o. oedipus[*]

Location	Number
Cecum	41
Ascending Colon	37
Transverse Colon	29
Descending Colon	46
Rectum	13
Unspecified	3
Multiple	49

[*] number of animals, 81.

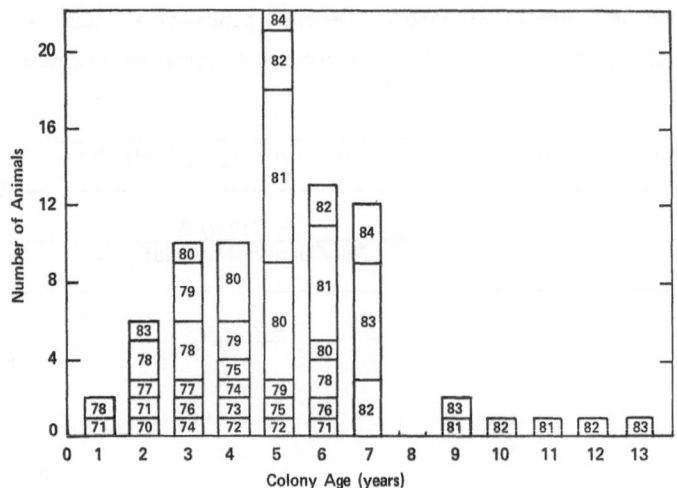

FIGURE 1. Colon cancer deaths by colony age in S. o. oedipus at ORAU, 1970-July, 1984.

Colonic carcinomas have been diagnosed in cotton-top tamarins from four different colonies in the United States and England despite different environments and different dietary and husbandry protocols (Table 4). This wide geographic dispersion suggests that this species has a hereditary component to its susceptibility to cancer. (The first colon cancer in a zoo-maintained S. o. oedipus colony was recently reported to us from Buffalo Zoological Gardens, Buffalo, NY; Dr. Allen Prowten, personal communication, 1984).

Table 4. Colonic Carcinomas Diagnosed in Different S. o. oedipus Colonies

Colony Site	Number of Cases
ORAU[*] -(Oak Ridge)	81
-NCI Animals (Currently at Oak Ridge)	3
NERPRC	29
Bristol, England	1

[*] ORAU - Oak Ridge Associated Universities; NERPRC - New England Regional Primate Research Center

Histology

Tamarin colon cancer develops in the base of the crypts in flat (nonpolypoid) mucosa altered by chronic colitis (4); most often the cancer cells are undifferentiated

34

and form structureless masses (Figure 2). The malignant cells invade the lamina propria and muscularis mucosae at vascular clefts, and then the mucosal lymphatics (Figure 3), through which they extend into the submucosa, the mesenteric lymphatic channels, and the mesenteric lymph nodes. The cancers are often multicentric and primary cancer foci can be found throughout most of the colon. These foci are almost identical in size and histological appearance (Figure 4). To date, the precancerous stage of the cancer has not been identified; the earliest recognized lesion consists of isolated crypts in which the hyperplastic epithelium abruptly forms cancer cells that "bud off" into the lumen of the crypt (4). Three such crypts are shown in Figure 5; a small cluster of cancer cells have invaded into the lamina propria.

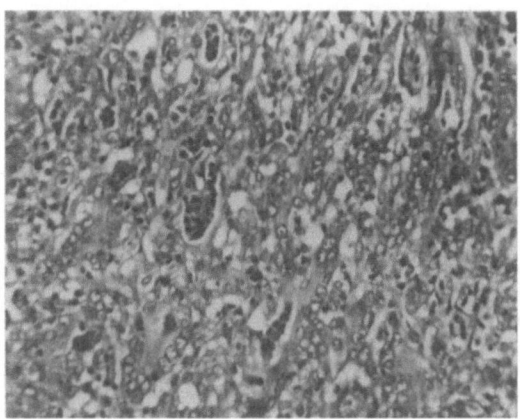

FIGURE 2. Undifferentiated rectal cancer. Cancer cells form glands very poorly. (PAS, 100x)

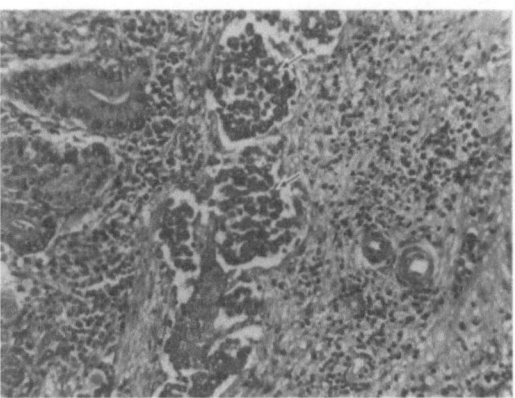

FIGURE 3. PAS-positive colonic carcinoma cells (arrows) in submucosal lymphatics. (PAS, 100x)

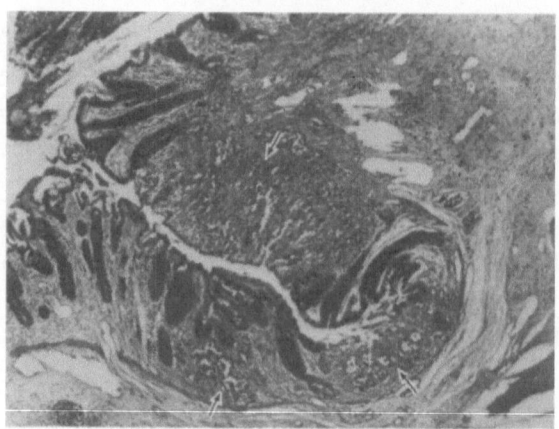

FIGURE 4. Multiple primary carcinomas in situ in the cecum. Cancers (arrows) are approximately the same size. (PAS, 25x)

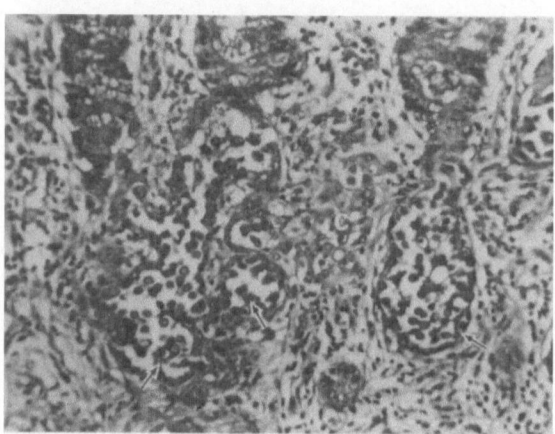

FIGURE 5. Carcinoma of the ascending colon. Three crypts (arrows) are budding cancer cells into the crypt lumen; a small cluster of cancer cells (c) infiltrates the lamina propria. (PAS, 100x)

Metastatic Potential

Although most chemically induced rodent tumors have a relatively low metastatic potential, 81% of the tamarin colon cancers metastasized to the regional lymph nodes (Figure 6). Whereas no liver metastases have been seen, metastases to the lung (Figure

7) have been diagnosed in 27%, to the pancreas in 15% and to the adrenal glands in 6% of the cases. The lack of hepatic metastases in tamarins, which contrasts with the high frequency of liver metastases in humans, may reflect anatomic differences in the lymphatic drainage of the large bowel, a lack of portal-vein invasion, or metabolic differences yet to be identified.

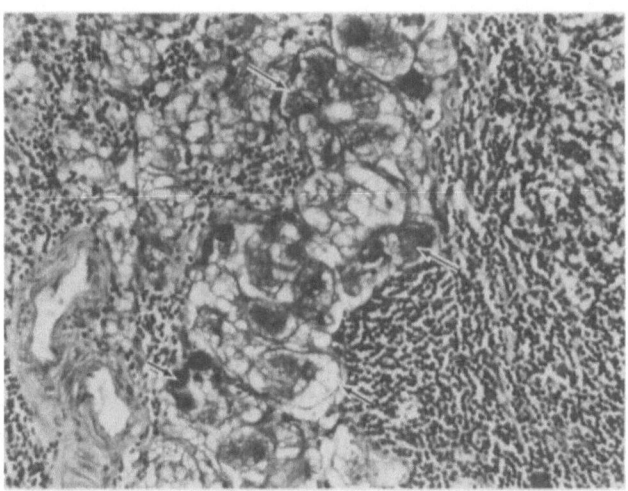

FIGURE 6. PAS-positive metastasis (arrows) from colon carcinoma to the mesenteric lymph nodes. (PAS, 100x)

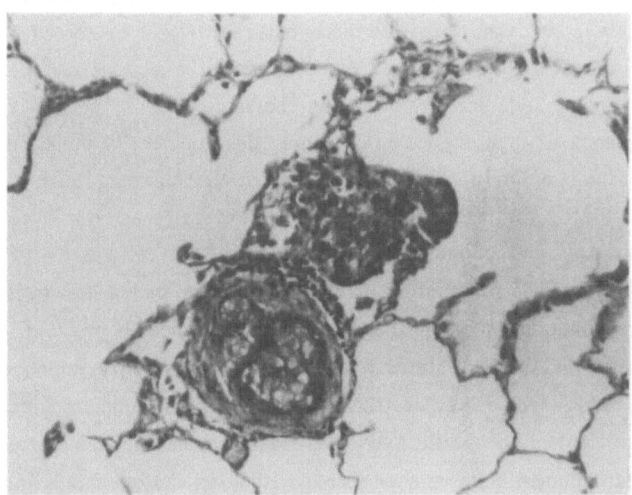

FIGURE 7. Metastasis from colon carcinoma to the lung. Cancer cells are seen in an arteriole and in alveolar septae (PAS, 100x).

Utilization of the periodic acid-Schiff (PAS) stain frequently shows mucin-producing cells from microscopic primaries in the lymphatics and regional lymph nodes, with no other cancer visible either grossly or microscopically. The level of mucin production, though it provides a usable diagnostic tool, is significantly lower in tamarin colon tumors than that observed in some human colon tumors. Large mucin lakes, however, are occasionally found in the tamarin lymphatics and other metastatic sites such as unmyelinated nerves.

DISCUSSION

One advantage of the tamarin as a potential model of human colon cancer is that the cancer and metastatic lesions usually can be diagnosed antemortem. A few cases have now been followed clinically for 12 to 15 months by barium-pneumoperitoneography (5). The metastatic lesions (i.e., enlarged lymph nodes) often are detected before clinical recognition of the primary site is possible (1-3,5); this suggests that metastases occur very early in the course of the disease. Several intriguing questions are raised regarding the observed metastatic patterns: 1) Why is the liver not a primary site of metastasis in the tamarin, as it is in humans? 2) Why does a tumor that metastasizes early fail, in most cases, to spread significantly beyond the local lymph nodes during the next several months? 3) Is the antigenicity of the tumor reflected in the aggressiveness and patterns of the metastases? 4) Can potential therapeutic strategies be tested in such a model system? The answers to these and other significant questions can help explain the developmental and biologic activity of tamarin colon cancer.

The frequency of spontaneous colon cancer development in the cotton-top tamarin makes it a potential animal model for the study of that disease. Such an animal model could be manipulated for mechanistic studies of causative agents, metastatic disease, diagnostic markers, and chemotherapeutic agents. Investigations of immunologic, anatomic, and physiologic parameters may help in understanding the development of this animal cancer. Since antemortem diagnosis of colon cancer is possible in the tamarin, factors affecting metastatic potential (e.g., tumor antigenicity, immune competence, etc.) can also be studied. Likewise, the contribution of inflammatory bowel disease to the expression of colonic neoplasia may be evaluated and better understood. We hope to better understand human colon cancer through studying and eventually manipulating the genetic and nutritional factors related to this spontaneous animal malignancy.

ACKNOWLEDGEMENTS

This report is based on work currently supported by Oak Ridge Associated Universities Corporation and National Cancer Institute, DHHS, Contract No. N01 CP 21004.

References

1.   Lushbaugh CC, Humason GL, Swartzendruber DC, Richter CB, Gengozian N: Spontaneous colonic adenocarcinoma in marmosets. In: Gengozian N, Deinhardt F (eds), Primates in Medicine, Vol. 10. Basel, New York, Karger, 1978, pp 119-134.
2.   Clapp NK, Lushbaugh CC, Humason GL, Gangaware BL, Henke MA: Natural history and pathology of colon cancer in Saguinus oedipus oedipus. Dig Dis Sci, 1985 (In press).
3.   Richter CB, Lushbaugh CC, Swartzendruber DC: Cancer of the colon in cotton-top tamarins. In: Montali RJ, Migaki G (eds), Comparative Pathology of Zoo Animals. Smithsonian Institute, Washington, DC, 1980, pp 567-571.
4.   Lushbaugh CC, Humason GL, Clapp NK: Histology of colon cancer in Saguinus oedipus oedipus. Dig Dis Sci, 1985 (In press).
5.   Clapp NK, Henke MA, Holloway EC, Tankersley WG: Carcinoma of the colon in the cotton-top tamarin: A radiographic study. J Am Vet Med Assoc 183: 1328-1330, 1983.

4

CLINICOPATHOLOGIC STUDIES ON MECHANISMS OF METASTASIS IN MAN AND OTHER VERTEBRATES

David Tarin

SUMMARY

Recent information on factors affecting metastatic spread of cancer in humans acquired from study of patients treated with peritoneovenous shunts for intractable malignant ascites is reviewed.   The evidence indicates that human tumors are heterogeneous in metastatic behavior, that this depends on intrinsic properties of the tumor cells, and that metastasis-competent cells can only colonize sites that are permissive to their presence and growth. The clinical indications for treating patients with peritoneovenous shunts and its complications are discussed, and its value in palliation as well as the absence of significant metastatic sequelae are stressed. The value of the procedure is that it significantly helps terminal patients who otherwise would have a poor quality of life, and it has the by-product of allowing, without distress or hazard, investigation of factors affecting the metastasis of tumors in humans. Already, it has provided direct validation of the applicability of several important observations in animal experiments to the behavior of human metastatic neoplasms.

INTRODUCTION

In this chapter, we review recently obtained information on the basic biology of human tumor metastasis and the use of peritoneovenous shunting for the palliation of malignant ascites resulting from inoperable abdominal cancer.   Traditionally, this condition was treated by paracentesis, but in some patients the reaccumulation of fluid is so copious and frequent (for instance, 250 liters were removed from one of our patients in six months) that its regular removal results in dehydration and depletion of proteins and essential minerals, which leads to severe metabolic imbalance. Added to this are the risk of other complications, such as implantation of tumor in the abdominal wall and peritonitis, together with the social dislocation that occurs when the patients have to be brought repeatedly to the hospital, sometimes from long distances, for this procedure.

Patients with malignant ascites, therefore, frequently face a miserable terminal illness, and it was to try to circumvent some of these problems, while still achieving some palliation of the pain and discomfort caused by the fluid accumulation, that the procedure of peritoneovenous shunting was first introduced by Pollock (1). In this procedure, the malignant ascites is returned to the circulation via a piece of plastic tubing containing a one-way valve (to prevent the reflux of blood) that opens at a pressure of 5 cm of water. The shunt does not contain a filter because this would rapidly block, and the suspended malignant cells are therefore infused directly into the blood as a steady trickle while the shunt remains patent. Because of this, many physicians are reluctant to risk possible massive metastatic sequelae, and the technique has taken a long time to gain acceptance, mostly because of the lack of systematic autopsy studies. Nevertheless, the excellence of the palliation in most patients, together with the recovery and symptom-free survival (median eight months in some centers - R. Lund, personal communication, October, 1984) of apparently moribund patients, are resulting in its more frequent use in suitable cases. The autopsy observations on the series of patients presented below endorse the clinical impression that this procedure does not expose the patient to clinically significant metastatic disease and, as a by-product, provide new and ethical observations on mechanisms of tumor spread in man.

The indications for peritoneovenous shunting are pain and discomfort resulting from accumulation of fluid in excess of two liters a week in patients with inoperable abdominal tumor, where antineoplastic therapy has failed, and diuretics cannot control the fluid production. Experience has indicated that some patients with ascites do not benefit from peritoneovenous shunting and some selection of patients is therefore necessary to avoid ineffective surgical intervention. Criteria for considering this as the treatment of choice are that the fluid should not be too viscous to flow along the tube and should not contain excessive coagulated fibrin or debris that would block the valve. Also the ascites should not be multiloculated, as this will interfere with drainage, and the patient should not be too debilitated to survive surgery and anesthesia (2).

The scientific interest of this mode of therapy relates to the ethically sound opportunities it provides for direct investigation in the living human of factors affecting tumor metastasis, without inconvenience, distress, or special clinical procedures. The observations have to be interpreted with caution because the mode of collecting information cannot be purpose designed. There is, therefore, considerable variation in length of patient survival, type of primary tumor, and other circumstances relating to each case, but the observations still provide information that, when pooled with laboratory studies on the cell biology of the same patient's tumor cells, can usefully be compared with results obtained from more controlled studies in experimental animals.

42

The findings on the first 15 cases (3,4) undergoing autopsy, now supplemented to 18, together with laboratory studies on the malignant cells of several more (4; unpublished observations, D. Tarin) lead to several conclusions considered below.

METASTATIC TUMOR DIVERSITY

Malignant human tumors show considerable diversity in their capability to form metastatic deposits, and mere entry of malignant cells into the circulation even in substantial numbers does not guarantee completion of the sequence of processes required to form metastases. The necropsy details provided in Table 1 show that some tumors in patients treated with this technique had speedily formed tiny seedlings in several organs (within one month), whereas others had not formed any detectable metastases despite survival of the patient for many months. As one of the main criteria for selecting patients for shunting was failure of other means of treatment, none received antineoplastic or anticoagulant therapy after shunt insertion, and differences in extent of metastasis among them, therefore, do not reflect differences in therapy. Failure to form detectable metastases was not solely a function of time, since their presence in some patients who survived very short intervals indicates that cells with the necessary potential can metastasize quickly. This heterogeneity among tumors with regard to behavioral potential is seen even among tumors of the same organs and histologic type (among 10 serous cystadenocarcinomas of the ovary in this study, 3 formed metastases, whereas 7 did not). As entry of substantial numbers of viable cells (4) into the circulation is guaranteed in all patients treated with this technique, the findings indicate that the metastatic competence of a tumor is determined by intrinsic properties of its constituent cells. These conclusions on human tumor behavior are extremely similar to earlier ones based upon our studies on naturally occurring mammary tumors in mice (5,6,7) and imply that metastasis is not a random process, but is the recurrent outcome of systematic disturbances in control of cellular activities.

SITES OF METASTATIC CELL COLONIZATION

Tumors cannot colonize all sites in which substantial numbers of viable tumor cells lodge, and this experimentally confirms, in living human subjects, Paget's deductions based on autopsy data (8). The findings also challenge the interpretations of Ewing (9) and others that the distribution of metastases is solely determined by the anatomic patterns of vascular and lymphatic drainage from the site of the primary tumor, although sieving effects exerted by the capillaries of the lung and the sinusoids of the liver can

43

Table 1. Summary of Clinical and Pathologic Findings

Patient	Sex	Age	Site of primary tumor	Survival time after shunting (months)	Distribution of metastases
Group 1: No hemato-genous metastases					
1. DG	F	53	Ovary	27*	None
2. EH	F	66	Ovary	2	None
3. RH	F	68	Stomach	1	None
4. DJ	M	60	Unknown	2.5	None
5. AR	F	57	Ovary and breast	7	None
6. HM	F	48	Ovary	2	None
7. JB	F	76	Ovary	4	None
8. BB	F	46	Ovary	1	None
9. GP	F	73	Ovary	2	None
Group 2: Hematogenous metastases present					
10. MM	F	49	Vagina	2.5	Lungs, liver
11. WA	F	82	Ovary	4	Several organs [†]
12. ER	F	55	Ovary	3.5	Lungs
13. FG	M	67	Pancreas	9	Lungs, liver
14. DJ	F	59	Unknown	5	Liver, vertebrate
15. WH	M	51	Bronchus [§]	1	Other lung
16. EJS	F	61	Colon	4	Lungs
17. EES	F	76	Ovary	5	Several organs [//]
18. FM	F	79	Colon	10	Liver, ovary [#]

* First shunt functioned for 5 months and second for 6 months, with an interim period of 16 months with intermittently functioning shunt.

† Lungs, liver, spleen, brain, choroid plexus, intestinal wall, adrenals; all tiny deposits.

‡ Large deposits before shunt inserted. Lungs and other organs completely negative.

§ Pleurovenous shunt.

// Adrenals, lungs, and liver.

No pulmonary metastases despite colonization of liver and ovary.

clearly reduce the tumor cell burden entering the systemic circulation and have some influence on whether metastases form outside the lungs.

All of the tumors in the patients listed in Table 1 had, to greater or lesser extent, succeeded in transcelomic metastasis and were therefore proven to be capable of growing in the peritoneum, but either failed to grow anywhere after hematogenous dissemination (Table 1; Group 1) or did so only in certain organs and not in others (Group 2). Three patients in Group 2 (two with colorectal cancer and one with an unknown primary tumor, probably gastrointestinal) are of particular interest. Patient 16 (EJS) and patient 18 (FM) both had well-differentiated mucin-secreting adenocarcinomas of the colon. The former patient (EJS) had formed microscopic metastases in the interstitial tissues of the lungs (Figure 1) within two months of shunt insertion. Although it cannot be categorically stated that these tiny secondary lesions resulted from the vascular infusion of tumor cells via the shunt rather than by spontaneous hematogenous metastasis, their uniformly small size makes it as certain as anything can be in clinical medicine that this was the case. In this patient, the liver had no microscopic or macroscopic tumor deposits, but tumor growth was extensive in the abdominal lymph nodes and in the lymphatics permeating the diaphragm. In contrast, patient FM had obvious macroscopic hematogenous metastases in the liver (Figures 2 & 3), but the lungs and other organs were free of hematogenous metastases, even though she had survived 10 months and small clumps of mucin-secreting tumor cells could be identified in the pulmonary vessels (Figure 4). In this patient, therefore, cells proven to be capable of hematogenous metastasis in the liver failed to form detectable metastases in the lung, although they were being infused directly into the capillaries of this organ in large numbers for several months. Similarly, the tumor in patient 14 (DJ), who had extensive hepatic and spinal metastases prior to insertion of the shunt, did not form any pulmonary secondary lesions in five months, although the cells were obviously viable and capable of hematogenous metastasis before the shunt was ever inserted. Laboratory studies confirmed that the cells in her ascites were 95% viable (4), and there can therefore be no reasonable doubt that large numbers of cells, proven in advance to be tumorigenic, reached the lungs through the superior vena cava, but, for one reason or another, did not grow there.

Again, the findings in humans are in direct agreement with our previous studies on naturally occurring murine mammary tumors (10). Using homologous techniques of intravascular infusion of tumor cells, we demonstrated that cells from tumors known to be capable of forming metastases in the lungs would not necessarily form hematogenous deposits in other organs, such as the liver, even if injected directly into the supplying vessels. Similarly, experiments on a transplantable mouse tumor (B16 melanoma) showed

45

that tumor cells known to grow preferentially in the lungs and ovaries still did so after intravenous inoculation, even when the organs were transplanted to an anatomically unusual location (11). The findings collectively indicated that in both species specific microenvironmental influences in the sites where tumor cells lodge can modulate whether cells with proven metastatic capability can express this potential. It may therefore be concluded that tumor cells, even of high growth potential in some sites, are not invincible everywhere and the results of this investigation demonstrate unambiguously that in humans, as in other animals (5,12,13), metastasis is not an inevitable consequence of tumor cell dissemination.

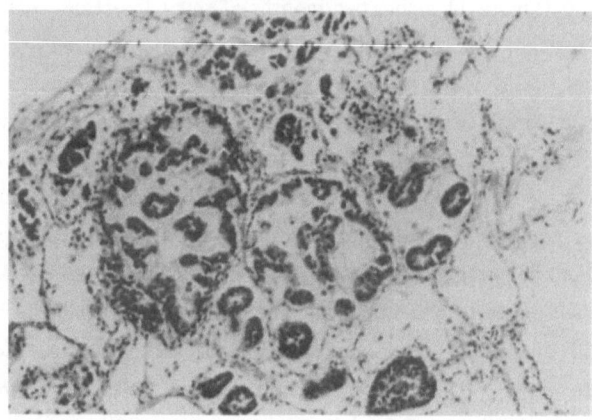

FIGURE 1. Patient 16 (EJS). Photograph of lung metastasis from mucin-secreting adenocarcinoma of the colon. (x 50)

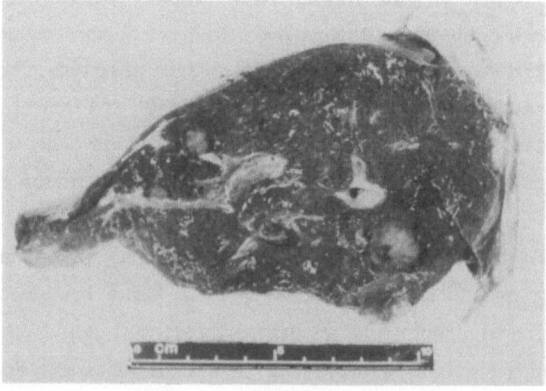

FIGURE 2. Patient 18 (FM). Section through liver showing hematogenous metastases.

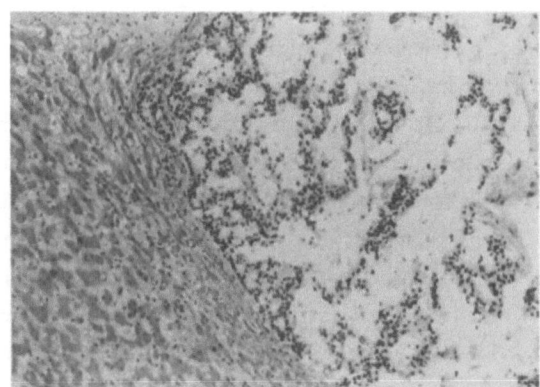

FIGURE 3. Patient 18 (FM). Photomicrograph of liver metastasis from mucin-secreting adenocarcinoma of the colon. (x 50)

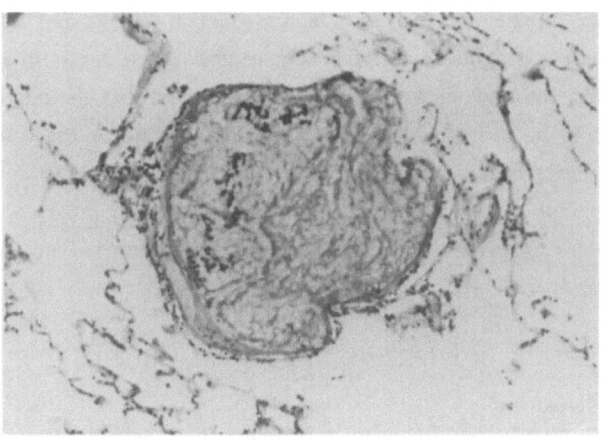

FIGURE 4. Patient 18 (FM). Photomicrograph showing sparse tumor cells in a pulmonary arteriole filled with mucus, but no tumor was growing extravascularly in the lungs. (x 50)

Such vindication of the "seed and soil" hypothesis of Paget has implications not only for clinical issues, such as knowing where to look for residual systemic disease after therapy, but also for understanding mechanisms underlying metastatic spread. Once it is accepted that tumors are composed of heterogeneous populations of tumor cells (see preceding section and reference 14) scattered more or less representatively throughout the body after mixing in the vortex of the blood (13) and that they reproducibly grow in some sites and not others, it follows that individual organs permit or inhibit secondary

47

tumor formation by metastasis-competent cells and hence that cells of normal organs can, on occasion, suppress or at least fail to support malignant growth. Verification of this interpretation requires demonstration of the mechanisms of the microenvironmental effects deduced to be operative in vivo, and recent work in this laboratory has been directed towards this aim. We found (15) that co-culturing mouse mammary tumor cells, which normally only form pulmonary metastases, with fragments of liver or thyroid results in the death of the tumor cells, whereas co-culture with pieces of lung results in increased survival and adherence of the tumor cells to the substratum, with most of the naturally-occurring tumors tested. Renal and ovarian fragments are occasionally facilitatory in vitro, but usually neutral, and it is interesting to note that occasional deposits are seen in these organs when cells from murine mammary tumors are inoculated via the aorta (13). The inhibitory effect can be dialyzed as well as transferred from one culture to another with cell-free media (15). Organ fragments co-cultured with fluorescein isothiocyanate (FITC)-labeled tumor cells are, on examination of frozen sections under an ultraviolet microscope, readily invaded. When lung fragments from these cultures are reimplanted in vivo, a high proportion form tumors that subsequently metastasize, whereas fragments of other organs less often result in implant-derived tumors (16). Thus, the findings with mouse tumors suggest that the microenvironmental effects deduced to be operative in vivo (3,4,10,11) are due to the release of soluble substances that exert organ-specific effects. Further studies using cells from human tumors and fragments of normal human organs are currently in progress, and the results show that similar organ-specific effects can be demonstrated in vitro (E. Horak, unpublished observations).

APPLICABILITY OF EXPERIMENTAL ANIMAL FINDINGS TO HUMANS

The similarity of the findings in humans to those in animal experiments, particularly those we have conducted using homologous techniques with naturally occurring mammary tumors (5,17,6,7), validates the applicability to human situations of conclusions based upon animal experimentation. They also indicate that at least some of the underlying mechanisms in the phenomenon of metastasis in higher vertebrates are shared and are amenable to systematic analysis. In particular, therefore, the evidence already available suggests that human tumors, like their murine counterparts, exhibit diversity of metastatic behavior (3,4) attributable to heterogeneity in the intrinsic properties of their constituent cells (18,19), that these properties are inherently unstable (20,21), and that the metastatic process is effected by a highly active subpopulation with special properties emerging from the primary tumor early in its development (7). The implications of the findings of Poste et al. (20), that the metastatic potency of a clone does not remain stable if it is isolated from others of the same tumor, are gloomy if, as seems likely, they are corroborated for human material. They indicate that as the cells scatter and multiply in isolation from each other, their progeny in metastases will generate new diversity in behavior and resistance to treatment.

CELLULAR IMMUNE RESPONSE

In no patient treated with peritoneovenous shunts was any significant cellular immune response observed to deposits of latent tumor cells. In particular, no features suggesting regression of tumor deposits (dying tumor cells or host lymphoid infiltration) were seen even in those patients who survived only for short periods. This is of particular interest in those patients with hematogenous metastases at the time of death. In one patient, occasional small groups of lymphocytes were seen in the vicinity of a few of the tumor cell clumps in the pulmonary vessels, but most of these clumps were neither associated with cells of the immune system nor were those in other organs. In animals, Hanna and Fidler (22) and Fidler et al. (23) have demonstrated that natural killer cells and macrophages can be involved in destruction of disseminating tumor cells or of small deposits in the interstitial tissues. However, despite much work in several laboratories over many years, there is yet no decisive evidence that the immune system usually exercises a dominant influence on metastasis of tumors in general. Currently available evidence indicates that immunologic mechanisms can, with appropriate stimulation, be mobilized to combat metastasis but are not necessarily functioning ab initio in sufficient force to stem the process.

SHUNT COMPLICATIONS

The autopsy findings established that, even in those patients in whom small deposits had formed, the metastatic sequelae of peritoneovenous shunting were not harmful because the patients died of their abdominal tumor load before metastases were clinically evident. This is of practical importance for the implementation of this form of treatment in patients with inoperable malignancy and intractable ascites.

Peritoneovenous shunting, although demonstrated by this study not to pose a hazard of clinically significant metastasis, is not completely free of complications, which primarily affect the efficiency of drainage and palliation (24). The most important complications encountered are listed in Table 2 together with the numbers of patients affected, and it can be seen that the most common complication was tube blockage

49

owing either to endothelial ensleevement of the venous end of the shunt, thrombosis around its tip, or occlusion of the lumen by tumor, fibrin, or mucus. The next commonest complication was embolization of thrombi or neoplastic cells, although neither led to clinically detectable symptoms. In this series, there was no evidence of disseminated intravascular coagulation as reported in other published studies, but one patient died of acute pulmonary edema almost immediately after drainage began, presumed to be due to anaphylactic shock.

Table 2. Complications of Peritoneovenous Shunt -Oxford Series*

Complication	Number of Patients
Blockage	14
Embolization - tumor	8
Embolization - thrombi	4
Tumor implantation in shunt canal	2
Sepsis	1
Deaths (fluid overload)	1
Disseminated intravascular coagulation (DIC)	0

* Number of patients treated, 43.

Implantation of tumor deposits in the track of the shunt (Figure 5) is an undesirable event and is potentially alarming for the patient. Although an infrequent event, it results from leakage of malignant ascites along the subcutaneous tunnel caused by slackening of the purse-string suture around the tubing of the shunt as it enters the peritoneal cavity. (The second patient in our series (FM) in whom the tumor cells grew subcutaneously was the one referred to above with an adenocarcinoma of the colon. Her cells did not establish metastases in the lungs.)

The observations on patients treated with peritoneovenous shunts for intractable malignant ascites have established that, with properly selected patients, it is an effective means of palliation, resulting in extended survival with better quality of life and no clinically significant problems related to tumor metastasis. As an incidental by-product, the technique offers opportunities of unrivaled power and interest for investigating factors affecting tumor metastasis in man, without inconvenience to the patients. The findings bridge the gap between clinical experience and data from controlled experiments in animals thereby allowing recognition of information pertinent to human disease.

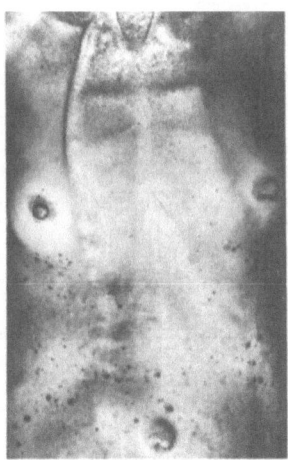

FIGURE 5. Patient 18 (FM). View of the body showing shunt in situ with adjacent nodules of tumor in the subcutaneous tunnel.

ACKNOWLEDGMENTS

This work was funded by the Cancer Research Campaign of Great Britain whose support is gratefully acknowledged. The author also wishes to thank Mr. M.G. Kettlewell, Dr. J.E. Price, and Mrs. P. Messer for their collaboration and help.

References

1. Pollock AV: The treatment of resistant malignant ascites by insertion of a peritoneo-atrial Holter valve. Br J Surg 62: 104-107, 1975.
2. Souter RG, Tarin D, Kettlewell MGW: Peritoneo-venous shunts in the management of malignant ascites. Br J Surg 70: 478-481, 1983.
3. Tarin D, Price JE, Kettlewell MGW, Souter RG, Vass ACR, Crossley B: Clinicopathological observations on metastasis in man studied in patients treated with peritoneovenous shunts. Br Med J 288: 749-751, 1984.
4. Tarin D, Price JE, Kettlewell MGW, Souter RG, Vass ACR, Crossley B: Mechanisms of human tumor metastasis studied in patients with peritoneovenous shunts. Cancer Res 44: 3584-3592, 1984.
5. Tarin D, Price JE: Metastatic colonization potential of primary tumor cells in mice. Br J Cancer 39: 740-754, 1979.

6. Price JE, Carr D, Jones LD, Messer P, Tarin D: Experimental analysis of factors affecting metastatic spread using naturally-occurring tumours. Invasion Metastasis 2: 77-112, 1982.
7. Price JE, Carr D, Tarin D: Spontaneous and induced metastasis of naturally-occurring tumors in mice: Analysis of cell shedding into the blood. J Natl Cancer Inst 73: 1319-1326, 1985.
8. Paget S: The distribution of secondary growths in cancer of the breast. Lancet i: 571-573, 1889.
9. Ewing J: Neoplastic Diseases, 3rd edn. WB Saunders Co, Philadelphia, 1928, pp 1127.
10. Tarin D, Price JE: Influence of microenvironment and vascular anatomy on "metastatic" colonization potential of mammary tumors. Cancer Res 41: 3604-3609, 1981.
11. Hart I, Fidler IJ: Role of organ selectivity in the metastatic patterns of B16 melanoma. Cancer Res 40: 2281-2287, 1980.
12. Juacaba SF, Jones LD, Tarin D: Organ preferences in metastatic colony formation by spontaneous mammary carcinomas after intra-arterial inoculation. Invasion Metastasis 3: 208-220, 1983.
13. Potter KM, Juacaba SF, Price JE, Tarin D: Observations on organ distribution of fluorescein-labeled tumor cells released intravascularly. Invasion Metastasis 3: 221-233, 1983.
14. Fidler IJ: Tumour heterogeneity and the biology of cancer invasion and metastasis. Cancer Res 38: 2651-2660, 1978.
15. Horak E, Darling D, Tarin D: Organ-specific effects on metastatic growth studied in vitro. (In press), 1985.
16. Horak E, Darling D, Tarin D: Organ-specific effects on metastatic tumour growth: studies involving transplantation techniques. (In press), 1985.
17. Tarin D: Investigations of the mechanisms of metastatic spread of naturally-occurring neoplasms. Cancer Metastasis Rev 1: 215-225, 1982.
18. Fidler IJ, Kripke ML: Metastasis results from pre-existing variant cells within a malignant tumor. Science 197: 893-895, 1977.
19. Kripke ML, Gruys E, Fidler IJ: Metastatic heterogeneity of cells from an ultraviolet light-induced murine fibrosarcoma of recent origin. Cancer Res 38: 2962-2967, 1978.
20. Poste G, Doll J, Fidler IJ: Interactions between clonal subpopulations affect stability of the metastatic phenotype in polyclonal populations of B16 melanoma cells. Proc Natl Acad Sci USA 78: 6226-6230, 1981.
21. Cifone MA, Fidler IJ: Increasing metastatic potential is associated with increasing genetic instability of clones isolated from murine neoplasms. Proc Natl Acad Sci USA 78: 6949-6952, 1981.
22. Hanna N, Fidler IJ: Role of natural killer cells in the destruction of circulating tumor emboli. J Natl Cancer Inst 65: 801-809, 1980.
23. Fidler IJ, Sone S, Fogler WE, Barnes ZL: Eradication of spontaneous metastases and activation of alveolar macrophages by intravenous injection of liposomes containing muramyl dipeptide. Proc Natl Acad Sci USA 78: 1680-1684, 1981.
24. Souter RG, Wells C, Tarin D, Kettlewell MGW: Surgical and pathological complications associated with peritoneo-venous shunts in management of malignant ascites. Cancer (In press), 1985.

5

METASTATIC COLORECTAL CARCINOMA: PATHOBIOLOGIC SUBSETS

Lewis A. Johnson

SUMMARY

The principal pathologic variables of colorectal cancer prognosis are reviewed. The interrelationship of the three variables, namely, tumor stage, tumor grade, and tumor cell type, is emphasized. Survival prognosis is very much influenced by the histologic/cytologic characteristics of the tumor with greater importance being placed on tumor grade and the predominant cell type present in metastatic colon cancer. The criteria, definition, and examples of the histologic grade and cell types are presented. The potential implications of these pathologic characteristics to therapeutic modalities are hypothesized.

PATHOBIOLOGIC VARIABLES

Survival following surgical resection of adenocarcinoma of the colon or rectum is related to three variables that are determined by microscopic laboratory assessment of the specimen. They are tumor stage, the extent of histologic spread from the mucosal primary site (1); tumor grade, the degree of histologic glandular differentiation of the tumor (2); and tumor cell type, mucinous versus nonmucinous cellular composition (3,4). Mucinous colorectal adenocarcinomas are associated with poorer survival prognosis than nonmucinous cell types (4). The three prognostic variables are interrelated; the higher the mucinous cell population and the higher the grade of the tumor, the greater the probability that the tumor will be a higher stage (1-5).

In metastatic colorectal adenocarcinoma, the stage prognostic variable becomes less critical in predicting survival than the tumor grade and predominant cell type variables. In the laboratory assessment of adenocarcinoma grade and predominant cell type composition of metastatic biopsy specimens, Eastern Cooperative Oncology Group (ECOG) pathologists utilize a histologic/cytologic classification scheme first proposed by Dukes (4). This scheme subdivides colorectal cancer into three glandular histologic grades, each with a predominantly nonmucinous or predominately mucinous cell type variant plus a nonglandular or undifferentiated grade with several probable pathobiologically different cell types (Table 1).

The standard for tumor histologic grade and cell type used by ECOG pathologists is that greater than 50% of the tumor in the metastatic site biopsy sample consists of that particular grade and cell type (5). Examples of the six glandular subsets are illustrated in Figures 1-6. An example of a large cell undifferentiated colorectal carcinoma is shown in Figure 7.

Table 1. Colorectal Carcinoma Pathobiologic Subsets.

Glandular Tumors (Nonmucinous or mucinous cell types)		
Numerical Grade	Descriptive Grade	Mucinous Cell Type Eponyms
1	Well Differentiated	Goblet cell
2	Moderately well differentiated	Colloid
3	Poorly differentiated	Signet ring cell

The descriptive types of undifferentiated nonglandular tumors are large cell (squamoid and transitional cell subtypes) or small cell.

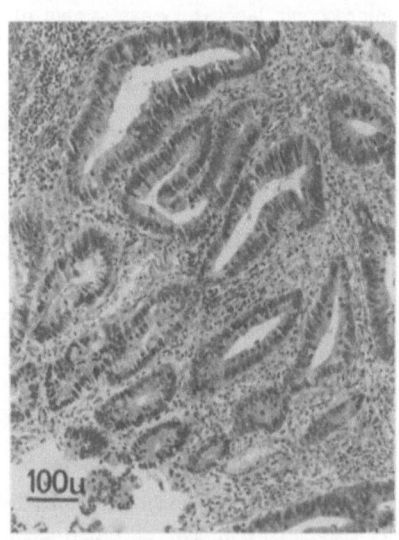

FIGURE 1. Grade 1 nonmucinous colon adenocarcinoma.

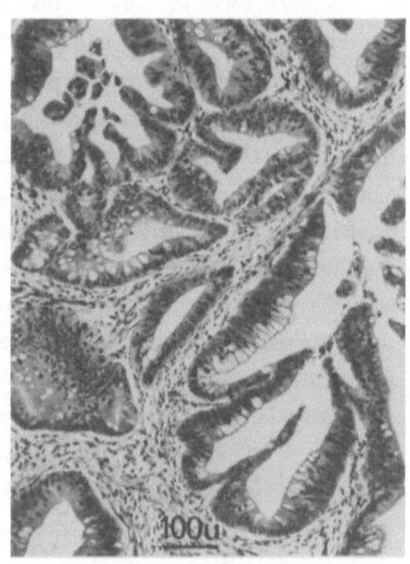

FIGURE 2. Grade 1 mucinous colon adenocarcinoma.

54

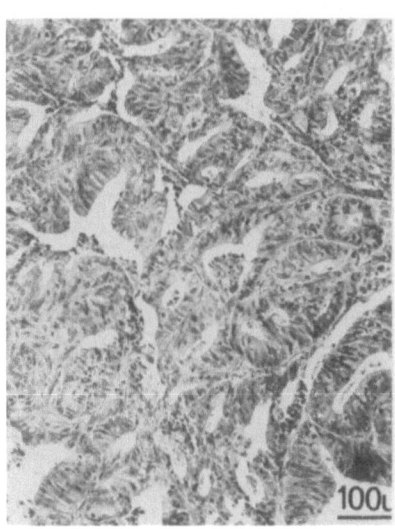

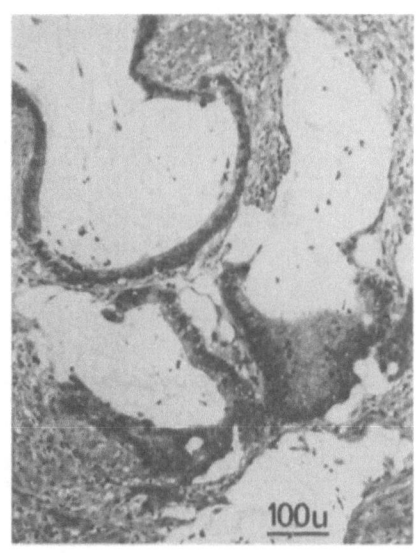

FIGURE 3. Grade 2 nonmucinous
colon adenocarcinoma.

FIGURE 4. Grade 2 mucinous colon
adenocarcinoma.

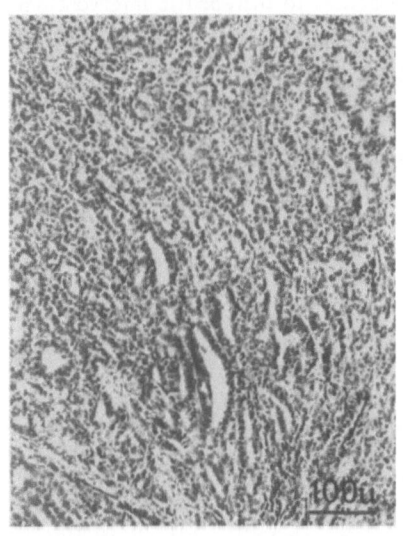

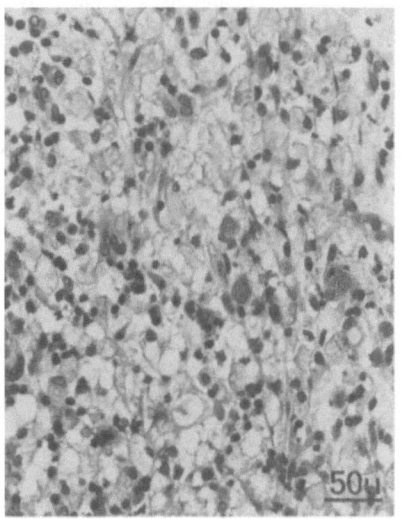

FIGURE 5. Grade 3 nonmucinous
colon adenocarcinoma.

FIGURE 6. Grade 3 mucinous colon
adenocarcinoma.

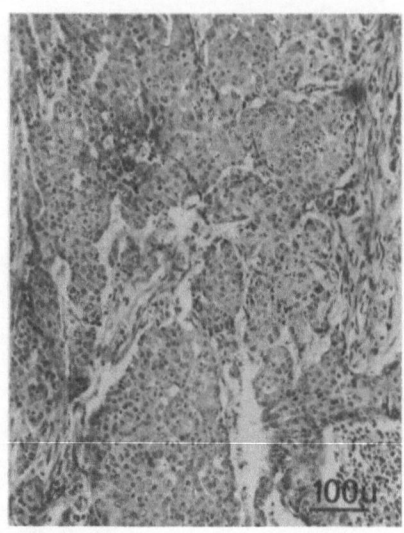

FIGURE 7.   Large cell undifferentiated colon carcinoma.

In addition to having different survival characteristics, these pathobiologic colorectal carcinoma subsets may have different responses to therapeutic interventions (5).   For example, metastatic colorectal small cell undifferentiated carcinoma may respond to treatment regimens devised for small cell undifferentiated lung carcinoma, whereas the other pathobiologic subsets may not (5).   In future colorectal carcinoma treatment investigations, ECOG pathologists will look for possible differential treatment responses by these histologic/cytologic subsets (5).

References

1.   Dukes CE, Bussey HJR: The spread of rectal cancer and its effect on prognosis. Br J Cancer 12: 309-319, 1958.
2.   Dukes CE: Histologic grading of cancer. Proc Roy Soc Med 30: 371-376, 1937.
3.   Symonds DA, Vickery AL: Mucinous carcinoma of the colon and rectum. Cancer 37: 1891-1900, 1976.
4.   Dukes CE: The surgical pathology of rectal cancer. J Clin Pathol 2: 95-98, 1949.
5.   Johnson LA, Masse SR, Simson IW, Barr JR, Nime F, Sumner H, Doos WG, Klaasen D, Mittelman A, Mansour EG, Douglas HO, Cooper HS, Geller SA: Standardized colorectal adenocarcinoma stage and grade data: Applications to future cooperative treatment research. In: A Gerard (ed), Progress and perspectives in the treatment of gastrointestinal tumors. Pergamon Press, Oxford, New York, 1981, pp 110-115.

6

THE USE OF LECTINS IN BIOCHEMICAL STUDIES
ON COLORECTAL CARCINOMA METASTASIS

Tatsuro Irimura, David M. Ota, Karen R. Cleary and Garth L. Nicolson

SUMMARY

Lectins have been used widely for investigating the structure and function of cell surface glycoproteins that are associated with metastatic behavior of tumor cells. Lectins have also been used for fractionating subpopulations of tumor cells that have altered metastatic capacities. We have initiated detailed histochemical and biochemical analyses of lectin-reactive glycoconjugates in colorectal carcinomas and their metastases. Among the nine lectins used, three blood group H-specific lectins have been useful in distinguishing normal colonic mucosa and adenocarcinoma from other types of cells. We found that Cytisus sessilifolius agglutinin binds to a highly differentiated portion of normal colonic mucosa, whereas Ulex europaeus agglutinin reactivity is occasionally seen in adenocarcinoma of the rectum or sigmoid colon. In some cases, the intensity of Ulex europaeus agglutinin binding is heterogeneous in primary tumors. By comparing the labeling patterns of heterogeneous primary tumors and their liver metastases, we may be able to elucidate the origin of cells that form liver metastases. Polyacrylamide gel electrophoresis of extracts of the tumor tissue followed by incubation with ^{125}I-labeled Ulex europaeus agglutinin indicates that a glycoprotein having a molecular weight greater than 500,000 is the only molecule with this lectin reactivity in primary colorectal carcinoma and liver metastases derived from this neoplasm.

INTRODUCTION

Successful tumor metastasis requires a series of complex interactions between tumor cells and their microenvironments (1,2). Cell surface and extracellular molecules produced by tumor cells, as well as by the host, play important roles in regulating these interactions (3). Three lines of evidence strongly suggest that glycoconjugate molecules at the tumor cell surface are significant in determining successful survival and colonization of specific distant organs in experimental animals. First, highly metastatic tumor cells selected for their organ colonization properties in vivo display alterations in their cell surface glycoconjugates (4-8). Second, enzymatic, metabolic, or other modifications of glycoconjugate molecules on the tumor cell surface resulted in reduced or increased colonization capacities (9-13). Third, tumor cell subpopulations or variants with altered cell surface glycoconjugates can be selected by use of lectins, carbohydrate-binding proteins (or glycoproteins) having cytoagglutinating or glycoconjugate-precipitating activities (14), and these selected cells possess different metastatic capacities (4,15,16).

Lectins have been used for structural characterization of glycoconjugates derived from tumor cells (6-8) and for the purification of certain classes of glycoconjugates (17,18). In addition, since most cell-surface components involved in regulating cell physiologic responses induced by extracellular stimuli are glycoconjugates, lectins have been used as probes for studying such responses. Lectins have also been used as cytochemical tools in order to differentiate and subfractionate heterogeneous tumor cell populations (19). Histochemical use of lectins has revealed tumor cells in tissue sections (20), and in some cases, the expression of lectin-reactive molecules at the cell surface appears to be related to normal cellular differentiation. In cancer, expression of certain metastatic phenotypes may also be related to the expression of particular glycoconjugate markers (3,10,11).

A few laboratories have attempted to use lectins in studies on human colorectal carcinoma; however, none of these studies have concentrated on mechanistic aspects of metastasis. In this chapter, we present some uses of lectins for studies on experimental metastasis and for observations on human colorectal carcinoma metastasis.

LECTIN-REACTIVE GLYCOPROTEINS AND TUMOR METASTASIS IN EXPERIMENTAL ANIMALS

Murine B16 melanoma cells were derived from a melanoma that spontaneously arose in a C57BL/6 mouse. A variety of B16 sublines have been selected in vivo, as well as in vitro, and these have been tested for their spontaneous metastatic and blood-borne experimental metastatic colonization properties. Most of the earlier attempts to discover specific differences in cell surface glycoproteins between nonmetastatic and metastatic cells proved unsuccessful (21), except those by Brunson et al. (22), who demonstrated a correlation between brain-colonizing ability of B16 variants and expression of a M_r ~ 90,000 cell surface component revealed by lactoperoxidase-catalyzed iodination. This correlation was further confirmed later by using clonal subpopulations of another brain-selected series of B16 (23).

Evidence that melanoma surface glycoproteins are important in blood-borne lung colonization came from a series of experiments that utilized an inhibitor of asparagine-linked carbohydrate chain formation in glycoproteins (10,11). After a 24 hr treatment with tunicamycin, lung-colonizing B16-F1 or B16-F10 melanoma cells had lowered incorporation rates of carbohydrate into macromolecules and altered morphologies. The treated cells lost cell surface lectin-binding sites, such as those that bind Ricinus communis agglutinin I (RCA$_I$), and adhesiveness to plastic culture substratum. At the same time, their ability to colonize lung following intravenous injection decreased dramatically (10,11). Since all melanoma cells recovered from the effects of tunicamycin within 24 hr after removal of this drug from the culture medium, the modified cell surface glycoconjugate must have affected early events in implantation that determine the fate of injected tumor cells. Indeed, for tunicamycin-treated cells, we found that the kinetics of adhesion to the endothelial monolayer, as well as to the endothelial extracellular matrix, decreased dramatically (10,11). Although the primary target of this antibiotic is carbohydrate chain formation, it is not known whether the carbohydrate portion of the cell surface glycoproteins (sialoglycoproteins as indicated by lectin-binding patterns) are directly involved in tumor cell implantation. Nonglycosylated proteins are highly susceptible to proteolytic enzymes. In addition, when glycoprotein turnover rates are altered, other physiological properties may also change. The primary function of the sialoglycoproteins might be to serve as a combining site for extracellular matrix components. We have purified this class of sialoglycoproteins by use of affinity chromatography on wheat germ agglutinin (WGA)-agarose and found that one of these glycoproteins possesses affinity to endothelial extracellular matrix (24).

We have concluded from studies using tunicamycin that the differences between the colonization abilities of low (B16-F1) and high (B16-F10) lung-colonizing sublines cannot be explained solely by tunicamycin-sensitive sialoglycoproteins. We could not find differences in the expression of this class of glycoproteins between F1 and F10, and these two B16 sublines were equally sensitive to the effects of tunicamycin. Therefore, we have been examining differences in other classes of cell surface glycoproteins. From the early studies on other cell types, such as human erythrocytes, we knew that single cells can synthesize multiple glycoproteins with entirely distinct carbohydrate chains (25-26). However, in the case of B16 melanoma sublines, the overall profiles of cellular glycoproteins and the presence of various glycoprotein classes were not known, and purification of each individual glycoprotein and determination of exact structural and

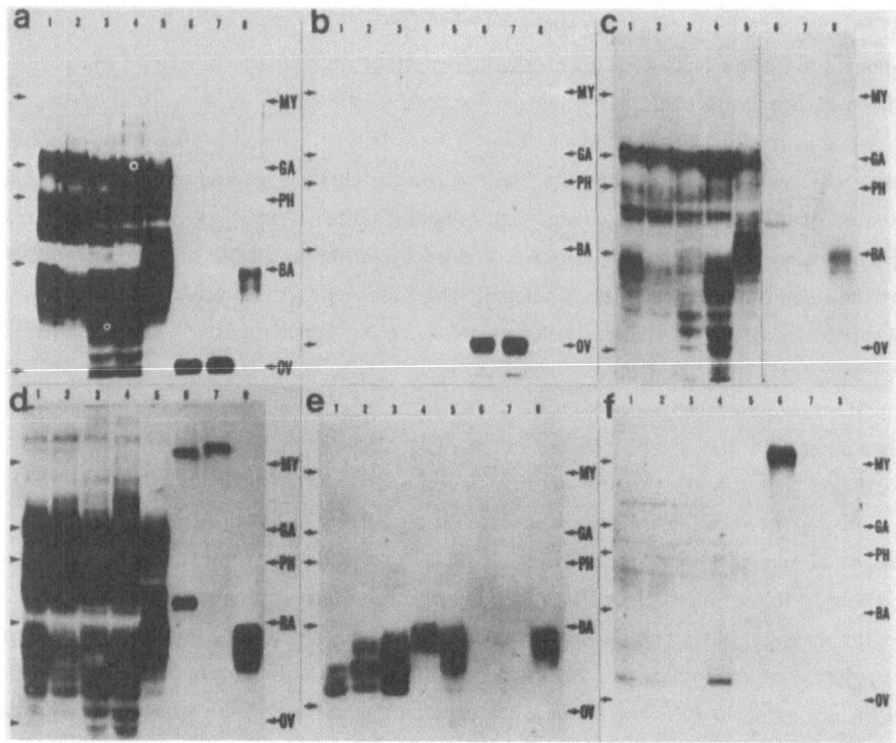

FIGURE 1. Glycoprotein profiles of various B16 melanoma sublines with different organ-specific colonization capacities (6,8,27). Nonionic detergent extracts of sublines B16-F1 (lane 1), high lung colonizing B16-F10 (lane 2), high basement membrane invasion B16-BL6 (lane 3), high ovary colonizing B16-O13 (lane 4), and high brain colonizing B16-B15b (lane 5) were analyzed electrophoretically in sodium dodecyl sulfate together with glycoprotein standards with known carbohydrate structures: porcine thyroglobulin, human transferrin and ovalbumin unbound to Con A-Sepharose (lane 6); bovine serum fibronectin and ovalbumin weakly bound to Con A-Sepharose (lane 7); bovine fetuin and ovalbumin strongly bound to Con A-Sepharose. The fixed gels were untreated (panels a,f), hydrolyzed with mild acid to remove sialic acid from the glycoproteins (panels b,d,e) or mild acid hydrolyzed followed by Smith degradation (panel c). The gels were finally stained with ^{125}I-labeled WGA (panels a-c), RCA$_I$ (panel d), PNA (panel e), or LCH (panel f) and processed for autoradiography. Migration positions of M_r markers are indicated at the right side of each panel, MY myosin, M_r ~ 200,000; GA, β-galacto-sidase, M_r ~ 116,000; PH, phosphorylase b, M_r ~ 93,000; BA, serum albumin, M_r ~ 66,000; OV, ovalbumin, M_r ~ 45,000. Panels (a-d) demonstrate that a group of sialoglycoproteins are revealed by the binding of ^{125}I-WGA, as well as by ^{125}I-RCA$_I$ after removal of sialic acid in situ. The backbone structure of the carbohydrate chains seems to be highly branched complex type. Another class of sialoglycoproteins are revealed by ^{125}I-PNA (Panel e).

functional characteristics, such as we performed with erythrocytes, were not possible. Instead, we have developed a technique in which various classes of carbohydrate chains on individual glycoproteins can be estimated by use of lectins (27,28). This method utilizes the binding reactions of ^{125}I-labeled lectins to glycoproteins that have been separated by polyacrylamide gel electrophoresis.

In order to estimate the structural features of the carbohydrate chains, the following points must be considered: binding reactions of standard glycoproteins with known carbohydrate structures have to be performed as positive controls; specific chemical modifications of carbohydrate chains, such as removal of sialic acid or Smith degradation, must be performed in situ; comparisons between lectins with similar but not identical carbohydrate specificities, such as RCA$_I$ to peanut agglutinin (PNA), and concanavalin A (Con A) to Lens culinaris hemagglutinin (LCH), should be examined (8,27). By employing the technique, we have obtained unique glycoprotein profiles from B16 melanoma sublines of differing abilities to colonize specific organs, such as lung, ovary, and brain (8). The results indicated that the in vivo-selected melanoma sublines had similar glycoproteins, but there were significant differences in the quantities of particular glycoproteins. For example, the intensity of M_r ~ 51,000 and ~ 56,000 bands, revealed by PNA binding, appeared to correlate with lung colonization ability. These glycoproteins are apparently sialoglycoproteins, but they are distinct from the RCA$_I$-reactive, major sialoglycoproteins described above (Figure 1). A M_r ~ 50,000 band revealed by LCH binding was most prominent on the ovary-colonizing B16 subline. Since all the B16 melanoma sublines used in this study had been selected in vivo by organ colonization, except B16-BL6, which was selected for tissue invasiveness, the glycoprotein differences found are very likely to be important in tumor cell implantation, survival, and metastasis formation. Other properties, such as enzymatic activities that degrade vascular basement membranes (29-34) and the cell cytoskeletal system that controls cell motility (35,36) are also important factors. Changes in various cell properties that the melanoma cells acquired through in vivo selection are probably involved collectively in determining the outcome of metastasis formation.

We have developed another animal model for studying metastasis of large cell lymphoma. The murine RAW117 large cell lymphoma/lymphosarcoma line was originally developed by transformation of BALB/c splenocytes with the Abelson leukemia virus. This lymphoma of B-cell lineage forms solid tumor nodules in liver, lung, and spleen of syngeneic mice after subcutaneous or intravenous inoculation (37). Various RAW117 sublines have been selected for enhanced liver or lung colonization (37). Similar analyses of the expression of certain cellular glycoproteins have revealed that decreased expression of RNA tumor virus envelope glycoprotein gp70 in cells of enhanced liver-colonization potential (4,5). Con A binding to the glycoprotein doublet bands at the M_r region between 70,000 and 80,000 clearly correlated with the amount of gp70 measured by radioimmunoassay. In addition, the high liver-colonizing RAW117 variant sublines possessed larger amounts of WGA-reactive sialoglycoproteins than the parental line (Irimura, T., Belloni, P.N., Nicolson, G.L., unpublished). This is a group of sialoglycoproteins of apparent M_r between 100,000 and 200,000, as assessed by polyacrylamide gel electrophoresis in the presence of sodium dodecyl sulfate, which does not appear to be biosynthetically related to gp70, but presumably does contribute to the net negative cell surface charge of RAW117 cells (38). These components could be adhesive receptors for liver parenchymal cells (39,40) and may protect tumor cells from macrophage cytotoxicity (41). Differences in the amounts of WGA binding to this class of glycoproteins between liver-colonizing RAW117-H10 and the parental line are not due to different sialylation of the glycoprotein carbohydrate chains, because the difference has also been observed with ^{125}I-RCA$_I$ after sialic acid removal from the glycoproteins in situ. Sialidase treatment of the RAW117 cells followed by polyacrylamide gel electrophoresis demonstrated that the desialized glycoproteins migrate at an identical position to that of the intact sialoglycoproteins (Figure 2). Thus, the extreme M_r range of the sialoglycoproteins is not due to sialylation.

Variants of RAW117 that show differing metastatic properties can be selected in vitro. For example, high liver-colonizing RAW117 variant cells can be selected by non-adherence to immobilized Con A on tissue culture dishes, and less-malignant RAW117 cells can be selected from the liver-colonizing RAW117-H10 subline by nonadherence to immobilized WGA (4). Indeed, most of the known selections using lectins yield tumor cells that are less malignant or as malignant as the parental cells, although most of these selections were for lectin-resistant mutants of tumor cells (15,16). Highly metastatic tumor cells may acquire the multiple properties required for metastasis through in vivo selection or adaptation. However, in vitro selection of tumor cells by means of lectin reactivity can result in tumor cell subpopulations with altered cell surface glycoconjugates, which is one series of the many biochemical determinants of tumor metastasis. Lectin-selected tumor cells might be more metastatic, but only if the function of the cell surface, lectin-reactive molecule is important in determining the ability to metastasize. For example, a RAW117 subline selected 10 times for nonadherence to Con A in vitro possessed similar cellular properties as the subline RAW117-H10, which had been selected in vivo for liver colonization (4). This suggests that in vitro selection of mixed populations of RAW117 cells can result in the isolation of a highly malignant preexisting subpopulation.

62

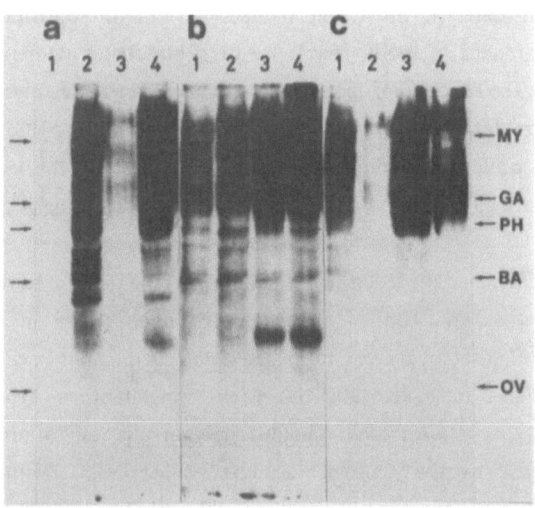

FIGURE 2. Sialoglycoprotein profiles of RAW117 lymphosarcoma sublines. Procedures are the same as in Figure 1. Nonionic detergent extracts of the RAW117 parental line (lanes 1,2) and RAW117-H10 (lanes 3,4) selected 10 times for liver colonization in vivo. Lanes 1 and 3 are lysates from intact cells, and lanes 2 and 4 are lysates from neuraminidase-treated gels. Panel a, stained with ^{125}I-RCA$_I$; panel b, the gel was treated with mild acid to remove sialic acid in situ and stained with ^{125}I-RCA$_I$; panel c, stained with ^{125}I-WGA.

THE USE OF LECTINS IN THE HISTOCHEMICAL AND BIOCHEMICAL ANALYSIS OF GLYCOPROTEINS OF COLORECTAL CARCINOMA METASTASES

Since experimental approaches utilizing tissue culture and experimental animals are not well established with colorectal carcinoma metastasis, we have initiated studies to elucidate the glycoproteins of tumor tissues. Various lectins have already been used for histochemically distinguishing various stages of differentiation of different epithelial cells. As it turns out, intestinal mucosa is one of the most extensively studied mammalian epithelial tissues. Etzler and Branstrator (42) examined the distribution of fluorescein-labeled RCA$_I$, WGA, Dolichos biflorus agglutinin (DBA), and Lotas tetragonolobus agglutinin (LTA) along the epithelium of adult rat small intestine. They found that the binding of WGA, RCA$_I$, and LTA occurs on the microvillar portions of epithelium, and the intensity of labeling decreases along the intestine. DBA reacted with 25-50% of the goblet cells, regardless of their location. The lectin-binding pattern of rat large intestine has been studied by Essner et al. (43), who used six different lectins to label cryostat sections. They found that certain lectins appear to be specific for

63

particular types of cells in the colon tissue. A similar approach by Freeman (44) demonstrated differences in lectin reactivity of goblet cells at different depths in the crypts. Changes in the subcellular localizations of lectin-reactive glycoconjugates during differentiation of goblet cells have also been demonstrated using RCA$_I$ and LCH (45). In addition, intensity of lectin binding appears to change along the length of the human colon, with soybean agglutinin (SBA) and DBA binding increasing in parallel with crypt differentiation.

Histochemical changes seen upon colon carcinogenesis have been studied in experimental systems, and similar changes have been noted in human specimens. Freeman (46) used dimethylhydrazine to induce colon carcinomas in rats, and he observed histochemical changes in carcinoma tissue by using lectins. He found decreased reactivity with WGA, RCA$_I$, and Limulus polyphemus agglutinin (LPA), and the appearance of PNA reactivity on surrounding goblet cells. Similar changes were observed in transitional mucosa adjacent to the carcinoma. The change in lectin reactivity on human colorectal carcinoma indicated disappearance of SBA and DBA binding and increased reactivity with PNA (47). The subcellular localization of PNA-reactive molecules also appeared to change (48), and these changes also occurred in precancerous tissues (49,50). A more complex pattern has been reported by Yonezawa et al. (51,52) using Ulex europaeus agglutinin I (UEA$_I$). According to their findings, carcinoma of the distal colon and rectum sometimes falsely expresses UEA$_I$ reactivity, which is similar to the blood group H-antigen. In contrast, occasional loss of UEA$_I$ reactivity was observed in carcinoma of the proximal colon, where reactivity is present on the normal mucosal surface. These results clearly demonstrate that there are changes in lectin reactivity of normal glycoconjugates during differentiation of colonic mucosa, and lectin reactivities are changed in colorectal carcinoma cells. However, relationships between the types of glycoconjugate markers and stage of the disease, which is commonly defined by the presence of metastasis, are unknown. Also, whether lectin reactivities correlate with the state of morphologic differentiation of the tumor is not known.

Since glycoprotein alterations can be detected along with the changes in metastatic capacity of some animal tumor cells, as described above, we have conducted studies on the reactivities of lectins with colorectal carcinoma of various stages in primary and metastatic lesions. Here we present our observations on Dukes' D stage carcinoma and its liver metastases.

Surgically resected specimens of neoplastic or nonneoplastic tissues from patients with Dukes' D stage colorectal carcinoma were fixed in formalin and embedded in paraffin using routine procedures. One micrometer-thick serial sections were cut and deparaffined, and endogenous peroxidase activity was destroyed with 0.5% hydrogen peroxide for 20 min. Rehydrated sections were first incubated with 5% bovine serum albumin in order to block nonspecific absorption of lectins, and they were incubated with biotinylated lectins (50 µg/ml) for 60 min in the presence of 2.5% bovine serum albumin. Lectins were previously biotinylated by use of the N-hydroxysuccinimide derivative of biotin for 4 hr at room temperature and isolated from unreacted reagents. After removal of excess biotinylated lectins, the sections were incubated with avidin-biotinylated peroxidase complex (Vector Laboratories, Burlingame, CA) followed by a substrate for peroxidase (53). The dehydrated specimens were mounted with Permount and examined under a Leitz Ortholux I (E. Leitz, Rockleigh, NJ) microscope equipped with an Orthomat camera.

Among the nine lectins tested, which included Con A, LCH, WGA, RCA_I, PNA, UEA_I, LTA, Cytisus sessilifolius agglutinin (CSA), and pokeweed mitogen (PWM), three blood group H-specific lectins were found to be useful. UEA_I reactivity with carcinoma tissue was often different from that with normal mucosa, but this was not always reproducible, which is consistent with the results of Yonezawa et al. (51).

We examined four cases of UEA_I-positive carcinoma and five cases of UEA_I-negative carcinoma among nine patients with Dukes' D stage disease. In Figure 3a and b serial sections of the primary carcinoma of the rectum from a 39-year-old woman whose blood type is O-positive show slight UEA_I reactivity with the apical surface of the lower portion of the crypt in the normal mucosa. No reactivity was observed with carcinoma tissue. This lectin reacts with the vascular endothelium and blood cells. Another blood group H-specific lectin, LTA, yields similar results to UEA_I. The third anti-H lectin used (CSA) interacts with the inner portion of the blood group H antigen (Figure 4) (54,55), and this lectin possesses different staining properties. As shown in Figure 3b, CSA reacts with the goblet cells of the upper crypt and the luminal surface in the colonic mucosa. These cells are considered to be terminally differentiated at the colonic epithelium. No reactivity was observed on carcinoma cells, including UEA_I-positive and -negative tumors. Therefore, loss of CSA reactivity appears to be a more consistent marker for neoplastic transformation than UEA_I reactivity.

We have observed heterogeneity in lectin reactivity within the tumors examined. Figure 3c shows the staining pattern of UEA_I to a primary tumor of the sigmoid colon from a 61-year-old man with O-positive blood type. The top portion of this picture contains the carcinoma cells in which UEA binding is seen at the apical and lateral surface. UEA_I binding, shown on the bottom-right side of the figure, is limited to the apical surface of the tumor cells. All the tumor cells in the liver metastasis in this patient appear to react similarly to the primary tumor cells, which stain strongly with

UEA_I (Figure 3d). In experimental systems, distant metastasis originates from a portion of a heterogeneous cell population within the primary tumor, and so the above staining profile suggests that the liver metastasis is derived from a portion of the tumor where UEA_I reactivity is high. It would be interesting if the localization of other metastasis-associated properties, such as degradative enzymes and specific adhesive molecules, are also present in cells with high UEA_I reactivity.

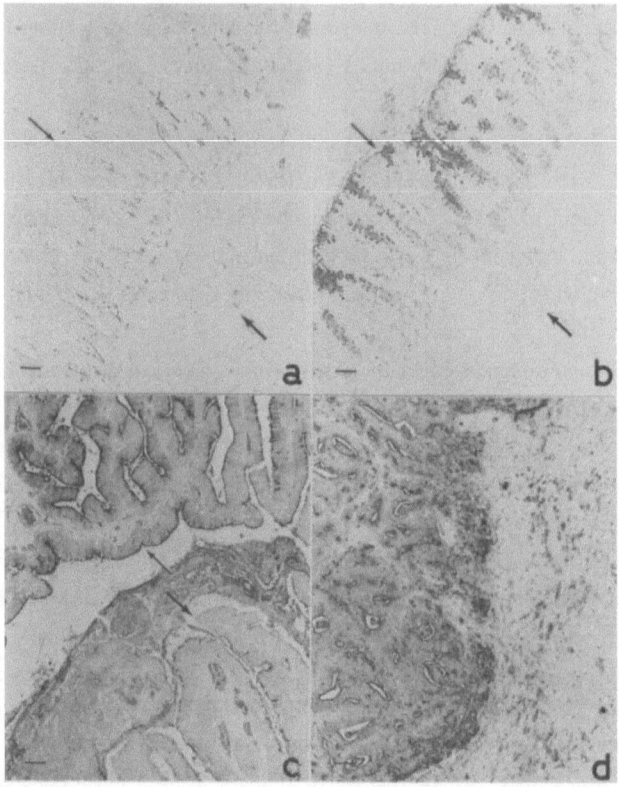

FIGURE 3. Distribution of biotinylated lectins on colorectal carcinoma tissue sections from patients with Dukes' D stage colorectal carcinoma revealed by avidin-biotin-peroxidase complex. Panel a, a section of rectal tumor tissue containing normal mucosa (thin arrow) and carcinoma (thick arrow) stained with biotinyl-UEA_I; panel b, the same portion of the tissue as in panel a, stained with biotinyl-CSA; panel c, a section of sigmoid colon adenocarcinoma heterogeneously stained with biotinyl UEA_I; panel d, a section of liver metastasis derived from the colon carcinoma shown in panel c. Bars indicate 100 μm.

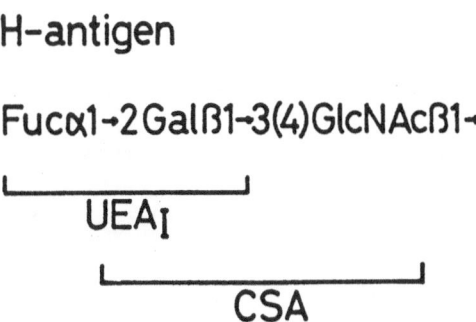

H-antigen

$$Fuc\alpha 1 \rightarrow 2 Gal\beta 1 \rightarrow 3(4) GlcNAc\beta 1 \rightarrow$$

UEA$_I$

CSA

FIGURE 4. Proposed carbohydrate specificity of UEA$_I$ and CSA (54,55).

Not all of the primary colorectal tumors examined possess heterogeneity in UEA$_I$ binding. UEA$_I$ staining of sections of a primary tumor (Figure 5a,b) and a liver metastasis (Figure 5c,d) from another 61-year-old man with O-positive blood type indicates apparent homogeneity in the binding of UEA$_I$. Tumor cells adjacent to the normal mucosa (Figure 5a) and cells that invaded blood vessels (Figure 5b) show the same UEA$_I$ reactivities. Similar results were obtained with a liver metastasis. All of the adenocarcinoma cells examined in the liver (Figure 5c), including tumor cells extravasating from a small blood vessel (Figure 5d) are similarly reactive with UEA$_I$. Thus, it is not likely that the presence or absence of these lectin-reactive molecules directly correlates with the metastatic capacity of colorectal carcinoma. However, a statistical evaluation based on a more accurate quantification of UEA$_I$-reactive glycoproteins may prove necessary. We have determined that there is a UEA$_I$-reactive glycoprotein of M_r higher than 500,000 in colorectal carcinoma tissue by using the techniques described above (Figure 6). The relative intensity of binding of ^{125}I-labeled UEA$_I$ to this glycoprotein extracted from tumor tissues is consistent with our histochemical observations. Other lectins, such as ^{125}I-labeled WGA, bind to the same high-molecular-weight glycoprotein, as do many other classes of glycoproteins from colorectal carcinoma. The UEA$_I$ reactivity of this high M_r glycoprotein is apparently due to differences in carbohydrate chains and not to the amount of glycoprotein molecules present in carcinoma cells.

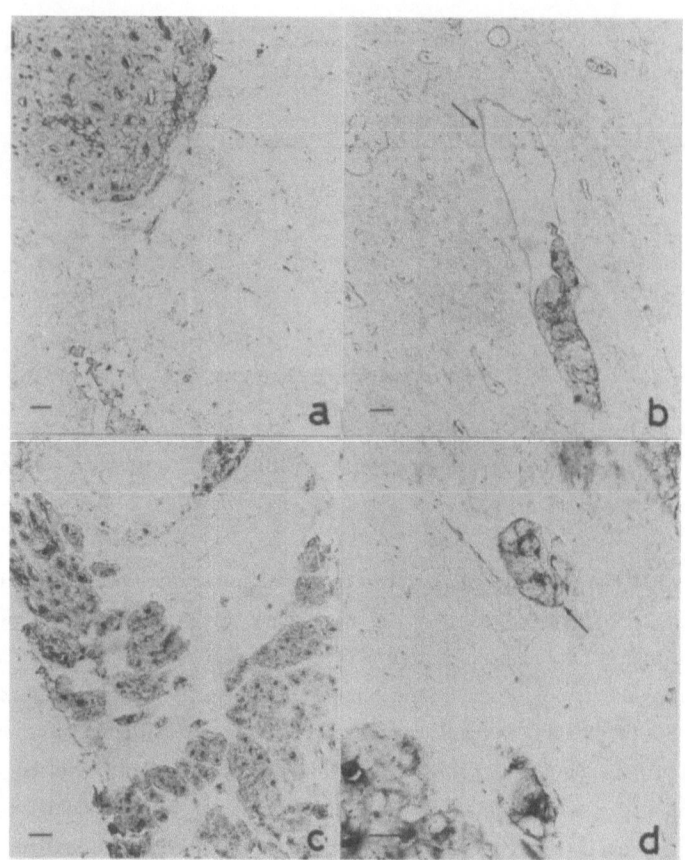

FIGURE 5. UEA$_I$ staining patterns of a sigmoid colon adenocarcinoma and its liver metastasis from a patient with Dukes' D stage carcinoma. Panel a, portion of the primary tumor where the growing edge of carcinoma is adjacent to normal colonic epithelium; panel b, bottom of the tumor where carcinoma cells are invading blood vessel, endothelial cells are also stained with this lectin (arrow); panel c, a section from the liver indicating widespread metastasis; panel d, higher magnification of a field in panel c where tumor cells appear to be extravasating from blood vessels (arrow). Bars indicate 100 μm, except in panel d, where the bar indicates 25 μm.

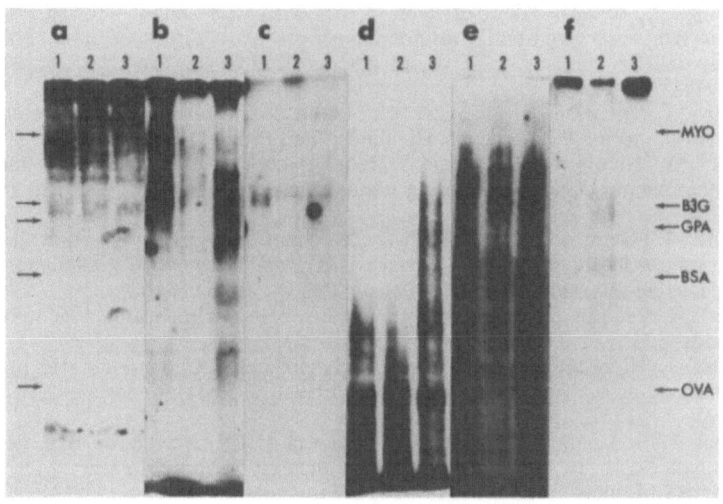

FIGURE 6. Glycoproteins profiles of primary colon carcinoma (lane 1), lymph node metastasis (lane 2), and liver metastasis (lane 3), taken out at the same time from the same patient. Sodium dodecyl sulfate-polyacrylamide gel electrophoresis of non-ionic detergent extracts was performed after sodium dodecyl sulfate treatment under reducing condition. The gels were stained with ^{125}I-WGA (panel a), ^{125}I-RCA$_I$ after removal of sialic acid (panel b), ^{125}I-PNA after removal of sialic acid (panel c), ^{125}I-Con A (panel d), ^{125}I-LCH (panel e), and ^{125}I-UEA$_I$ (panel f). Bound ^{125}I-lectins were detected by autoradiography. Arrows indicate migration distance of standard proteins and glycoproteins MYO: myosin, B3G: erythrocyte band 3, GPA: erythrocyte glycoprotein A, BSA: serum albumin, OVA: ovalbumin.

References

1. Nicolson GL, Poste G: Tumor cell diversity and host responses in cancer metastasis. I. Properties of metastatic cells. Curr Prob Cancer 7: 1-83, 1982.
2. Nicolson GL, Poste G: Tumor cell diversity and host responses in cancer metastasis. II. Host immune responses and therapy of metastases. Curr Prob Cancer 7: 1-43, 1983.
3. Nicolson GL: Cell surface molecules and tumor metastasis. Regulation of metastatic diversity. Exp Cell Res 150: 3-22, 1984.

4. Reading CL, Belloni PN, Nicolson GL: Selections and in vivo properties of lectin-attachment variants of malignant murine lymphosarcoma cell lines. J Natl Cancer Inst 64: 1241-1249, 1980.

5. Reading CL, Brunson KW, Torrianni M, Nicolson GL: Malignancies of metastatic murine lymphosarcoma cell lines and clones correlate with decreased cell surface display of RNA tumor virus envelope glycoprotein GP70. Proc Natl Acad Sci USA 77: 5943-5947, 1980.

6. Irimura T, Nicolson GL: Sugar chains on lectin-binding glycoproteins from metastatic murine B16 melanoma sublines. Fed Proc 41: 1159, 1982.

7. Steck PA, Nicolson GL: Cell surface glycoproteins of 13762NF mammary adenocarcinoma clones of differing metastatic potentials. Exp Cell Res 147: 255-267, 1983.

8. Irimura T, Nicolson GL: Carbohydrate chain analysis by lectin binding to electrophoretically separated glycoproteins from murine B16 melanoma sublines of various metastatic properties. Cancer Res 44: 791-798, 1984.

9. Fidler IJ: General considerations for studies of experimental cancer metastasis. Methods in Cancer Res 15: 399-439, 1978.

10. Irimura T, Nicolson GL: The role of glycoconjugates in metastatic melanoma blood-borne arrest and cell surface properties. J Supramol Struct Cell Biochem 17: 325-336, 1981.

11. Irimura T, Gonzalez R, Nicolson GL: Effects of tunicamycin on B16 metastatic melanoma cell surface glycoproteins and blood-borne arrest and survival properties. Cancer Res 41: 3411-3418, 1981.

12. LeGrue SJ: 1-Butanol extraction and subsequent reconstitution of membrane components which mediate metastatic phenotype. Cancer Res 42: 2126-2134, 1982.

13. LeGrue SJ: Extraction of immunogenic and suppressogenic antigens from variants of B16 melanoma exhibiting low or high metastatic potentials. Cancer Res 43: 5106-5111, 1983.

14. Goldstein IJ, Hughes RC, Monsigny M, Osawa T, Sharon N: What should be called a lectin? Nature 285: 66, 1980.

15. Tao TW, Burger MM: Lectin resistant variants of mouse melanoma cells. I. Altered metastasizing capacity and tumorigenicity. Int J Cancer 31: 239-247, 1983.

16. Kerbel RS: Immunologic studies of membrane mutants of a highly metastatic murine tumor. Am J Pathol 97: 609-622, 1978.

17. Lotan R, Nicolson GL: Purification of cell membrane glycoprotein by lectin affinity chromatography. Biochim Biophys Acta 559: 329-376, 1979.

18. Nicolson GL: Lectin interactions with normal and tumor cells and the affinity purification of tumor cell glycoproteins. In: S Sell (ed), Cancer markers. Humana Press, Clifton, New Jersey, 1980, pp 403-443.

19. Irimura T: Histochemical application of lectins. In: T Osawa (ed), Lectins and cell biology. Kodansha, Tokyo, 1985, pp 128-145.

20. Irimura T, Nakajima M: Use of lectins in tumor biology. In: T Osawa (ed), Lectins and cell biology. Kodansha, Tokyo, 1985, pp 171-213.

21. Raz A, McLellan WL, Hart IR, Bucana CD, Hoyer LC, Sela B-A, Dragsten P, Fidler IJ: Cell surface properties of B16 melanoma variants with differing metastatic potential. Cancer Res 40: 1645-1651, 1981.

22. Brunson KW, Baettie G, Nicolson GL: Selection and altered tumor cell properties of brain-colonizing metastatic melanoma. Nature 272: 543-545, 1978.

23. Miner KM, Kawaguchi T, Uba GW, Nicolson GL: Clonal drift of cell surface, melanogenic, and experimental metastatic properties of in vivo-selected brain meninges-colonizing murine B16 melanoma. Cancer Res 42: 4631-4638, 1982.

24. Irimura T, Nicolson GL: Affinity isolation of cell surface sialoglycoproteins from metastatic B16 melanoma cell and their interaction with endothelial cell basal lamina. J Cell Biol 91: 118a, 1981.
25. Tsuji T, Irimura T, Osawa T: The carbohydrate moiety of band-3 glycoprotein of human erythrocyte membranes. Biochem J 187: 677-686, 1980.
26. Irimura T, Tsuji T, Tagami S, Yamamoto K, Osawa T: Structure of a complex-type sugar chain of human glycophorin A. Biochemistry 20: 560-566, 1981.
27. Irimura T, Nicolson GL: Carbohydrate-chain analysis by lectin binding to mixtures of glycoproteins, separated by polyacrylamide slab-gel electrophoresis, with in situ chemical modifications. Carbohydr Res 115: 209-220, 1983.
28. Irimura T, Nicolson GL: Interaction of pokeweed mitogen with poly(N-acetyllactosamine)-type carbohydrate chains. Carbohydr Res 120: 187-195, 1983.
29. Nakajima M, Irimura T, DiFerrante N, DiFerrante DT, Nicolson GL: Heparan sulfate degradation: Relation to tumor invasive and metastatic properties of mouse B16 melanoma sublines. Science 220: 611-613, 1983.
30. Irimura T, Nakajima M, DiFerrante N, Nicolson GL: High-speed gel-permeation chromatography of glycosaminoglycans: Its application to the analysis of heparan sulfate of embryonic carcinoma and its degradation products by tumor cell derived heparanase. Anal Biochem 130: 461-468, 1983.
31. Irimura T, Nakajima M, Nicolson GL: Metastatic tumor cell attachment to vascular endothelial cells and destruction of their basal lamina-like matrix. Gann Monogr. Cancer Res 19: 35-46, 1983.
32. Nakajima M, Irimura T, DiFerrante N, Nicolson GL: Metastatic melanoma cell heparanase: Characterization of heparan sulfate degradation fragment produced by B16 melanoma endoglucuronidase. J Biol Chem 259: 2283-2290, 1984.
33. Liotta LA, Rao NC, Terranova VP, Barsky S, Thorgeirsson U. Tumor cell attachment and degradation of basement membranes. In: GL Nicolson and L Milas (eds), Cancer invasion and metastasis: Biologic and therapeutic aspects. Raven Press, New York, 1984, pp 169-176.
34. Sloane BF, Dunn JR, Honn KV: Lysosomal cathepsin B correlation with metastatic potential. Science 212: 1151-1153, 1981.
35. Hart IR, Raz A, Fidler IJ: Effect of cytoskeletal-disrupting agents on the metastatic behavior of melanoma cells. J Natl Cancer Inst 64: 891-900, 1980.
36. Volk T, Geiger B, Raz A: Motility and adhesive properties of high- and low-metastatic murine neoplastic cells. Cancer Res 44: 811-824, 1984.
37. Brunson KW, Nicolson GL: Selection and biologic properties of malignant variants of a murine lymphosarcoma. J Natl Cancer Institute 61: 1499-1503, 1978.
38. Miner KM, Walter H, Nicolson GL: Subfractionation of malignant variants of metastatic mure lymphosarcoma cells by counter-current distribution in two polymer aqueous phase. Biochemistry 20: 6244-6250, 1981.
39. Nicolson GL, Mascali JJ, McGuire EJ: Metastatic RAW117 lymphosarcoma as a model for malignant normal cell interactions: possible roles for cell surface antigens determining the quantity and location of secondary tumor. Oncodev Biol Med 4: 149-159, 1982.
40. McGuire EJ, Mascali JJ, Grady SR, Nicolson GL: Involvement of cell-cell adhesion molecules in liver colonization by metastatic murine lymphoma/lymphosarcoma variants. Clin Exptl Metastasis 2: 213-222, 1984.
41. Miner KM, Nicolson GL: Differences in the sensitivities of murine metastatic lymphoma/lymphosarcoma variants to macrophage-mediated cytolysis and/or cytolysis. Cancer Res 43: 2063-2067, 1983.
42. Etzler M, Branstrator M: Differential localization of cell surface and secretory components in rat intestinal epithelium by use of lectins. J Cell Biol 62: 329-343, 1974.

43. Essner E, Schreiber J, Griewski RA: Localization of carbohydrate components in rat colon with fluoresceinated lectins. J Histochem Cytochem 26: 452-458, 1978.

44. Freeman HJ, Lotan R, Kim YS: Application of lectins for detection of goblet cell glycoconjugate differences in proximal and distal colon of the rat. Lab Invest 42: 405-412, 1980.

45. Thomopoulos GN, Schulte BA, Spicer SS: Light and electron microscopic cytochemistry of glycoconjugates in the recto-sigmoid colonic epithelium of the mouse and rat. Am J Anat 168: 239-256, 1983.

46. Freeman HJ: Lectin histochemistry of 1,2-dimethylhydrazine-induced rat colon neoplasia. J Histochem Cytochem 31: 1241-1245, 1983.

47. Boland CR, Montgomery CK, Kim YS: Alterations in human colonic mucin occurring with cellular differentiation and malignant transformation. Proc Natl Acad Sci USA 79: 2051-2055, 1982.

48. Cooper HS: Peanut lectin-binding sites in large bowel carcinoma. Lab Invest 47: 383-390, 1982.

49. Boland CR, Montgomery CK, Kim YS: A cancer-associated mucin alteration in benign colonic polyps. Gastroenterology 82: 664-672, 1982.

50. Cooper HS, Reuter VE: Peanut lectin-binding sites in polyps of the colon and rectum: Adenomas, hyperplastic polyps, and adenomas with in situ carcinoma. Lab Invest 49: 655-661, 1983.

51. Yonezawa S, Nakamura T, Tanaka S, Sato E: Glycoconjugate with Ulex europaeus agglutinin-I-binding sites in normal mucosa, adenoma, and carcinoma of the human large bowel. J Natl Cancer Inst 69: 777-785, 1982.

52. Yonezawa S, Nakamura T, Tanaka S, Murata K, Nishi M, Sato E: Binding of Ulex europaeus agglutinin-I in polyposis coli-comparative study with solitary adenoma in the sigmoid colon and rectum. J Natl Cancer Inst 71: 19-24, 1983.

53. Hsu SM, Raine L: Versatility of biotin-labeled lectins and avidin-biotin-peroxidase complex for localization of carbohydrate in tissue sections. J Histochem Cytochem 30: 157-161, 1982.

54. Matsumoto I, Osawa T: On the specificity of various heterologous anti-H hemagglutinins. Vox Sang 21: 548-557, 1971.

55. Matsumoto I, Osawa T: Specific purification of eel serum and Cytisus sessilifolius anti-H hemagglutinins by affinity chromatography and their binding to human erythrocytes. Biochemistry 13: 582-588, 1974.

SECTION II.

CONTROVERSIES IN THE MANAGEMENT OF
PATIENTS WITH COLORECTAL CANCER METASTASIS

7

QUALITY OF LIFE: A CEREBRAL AFFAIR

Frank Adams and Theresa Adams

To look into the heart is not enough;
One must also look into the cerebral cortex.

-- T. S. Eliot

INTRODUCTION

Remarkable progress has been made in the treatment of cancer over the past quarter of a century, with notable prolongation of patient survival. But, the idea that biologic existence, though necessary, is not necessarily sufficient to ensure quality of life is slowly taking root in oncology. Patients, their families, and many physicians now accept the fact that the pursuit of cure for the "scourge of scourages" has not been without considerable price. As a result, there is growing recognition that therapeutic success all too frequently, and tragically, is characterized by life, that is, so to speak, unfit for human consumption.

Attention to the quality of life of cancer survivors has recently caught the attention of research investigators. To date, however, the efforts have little scientific merit or clinical worth. On the one hand, narrow psychosocial measures are extolled endlessly, with theory, inference, and speculation substituting for sound clinical decision making. On the other hand, sundry computer schemes and elaborate mathematical formulae obfuscate the obvious. The former reflects the persistent tendency in American medicine to treat behavior and emotions in a vacuum, devoid of neurobiologic correlates and processes. The latter approach represents far-fetched attempts to give scientific credibility to the elusive task of quantitating the qualitative. Meanwhile, simplistic quality of life questionnaires threaten to reduce a noble pursuit to the level of a trivial consumer satisfaction survey.

Since quality of life is a complex, multidetermined human experience, understanding it requires that physicians draw from as broad a domain of evidence as possible. But thus far, attempts at evaluating quality of life in patients with cancer have been seriously incomplete, reflecting, among other things, an almost total neglect of recent dramatic advances in neuroscience. Ignorance of the subtle and even not so subtle effects of cancer and its treatments on the brain, the principal organ responsible for the conduct of human experience, has resulted in the failure to recognize that:

1. neurobehavioral disorders occur at some point during the treatment of most patients with malignancies;

2. most social and phychological dysfunctions measured by current quality of life scales are the consequence of unrecognized cognitive deficits resulting from cerebral pathology;

3. there is a staggering prevalence of unsuspected cerebral impairment among patients with advanced and aggressively treated cancer, secondary to direct and indirect influences upon the brain by the disease or its treatment.

These comments should make it clear that the quality of life issues facing oncologists are more complex than those over-simplified approaches currently in vogue would lead us to believe.

Patient evaluation

Attention to the higher neurologic functions of patients at The University of Texas M. D. Anderson Hospital and Tumor Institute at Houston is the major clinical pursuit of the Section of Neuropsychiatry. All patients referred to the Section undergo a neurobehavioral examination that we developed, utilizing the principles and methodologies of behavioral neurology. The examination is thus both quantitatively and qualitatively sensitive to a broad range of higher neurologic functions. It is also more discriminating than the electroencephalogram (EEG) of brain changes resulting from toxic, metabolic, or cerebral metastatic events. The examination emphasizes the neurodynamic rather than the psychodynamic meaning of patients' signs and symptoms.

Study Results

Our studies to determine the array of organic brain syndromes (OBS) that present with clinically deceptive features of depression have shed considerable light on the clinical problems associated with quality of life. We first examined the records of 20 patients with head and neck cancer (1). All had been referred by head and neck surgeons for evaluation of significant symptoms of depression. There were 9 men and 11 women in the study, and their ages ranged from 17-76 years, with a median age of 60.

By traditional psychiatric mental status interview standards, 16 of the 20 patients studied presented with a range of symptoms significant for the diagnosis of depressive disorder. However, detailed neurobehavioral examination revealed that for 12 of the patients (60%) the symptoms were secondary to OBS and were unsuspected by the primary physicians. These patients demonstrated an array of notable cognitive deficits ranging from temporal disorientation, to difficulties with simple calculations, spoken and written language, left-right orientation, short-term verbal and visual memory, visuospatial organization, motor-imitative tasks, and simple and complex information processing. The neurobehavioral findings were verified by EEG or computed tomographic (CT) scan of the brain in 10 of the 12 patients, disclosing brain necrosis, cerebral atrophy, or brain metastasis. The remaining two patients were diagnosed with OBS solely on clinical grounds. Only four patients (20%) were diagnosed as having depression treatable with tricyclic antidepressants.

Interpretation and Application of Study Findings

If we review our results from a quality of life perspective, a number of important points emerge. One is the necessity to pay attention to the ages of cancer patients. Fifty percent of the study patients were 65 years of age or older, a finding consistent with national statistics that show that cancer is mostly a disease of the elderly. The finding of senile dementia Alzheimer's type (SDAT) in four (20%) of the eight dementia patients strengthens concerns about the lack of geriatric sensitivity in oncology. Missing is an awareness that elderly patients with cancer are at special developmental and biologic stages of life. Yet, what oncology fellowship program provides training in geriatric medicine? What cancer center has a staff of geriatricians? How many oncologists consider age in their diagnosis and treatment options?

A quite incidental finding in this study is the positive contribution that a diagnosis of dementia can have on a patient's quality of life. We are struck by the psychotherapeutic benefits experienced by patients who almost universally feel unburdened by someone validating the abnormal mental state they were too afraid or embarrassed to reveal. The gentle exposure of their failing cognitive skills, with discussions of diagnosis and outcome, is more often than not greeted by the patients with relief. It is wrong to assume that patients with dementia cannot profit personally from learning about their diagnosis or participate meaningfully in decisions about their care or their future. Only profound mental incompetency, on rare occasions, prevents this form of dialogue. Moreover, dementia does not contraindicate aggressive chemotherapy or radical surgery if there are benefits to the patient. But, the additional diagnosis brings more sharply into focus the need to rebalance quality of life and treatment plans.

Seven of our patients (30%) had irreversible OBS of varying degrees. Apprised of this, surgeons were able to modify their diagnostic and proposed therapeutic approaches. Radical surgery was carried out only if it was felt the procedure would enhance existence. In one case the decision was for surgery for palliation only and in another, the scheduled procedure was replaced by better narcotic pain control and discharge home, in compliance with the patient's wishes.

77

It is not unusual after a brain-impaired patient has been diagnosed to discover that the patient has been submitting to cancer treatment to make the family feel better. The diagnosis of a second serious illness often provides the patient with the strong and compelling reason to decline further aggressive therapy in favor of supportive care and discharge home for whatever time remains. Here the intelligent and compassionate use of the appropriate narcotics for pain, neuroleptics for relief of neurosensory and behavioral distress, or neurostimulants to increase alertness, mood, appetite, and energy are indicated. These are chemical strategies to improve quality of life with high yield, and we frequently are able to enhance cognitive and social functioning for a number of months in selected patients.

The importance of establishing the quality of brain functions in the mentally failing cancer patient is best illustrated by the fact that 5 of 12 (25%) patients with OBS had treatable and reversible disorders. Their quality of life was restored following appropriate treatment, and they were able to continue with cancer therapy, freed of neurologic problems, or if cured of their malignancies, to enjoy normal lives. One case will suffice to illustrate this practice, based on our philosophy that the diagnosis and treatment of the complications of cancer and its treatments warrants the same aggressive approach as the treatment of the malignancy.

A 73-year-old man was admitted to the hospital for failure to thrive. Six months earlier, at another hospital, he underwent surgery and postoperative radiation therapy for basal cell carcinoma of the right ear. Then, free of disease, he vegetated at home, where he had become irritable and withdrawn, at one point putting a revolver to his head intending to kill himself. The patient was adamant that he was not depressed. Rather, he said he was disgusted with the loss of physical vitality and mental acuity. Without quality of life, he informed us, death was a welcome alternative.

This retired high school mathematics teacher could no longer do even simple two-step calculations. Neurobehavioral examination was significant for a diffuse cortical abnormality, the pattern of impairment suggesting a predominantly right hemisphere dysfunction. This was confirmed by EEG, which showed marked right cerebral slowing, probably the result of previous radiation therapy (7500 cGy) to that side of the head. He was placed on a total of 80 mg/day of methylphenidate in three doses, with slow but dramatic improvement in activity, mood, and cognition within the first week. After six months of treatment with the high-dose stimulant, he had gained 40 pounds, and his cognitive functions and EEG returned to normal. Free of malignancy and restored to neurobiologic health, he was well enough to return to part-time tutoring of mathematics students.

The retrospective analysis of the head and neck patients was followed up by a prospective study of all patients referred for evaluation of depression over a two-month period. There was a total of 101 medical and surgical patients between the ages of 18 to 74 years, with a median age of 54 years. The sample was almost evenly divided between men and women. Neurobehavioral examination uncovered unsuspected cerebral disorders in 74 of the 101 patients, 62 of which were verified by EEG, CT brain scan, or lumbar puncture. It is noteworthy that only nine patients were diagnosed as having depressive disorder according to the commonly accepted clinical criteria, which strengthens our clinical impression that depression is an uncommon disorder in patients with cancer.

Now that we know that neurobehavioral disorders contribute to morbidity, we need to determine if and how they contribute to mortality. In one study of general hospital patients with a variety of chronic illnesses, one-third of the patients examined and diagnosed with cognitive disorders were dead within three months (2). In our study of the 101 patients, 31 of those with neurobehavioral disorders (42%) were dead at three-month follow-up. Neurobehavioral disorders, it would seem, not only destroy quality of life, but may also destroy life as well.

DISCUSSION

The neurobehavioral approach to quality of life addresses a major deficiency in current evaluative efforts. This is not to dismiss the obvious importance of the many social and psychological measures currently in use, or to attempt to replace them. However, systematic examination of higher neurologic functions is not only an additional, but for most patients, is a superior clinical method for arriving at a fuller understanding of the rich and complex human dimensions of cancer. It can provide highly reliable information that can guide patients and physicians in moments of critical decision making.

The integrity of the cerebral correlates of behavior, emotion, and complex thinking must receive primary attention if optimal decision making by physicians and patients is to take place in oncology. It is unequivocal that the major determinant of quality of life is the condition of the human brain. The patient with undetected and untreated impairments of a faltering mental apparatus is destined to endure a state of imponderable hopelessness until death.

Quality of life is not only a clinical problem, but also a sociologic phenomena. Thus, it would be an error for physicians not to recognize that it is the most powerful social force directed at medicine in this century. As a major paradigm shift, it represents the end of an old era, where the physician's word was perceived as immutable truth, and the beginning of a new era, where the authoritarian style of medicine will be replaced by one responsive to a new consumer-directed, political, legal, and economic reality.

It is inescapable that the future principles and practices of the health-care industry will be shaped, not so much by physicians, as by the public. But, while a public more intelligently involved in decisions about its medical care is overdue, it is not without certain dangers. Though quality of life is simply one facet of a movement against professions generally in America, its sentiments run deeper in medicine. Here it is fueled by a resentful public seeking to redress its current alienation from vital decision-making processes in matters of its health.

This outrage is already manifest in psychiatry where, in a number of states, consumer advocates have obtained court orders limiting the doses of psychotropics that can be administered. Electroconvulsive therapy for the critically mentally ill is suffering a similar fate throughout the United States. It is not difficult to see how consumer-initiated judicial medicine could just as easily be applied to chemotherapy, radical surgery, radiotherapy, or use of intensive care units.

Franz J. Ingelfinger, editor emeritus of the New England Journal of Medicine, blames public disenchantment with quality of life issues on four factors (3). The first is economic, the high cost of medical care. The second is deceit, the unwarranted overselling of medicine's capabilities. The third is public self-delusion, the naive expectation that the physician will be both ultrascientific and as empathetic as the old-time family doctor. The fourth is the medical profession's capacity for self-delusion, poor recognition that the so-called curing of one disease in a high-risk group exposes that group to a further dilemma.

"Quality of life" is a protest, an outcry against medical practices which ignore the increasing sentiment for attention to human values. It is a recognition of the need for better rather than for more. For patients with cancer, it is a new climate of opinion compatible with Benjamin Franklin's conclusion that the ideal is to live well, rather than too long. It is a demand that medicine undergo a radical transformation of its Cartesian posture and become servant to the deepest aspirations of the people. It is an accusation that, though medicine has become brilliantly scientific, its priesthood has been found wanting in the stewardship of the new technical knowledge. It is a notice that the members of this priesthood are no longer regarded as privileged models of understanding, action or hope in human affairs, and are thus demoted from sacred to secular status. Quality of life challenges medicine to become a source of useful cultural wisdom in man's unceasing struggle against pain and suffering. Ultimately, quality of life is an anguished plea for help by a public bereft of consoling theologies or comforting high priests at the most profound moments of life and death.

ACKNOWLEDGMENTS

The author wishes to thank Martha Clayton for invaluable research, administrative assistance, and manuscript preparation.

References

1. Adams F, Larson D, Goepfert H: Does the diagnosis of depression in head and neck cancer mask organic brain disease? Otolaryngol Head Neck Surg 92: 618-624, 1984.
2   Robins PV, Folstein MF: Delirium and dementia: Diagnostic criteria and fatality rates. Br J Psych 140: 149-153, 1982.
3. Inglefinger FJ: Medicine: meritorious or meretricious. Science 200: 942-946, 1978.

Further Reading:

Luria AR: Higher cortical functions in man, 2nd ed. Basic Books, New York, 1980, pp 634.
Restak RM: The Brain: The last frontier. Doubleday and Co., Garden City, New York, 1979, pp 418.
Stoll BA: Cancer treatment: End point evaluation. John Wiley and Sons, New York, 1983, pp 520.
Strub RL, Black FW: Organic brain syndromes: An introduction to neurobehavioral disorders. WB Saunders, Philadelphia, 1981, pp 423.
Sugarbaker PH, Barofsky I, Rosenberg SA, Gianola FJ: Quality of life assessment of patients in extremity sarcoma clinical trials. Surg 91: 17-23, 1982.
Taylor DC: The components of sickness: Diseases, illnesses and predicaments. Lancet 2: 1008-1010, 1979.

8

QUALITY OF LIFE AND COST EFFECTIVENESS ISSUES IN THE MANAGEMENT OF PATIENTS WITH HEPATIC METASTASES FROM COLORECTAL CANCER

Paul H. Sugarbaker, Martin A. Adson, Ivan Barofsky, Edward M. Copeland, III, Sallie Martin Foley, Kevin S. Hughes, Frank Jones, M. Margaret Kemeny, Bernard Levin, Philip D. Schneider, Marshall Urist and Paul V. Woolley, III

SUMMARY

The intent of this chapter is to focus on relevant quality of life and cost effectiveness issues of new treatment strategies for patients who have colorectal cancer that has metastasized to the liver. At the present time, there is no potentially curative treatment except surgical excision of metastatic lesions. There is a danger of rediscovering limitations of old treatments by use of new technologies, unless carefully designed trials are performed. Unless treatment results in prolonged survival, the detrimental effects on quality of life that often accompany these chemotherapeutic regimens argue strongly against their use. It may be that the current strategy for clinical and research efforts in this field should be re-examined. The optimum management of the patient with hepatic metastases may not be part of routine cancer therapy and may still be an important area to investigate. Is it advisable that no more patients with hepatic metastases should be treated by infusion techniques unless they agree to participate in an experimental protocol? Also, should a no-treatment control arm be required in all therapeutic trials? Only with a no-treatment control arm can the survival, quality of life, and cost of these treatments be assessed properly.

The treatment history presentation of a patient with hepatic metastases will focus the discussion on differences in therapeutic strategies for patients with this disease. Through comments on patient management, the opinions of the participants representing several medical fields, will be presented. It is our intent to develop this discussion concerning quality of life issues so that physicians can see how these important concerns can be integrated into treatment plans for patients with incurable cancer.

INTRODUCTION

One may question why quality of life and cost effectiveness are being discussed along with the infusion therapies done for patients who have hepatic metastases from colorectal carcinoma. However, there are definite relationships because all treatment involves some cost and affects, in some way, quality of life. The optimal goal of treatment is to maximize survival and minimize adverse side effects. Therefore, the quality of life must be considered to be an important part of prospective clinical trials. Treatments are compared so that an optimal treatment plan can be identified. This plan is the one that cures a greater number of people, has the least adverse side effects, restores the quality of life, or maintains quality of life relative to some disease-dependent level. Rarely are these issues explicitly measured. Rather, assumptions are too often made about the quality of extended life. The adverse side effects that may have a short- or long-term detrimental effect on the quality of life are often enumerated; however an equation that includes treatment-related problems (debits of a treatment plan) is seldom, if ever, calculated. In the discussion that follows, we have assumed that all treatment-related decisions have an impact on quality of life and should, therefore, be discussed as one integrated issue.

In order to facilitate our discussion, the case of a patient with hepatic metastases is presented. The clinical history is presented followed by comments that may clarify treatment or quality of life decision making for this patient and for other patients with this disease.

PATIENT PRESENTATION AND PANEL DISCUSSION

In planning this program, the committee discussed many aspects of hepatic metastases among themselves. They recognized many questions concerning treatment of this problem that were unanswered. This program can not address, much less answer, all the patient-related problems that exist for patients with hepatic spread of colorectal cancer. The case presentation was designed to focus agreements and disagreements concerning patient care. The discussion panel members were encouraged to point out problems and controversies in patient management and to share their differences of philosophy and treatment strategy that are sure to be present, in view of the many institutions represented at the meeting.

Patient Presentation

Paul H. Sugarbaker, Bethesda, MD: Patient T.M.B. is a 57-year-old man from Boca Raton, Florida with hepatic metastases from colorectal cancer. In January of 1983 he underwent a left colectomy for a Dukes' stage B2 perforated sigmoid colon cancer. At the time of surgery, a single nodule was seen on the dome of the right lobe of the liver.

Biopsy results were positive for adenocarcinoma. One month later, the patient was referred to the National Institutes of Health in Bethesda, Md. A computed tomographic (CT) scan of the abdomen showed three nodules in the right lobe of the liver. Carcinoembryonic antigen (CEA) at that time was 14 ng/ml. The referring surgeon reported that the left colon lesion had been resected and the margins were negative for disease. An extensive radiologic workup for extrahepatic disease was also negative. We thought that there were four treatment options open to this young, healthy patient: (1) no treatment, (2) systemic chemotherapy, (3) pump perfusion of the liver with floxuridine (FUdR) via the hepatic artery using the Infusaid pump method, and (4) surgical resection of tumor from the liver.

Edward M. Copeland, III, Gainesville, FL: As moderator, the first question that I want us to address is what treatment should be recommended for this patient and why? Remember, at the present time, the patient is totally asymptomatic.

Marshall M. Urist, Birmingham, AL: The approach should begin with a complete discussion with the patient regarding his prognosis and options for therapy, including benefits, risks, and costs. He presented with a perforated carcinoma of the colon and therefore has a high probability of developing intraperitoneal and regional metastases, in addition to the hepatic metastases already noted. If we assume that the bilirubin is less than 0.5 mg/dl and the alkaline phosphatase is less than 100 U/L, then his estimated median survival without treatment would be 14 months. If he wishes to consider treatment at this time, I would recommend that he undergo exploratory celiotomy with careful attention to the detection of extrahepatic disease metastases. This involves the customary inspection of all areas and routine biopsy of celiac, portal, and possibly, retropancreatic nodes. If extrahepatic disease is not detected, the liver should be examined for the presence of metastases that were not demonstrated on the CT scan. We have observed this many times because lesions less than 2 cm are not reliably detected or are missed between cuts of the CT scan. If the metastases appear to be isolated to one side of the liver, then resection of this area is the one treatment with a chance for cure. If additional metastases are found in other areas of the liver, then regional chemotherapy by continuous infusion would be recommended. Previously untreated patients should be entered into the prospective randomized protocols that are available in many areas of the country.

Martin A. Adson, Rochester, MN: In our recent study of this subject, the median survival of untreated patients with three hepatic metastases was approximately 15 months (1). This means that this patient has a 50% chance of living nearly 1 1/2 years essentially free of symptoms from his disease, if he elects to forego the rigors of surgical resection or the use of biologic manipulations that may be noxious in some way. My thoughts about this specific patient relate to the size of the multiple lesions seen on CT scan. In our studies, we have found a difference between small and large metastases. More than one-third of patients who had multiple unilobar metastases greater than 4 cm in size removed lived five years or more, but no patient who had three small unilobar metastases removed lived five years.

The biology (or more likely the anatomic distribution) of small metastases is such that the presence of other small unseen metastases, both within the liver and at extrahepatic sites, is the rule. I think that these small metastases are not local descendants of a solitary blood-borne metastasis, but rather evidence of multiple "pioneer metastases" from the primary tumor. I think that the size and time of appearance of these multiple metastases is likely evidence of widely disseminated cancer that simply cannot be seen. Therefore, I would not recommend extirpation for this patient. For him, procrastination is not an evil, and surgery may cause more trouble than it is worth. If one waits for three to six months and still only three hepatic metastases are seen without evidence of extrahepatic metastases, an anatomically or biologically favorable type of cancer may exist and may be treated by resection. My recommendation is to delay surgery and to see what the patient's disease is doing and at what rate.

Bernard Levin, Houston, TX: My first move would be to ask the surgeons to see this patient. If they consider him a candidate for resection, I would proceed with surgery. If they did not wish to attempt potentially curative surgery in this asymptomatic 57-year-old man, the natural history of this disease must be taken into consideration. There are, at present, no effective systemic chemotherapeutic agents for patients with metastatic colon or rectal cancer. The agents available at this point are phase II study agents. If the patient is eager to have treatment and the disease is evaluable, I would recommend entering him into a phase II study in which he would be carefully followed up in a clinical research setting. The drugs used could either be a single agent or combination chemotherapy, or he might be a candidate for the randomized intra-arterial study of the inter-institutional Hepatic Tumor Study Group.

I should emphasize that I would be quite happy not treating this patient at this time, but rather wait for early development of symptoms before instituting therapy. However, if the patient desires treatment, there are treatment protocols available that have some potential for helping the patient and would, in a real way, advance our knowledge concerning chemotherapy for this problem. Certainly the wishes of the patient with incurable cancer must always be considered in every therapeutic decision. In summary, I would be very happy to follow the patient for several months and try to determine the rate at which his disease is progressing; when he becomes symptomatic there are treatment protocols available that may be of some benefit.

Sallie Martin Foley, Ann Arbor, MI: An important aspect of this patient's care involves the disruption of his lifestyle that these treatments may cause. He may live a long distance from where his treatments are to be administered. If so, the treatment will result in much time away from home, much time lost from meaningful pursuits like work, and much time spent away from his family. Although the majority of patients do want to pursue treatment, it is important that the patient be fully informed about the treatment and accept if before it is begun.

We must also determine if the patient and his family have sufficient knowledge upon which to base the multiple decisions that they will be required to make. As a social worker, I would want to know what this man's values are, what he expects to receive from his treatment, and if his expectations are likely to be fulfilled by the treatments offered.

Philip D. Schneider, Sacramento, CA: There is, I suspect, a low likelihood of curing this patient by means of a hepatic resection. But, we cannot assume that all the lesions seen on CT scan are hepatic metastases. The surgeon who operated reported and took a biopsy of only one lesion. It is completely possible that this is his only disease. The other lesions may be malignant or benign. If they are benign, he has a good chance of benefiting from surgery. I would be comfortable in waiting perhaps three months before treating him. Drs. Cady and McDermott in Boston have suggested that one biologic indicator of tumor behavior or determinant of survival is failure of the disease to disseminate (2). I think waiting three months will not prejudice the patient's chance for prolonged survival, should a hepatic resection be indicated.

I was asked to comment on cost effectiveness of infusion treatment for hepatic metastases. The cost of a treatment is not generally figured into the treatment equation. However, this may change, and treatment cost is very likely to influence treatment selection in the future. It one compares continuous systemic infusion of chemotherapy as an inpatient to hepatic perfusion chemotherapy with catheters placed by angiographers or surgeons, the costs are not much different. However, if one compares outpatient chemotherapy to hepatic perfusion there is a tremendous cost difference. Of course not treating the patient is undoubtedly the least expensive strategy and if it were shown to be "equally ineffective" it might be the treatment of choice.

Frank E. Jones, Milwaukee, WI: Cost of treatment must be a concern that is definitively addressed when making a therapeutic recommendation. Most older physicians and many patients today may believe that all care should be available to all patients, regardless of cost. Reality is quite different. Whether or not an individual physician regards his therapeutic regimen as being state-of-the-art medicine may play little or no role in insurance company payment decisions. A treatment regimen may be declared experimental, sometimes on rather arbitrary grounds, and charges disallowed by the companies. On the other hand, even though the treatment is acceptable, the patient's allowed benefits may be exhausted. A considerable proportion of patients referred to our institution for investigational therapies are patients whose insurance coverage has expired; the referring physicians assume that our experimental therapies will involve no cost to the patient. Even for the investigator to waive his professional charge is no solution, since the professional fee is a minor fraction of the total cost of any treatment regimen for advanced cancer. For many patients, any active treatment program involves a major financial burden.

Many physicians respond defensively if the patient decides against accepting the treatment recommendations. The patient may be sent to someone who is known to provide alternative therapy, or the patient may be abandoned, occasionally, because the patient "will not accept medical advice." In such situations, I believe that we physicians must maintain our humility. The patient's goals for the remainder of his lifetime may be quite different from ours. If the patient's original choice does not turn out well, the physician who remains involved may continue to exert his influence and repeat his recommendation of more effective therapy. On the other hand, when patients are able to accomplish their own goals, management results may be seen as being dramatically successful regardless of disease progression. Occasionally, a patient may do exceptionally well on "inadequate" or no therapy; we all are aware of occasional patients who were given only a few months to live, but were seen many years later with dormant disease. This uncertainty in making recommendations to individual patients must be kept in mind when patients disagree with us. Regardless of their situations, all patients are better off being followed up by a skilled, caring physician than being left on their own.

M. Margaret Kemeny, Duarte, CA: This patient would fit nicely into a protocol currently in progress at the City of Hope Hospital. The protocol is designed to treat patients who have multiple, but resectable hepatic metastases. Patients similar to this one are randomized into one of two arms of the protocol. One treatment is hepatic perfusion using the Infusaid pump; the other treatment is resection of hepatic metastases followed by Infusaid pump perfusion. The hepatic lesions are resected with a margin of normal tissue of at least 1 cm. Colorectal metastases are quite firm, and their edges are easy to identify, which facilitates surgery. Resection of multiple small metastases almost never require a formal hepatic lobectomy. By the fall of 1984, we had studied 18 patients on this protocol; 10 patients received perfusion alone, and all had a complete response in the liver, but 7 of the 10 patients developed extrahepatic disease. In eight patients treated with resection plus hepatic perfusion, five currently remain free of disease. Follow-up in both groups has been 12-30 months. Three patients in the surgery plus chemotherapy arm have died. Postmortem examinations showed no evidence of disease within the liver, but presence of extrahepatic disease in all three.

I think that all patients with multiple hepatic metastases should be treated according to established protocols so that a more effective therapy can be found.

Paul V. Woolley, III, Washington, D.C.: In my opinion, it is unwise to shift the burden for treatment selection from the physician to the patient. This can create great anxiety for the patient and family when they are not equipped to choose a treatment plan on the basis of the data available. There is an important distinction between informed consent and actually asking patients to make medical decisions. Secondly, patients come to our institutions for treatment and the expectation that something will be done, if at all possible, to help them. Simply telling patients to wait may be for them an intolerable option. Many patients prefer knowing that active treatment is being pursued in order to be comfortable with the efforts of a physician and an institution.

If a protocol exists that will determine response to therapy of the hepatic metastases, it may be the most desirable plan in a particular patient's course. Even if disease recurs in the pelvis or the lung, the patient may still have benefited by treatment of the hepatic disease, and the treatment will have been tested in a protocol setting. At our institution we would obtain a hepatic arteriogram, insert a catheter into the hepatic artery, and start continuous infusion of 5-FUdR at a dose of 0.1 or 0.15 mg/kg/24 hours.

In summary, since this group cannot agree on the proper treatment in this discussion, how can we expect the patient to arrive at a rational decision without any formal training? The effectiveness of hepatic perfusion needs to be subjected to protocol studies and the results presented to patients in an organized fashion in clinical situations similar to this case. If an uncertain plan of action is presented to a patient it may severely damage his ability to cope.

Dr. Jones: In Wisconsin in 1984, patients were accepting and demanding a more active role in selecting their treatment regimens. Actually, all a physician ever can do is recommend treatment; it is up to the patient to decide if he is going to accept that recommendation. In order to assist the patient in his decision, the physician must address a number of issues. First, the goal of treatment must be defined. When cure is not a reasonable goal, the physician must inform the patient of this and must guide the patient to ask the questions that allow him to decide what he wants to accomplish in his remaining lifetime. Next, each and every treatment option needs to be briefly, but adequately, explained. Reasonably expected good results, as well as side effects and complications (indicating those that occur commonly and rarely), must be described. Financial consequences for each option must be defined. If conventional therapy has been exhausted, or if no effective conventional therapy exists, the patient should be informed of research protocols that address his problem. Once all of this has been done, it is imperative that the physician give a definite and unequivocal recommendation for management and the rationale behind that recommendation.

Ms. Foley: There are many people who interact with a patient and his family. Yet there is an essential interaction that must take place directly between doctor and patient. After years of listening to patients, I think the physician gains a sense of how to communicate information specifically for an individual patient and when and how to inform the patient about his medical condition.

Currently, Dr. Andrew Salyer, a psychologist, and I are performing a study at the University of Michigan to compare attributes of psychological adjustment in patients receiving systemic chemotherapy versus those receiving hepatic artery infusion. The initial results are quite interesting. Patients who have participated in the selection of their treatment seem to have a more positive attitude towards their treatment course. Patients with implanted infusion pumps report significantly less interference with leisure activities, daily routine, and sexual functioning, than those receiving systemic chemotherapy.

I would like to emphasize the possible role of the social worker in helping patients and their families adjust to selected treatments. It is essential that the social workers be well informed about the treatments and that they make daily rounds with the medical oncologists. Because of the different perspective of the social worker, he or she can act as a third person to inform the surgeon of the patient's problems and discuss with the patient the psychological adjustment and quality of life issues related to the medical problem.

Dr. Urist: The issue of quality of life is especially important in asymptomatic patients with hepatic metastases. At the University of Alabama, we have included a rehabilitation and quality of life evaluation in our regional chemotherapy study (3). The patients in this study were evaluated by an independent observer for their status prior to pump implantation and again after four months of therapy. At the time of pump implantation, one-third of the patients were symptomatic and two-thirds had no symptoms that were directly relatable to the liver tumor. Over the following four months, approximately one-half of the symptomatic patients improved or became asymptomatic. One-third continued to be symptomatic because of drug toxicity or tumor symptoms. These patients all maintained a fairly normal level of physical activity.

90

Approximately 15% of the symptomatic patients became worse and this was usually due to progression of the tumor. Among the patients who were asymptomatic or had mild symptoms before therapy, approximately 60% remained asymptomatic four months later. One-third had moderate symptoms that were usually due to drug toxicity. Six percent of patients had symptoms that were severe and that lessened their quality of life. Seventy-two percent of patients who were employed prior to pump implantation returned to either part-time or full-time employment.

These results show that regional chemotherapy for asymptomatic patients has a significant chance of causing symptoms during a period in which they might otherwise have been asymptomatic. It is very important that patients understand these risks before undergoing infusion pump therapy. On the other hand, there does appear to be a survival advantage to regional chemotherapy in phase II trials. Since ours was a nonrandomized study, and infusion pump patients were compared to a controlled population matched for significant prognostic factors (tumor location and bilirubin and alkaline phosphatase levels); only limited conclusions regarding survival can be made.

I agree wholeheartedly with the recommendations that studies of the quality of life be included with measurements of the quantity of life when various treatment approaches are evaluated.

Dr. Adson: In a way, it is difficult to know what to tell the patient at this point, for there is really nothing good to say. Still, I think that patients may tolerate the truth better than they may tolerate some treatment that is ill advised. In this instance, I would spend a lot of time explaining the limitations of aggressive treatment to the patient and an equal or greater amount of time emphasizing the hope that can be derived from knowledge of the natural history and capriciousness of cancer and the availability of therapies that might well be useful if the disease becomes asymptomatic.

Dr. Sugarbaker: The treatment instituted at the National Institutes of Health (NIH) for the patient under discussion consisted of surgical exploration of the abdomen and then the right chest through a thoracoabdominal incision. Three hepatic metastases were found. Two were in the right lobe of the liver and one in the left. These metastases were resected and the patient randomized on protocol to receive intraperitoneal 5-fluorouracil (5-FU). In April of 1983, the intraperitoneal 5-FU was begun. CEA had fallen to 2 ng/ml following the resection. However, from July to December of 1983, despite intraperitoneal 5-FU, there was a progressive rise in CEA from 2 to 14 ng/ml. SGPT and SGOT were minimally elevated. In February of 1984 a repeat CT scan showed two nodules in the right lobe and one in the left. At this time, the patient was again taken to surgery, and five metastases were found in his liver. He was randomized to FUdR via hepatic artery infusion on a protocol in which the other arm was FUdR via a systemic vein. With hepatic artery infusion, his CEA again decreased to less than 2 ng/ml from its high of 22 ng/ml. The patient experienced moderate chemical hepatitis that resolved when the dosage was decreased. He had some symptoms of gastritis and duodenitis, which were treated with cimetidine and antacids. His symptoms with this treatment were minimal. In October of 1984, six months after insertion of the hepatic artery pump, his CEA level again began to increase. CT scan showed no new nodules in his liver, and we suspected extrahepatic disease.

At this point, I would like someone to comment on what it means for a patient with hepatic metastases to have a complete response to hepatic artery infusion chemotherapy. Should treatment be altered?

Dr. Levin: I would think that a salutary response indicates that treatment should not be changed at that point. The intra-arterial FUdR infusion should be continued. I would watch the dose of drug and be conservative with the drug treatment once the patient achieved complete response. Most important, I would not treat when there is evidence of hepatitis.

I would like to know how no-treatment control arms of protocols can be used in 1984 with patients who demand to be treated?

Dr. Sugarbaker: The pressure to treat with the infusion pump seems to be diminishing. It is now possible to treat patients by observation only when they do not have resectable metastases. At the NIH, we have contemplated reusing our protocol so that there would be three arms: an intra-arterial FUdR treatment, an intravenous continuous perfusion FUdR treatment, and a no-treatment control arm. In the third arm, patients would only be treated when they become symptomatic. If patients in the control group develop bulky hepatic metastases, painful hepatic metastases, or there seems to be an inordinately rapid progression of disease within the liver, pump infusion treatments might be instituted at that time. This delayed treatment plan is designed to prolong optimal quality of life, but to treat when symptoms develop. If we are clever enough, we should be able to assess the quality of life quantitatively in patients in the three arms of this trial. A comparison would tell us which patients have maintained good quality of life for the greatest time period. It is completely possible that the delayed treatment groups of patients might have the best quality of life and no shorter survival.

William D. Ensminger, Ann Arbor, MI: It may not be so important to do a quality of life study as it is to manage the drug judiciously so that there are fewer adverse quality of life consequences.

Dr. Schneider: There is a pressing reason to have a no-treatment control group in ongoing studies. In results of trials to date, the systemic continuous FUdR infusion-treated patients seem to be doing as well as those receiving intra-arterial pump infusions of FUdR. In the NIH studies, the median survival is over two years in both arms of the trial. This unexpectedly prolonged survival and lack of difference in survival is the important reason for including no-treatment control arms in hepatic metastases protocols. Modern staging using CEA and CT scans are able to select patients in favorable prognostic groups. This group of patients may do well no matter what treatment is used.

Dr. Jones: I agree that it is imperative to conduct appropriately controlled trials of new and, in some cases, old treatments for liver metastases from large bowel cancer. I agree that in the early asymptomatic phase of this condition, at least, it is imperative to include a "no immediate additional treatment" control group in order to prove both therapeutic and quality of life benefit of the experimental treatment. There is another reason, which is addressed by few investigators, to conduct such a trial. That is to document the economic effects of a management regimen. On a national scale, the resources consumed in managing these patients are enormous.

As an example, consider the adjuvant therapy for Dukes' stage C large bowel cancer with systemic 5-FU, an inexpensive drug, administered weekly by intravenous injections. In my institution, this "inexpensive" treatment program could easily cost $7,000 per patient over a two-year period. Nationally, the potential expense of this treatment for 60,000 patients (50% of the 130,000 new cases of large bowel cancer in 1984) exceeds $400,000,000 per year. If my community is typical, the majority of Dukes' stage C colon cancer patients receive this treatment even though most investigators believe that therapeutic benefit has never been proven. Nevertheless, this therapy is accepted and its costs reimbursed by health insurance companies. It seems to me that these companies would be extremely interested in supporting investigations to document the therapeutic advantage of such regimens in order to avoid paying for ineffective therapy.

In Wisconsin, the treatment of hepatic metastases by intrahepatic artery infusion of chemotherapy with an implantable pump is considered an investigational treatment by most insurance companies. Nevertheless, if each case is presented for payment on an individual basis, there is a very good chance that each patient's bill will be paid on a fee-for-service basis, when provided as active and specific treatment by a community practitioner. On the other hand, if our referral centers wish to be reimbursed for service administered to patients enrolled in a trial in which the patients may be randomized to receive no additional treatment, it is very difficult to receive reimbursement from the insurance companies. It seems that our current medical reimbursement system is organized so that investigation of significant therapeutic approaches is inhibited rather than supported.

Given the present difficulty with funding appropriate clinical trials and in the accrual of adequate numbers of patients for these trials, it makes a great deal of sense to me for health insurance companies to support well-designed trials by refusing to pay for certain treatments unless the patients are entered into a formal protocol. Were this policy adopted, I would hasten to suggest that the many well-trained community surgical, medical, and radiation oncologists be encouraged to participate in these trials. Such participation should dramatically facilitate patient accrual and confirm the therapeutic advantage of such treatment regimens, even when taken out of the academic setting and applied on a large scale in the community. It seems to me that such a policy would be the most efficient means of conserving resources otherwise wasted on ineffective treatment, as well as accelerating the process of bringing therapeutic advances to the general public.

James Foster, Hartford, CT: I always talk at considerable length with my patients who are candidates for hepatic resection and with their family members. I find that there is a great fear of chemotherapy. I tell patients quite frankly that after two decades of experimenting with 5-FU, I do not think that it prolongs survival. Also, no combination of other drugs has prolonged survival.

The tremendous enthusiasm for intra-arterial pump infusion has begun to diminish. With new knowledge about the natural history of the disease, I do not think that people should be treated with infusions or any other chemotherapy unless it is part of a protocol that includes a no-treatment control arm. We must remember that there are negative aspects to chemotherapeutic infusion. The increasing number of mutations caused by the chemotherapy may actually increase the rate at which systemic metastases occur. This is but one example of possible adverse effects of chemotherapy, and this is why the no-treatment study arm is essential.

I think that the physician who has the courage to tell patients that curative surgery is not an option, that pump perfusion is not necessary, and that the survival without treatment is longer than expected provide a great comfort to patients with hepatic metastases and to their families as well. We should not feel compelled to treat, and I do not feel as though we burn bridges if we wait until symptoms appear. One must remember that palliation is very difficult in the asymptomatic patient. The average cancer hospital in the average community does not need these high-powered treatment options in 1984. If patients want to be referred to a university center for treatment on protocols, the option is always open.

Dr. Woolley: It is important to realize that treatment control arms do not necessarily mean ultimately no treatment at all. After a period of observation, when the patient's disease progresses, other palliative treatments can be instituted. Therefore, the patient does not have to fear being deserted as a result of his randomization to an observation arm.

DISCUSSION

The goals of cancer treatment are to: (1) cure, (2) prolong life, (3) maintain or restore quality of life, and (4) gain information. In some patients, a cure is possible. When this goal is pursued, the treatments are instituted despite the adverse consequences in quality of life. Alternatively, treatments may be designed to maintain or restore the predisease quality of life of a patient who is suffering from cancer. Often patients in phase I studies gain little from the treatment. However, results of the patient's participation can provide important information that will aid the design of future treatment plans. When goals two, three, or four are being pursued, it is important that the adverse side effects and detriment to the quality of life be weighed against the benefits for the patient. It becomes clear that where curative treatments are involved, treatment-related decisions are easy. The possibility of a cure is the overriding consideration and adverse quality of life effects are, for the most part, disregarded. However, where palliative treatments are concerned, decisions regarding survival time and quality of life become important.

For some patients, prolonging life with a lesser quality is reasonable. Other patients may not want to sacrifice quality of life for an increase in its length. Decisions regarding the use of palliative treatments can be very difficult under these circumstances. Especially when dealing with palliative treatments for cancer patients, physicians are often forced to make judgements without adequate data. Recommendations are often based on intuition, compassion, current fashionable trends, institutional biases, and legal ramifications. Physicians often decide to treat, as opposed to doing nothing, feeling that it is better to offer some hope than allow the patient to think that nothing can be done. It can be very hard not to do anything. This may be true even though the treatment offers nothing in terms of prolonged life, but may add considerably to a deterioration in the quality of life. Clearly, more quantitative information is required regarding detrimental effects of prolonging life and on the quality of that life resulting from cancer treatments before rational judgements concerning palliative treatments can be made consistently.

Table 1 presents the credits and debits of treating hepatic metastases by regional perfusion chemotherapy. Quantitative data regarding these credits and debits need to be gathered from prospective clinical trials. If hepatic artery perfusion prolongs the life of cancer patients, then the detrimental effects that this treatment has on function and quality of life can be tolerated. If a symptom-free existence is maintained for an extended time period, even if survival is not prolonged, the adverse side effects of chemotherapeutic treatment are worth the price. However, before infusion treatments are used as routine parts of the oncologist's armamentarium, either a prolonged survival or a longer symptom-free existence must be demonstrated. Only as infusion treatments are compared to no-treatment control subjects can these judgments be made. One must accept the fact that the operative morbidity and mortality associated with pump insertion and with drug perfusion are realities.

Table 1. Treatment of hepatic metastases by regional infusion chemotherapy

CREDITS	DEBITS
Prolongation of life	Operative morbidity and mortality
Maintenance or restoration of quality of life	Treatment-related morbidity and mortality
Information gained that will benefit future patients	Changes in the natural history of the disease resulting in a more painful demise
	Expense

It is completely reasonable that if the treatment of hepatic metastases is purely palliative, it should only be used to palliate disease. That is, treatment should only be instituted when patients are suffering as a result of progressive cancer. At present, asymptomatic patients are generally the ones treated by infusion. If no prolongation of survival or maintenance of a symptom-free existence can be demonstrated, then infusion should be withheld until the patient becomes symptomatic. Indication for hepatic artery perfusion would be a mass effect, such as tumor necrosis that causes pain, discomfort, respiratory distress, or night sweats and fever. For patients with hepatic metastases from colorectal cancer, this means treating advanced bulky intrahepatic disease only. Certainly this would mean a profound decrease in the number of patients receiving this form of treatment.

CONCLUDING REMARKS

Quantitative quality of life data are needed in order to improve the end points of clinical trials. A great deal of intuitive clinical information can be turned into data if a quantitative assessment of a particular observation can be made. Quantitation of quality of life data would greatly improve one's ability to make clinical decisions. Quality of life data would be especially relevant if there were similar survival statistics provided in two different treatment plans within a clinical trial. Then, the treatment that had the lowest morbidity and allowed for the best quality of life would be recommended for broad application.

Should investigators attempt to make the quality of life assessment a part of hepatic perfusion clinical trials? We have argued in the past that quality of life assessment should be part of all clinical trials (4). Palliation has as a principal objective, optimization of quality of life so that it's a reasonable objective. Use of a control group can be justified on the grounds that chemotherapeutic regimens have a high probability of disrupting function, even if they produce local and regional control of disease. Local and regional control of disease may or may not extend survival or relieve symptoms. Thus, if the control group has a better quality of life and a comparable survival to treated patients, then a realistic assessment of the efficacy of alternative treatments can be made.

At present, several instruments are available that permit quantitation of quality of life data. The Karnofsky scale has been utilized frequently to stratify patients in controlled chemotherapy trials (5). Recently Spitzer reported the use of a new quality of life self-assessment for use with patients by physicians (6). Schipper and colleagues developed the patient-based Functional Living Index for Cancer (FLIC) (7). This has been useful in clinical trials of cancer patients receiving chemotherapy. Alternatively, protocol-specific quality of life assessments may be required, if those mentioned are inadequate. We have used the Treatment Trauma Scale, which permits patients to place a numerical quality of life value on adverse side effects, emotional stress, interference with function, economic hardships, and other problems (8). A treatment trauma scale could be designed by the clinician for specific use within a protocol based on his clinical experience, knowledge of the natural history of the disease, and knowledge of the effects of the treatment. It may be necessary to assess quality of life many times over a period of several years. Detriment to the quality of life caused by a particular treatment would be expected to change over time. These data, gathered over an extended period, would be invaluable when evaluating clinical trials.

Finally, we recommend that the quality of life assessment be a part of controlled clinical trials; that better and more easily measured quality of life instruments be developed; that more emphasis be placed on quality of life as an outcome of treatment; and that the necessary expenditure of personnel time and institutional money be directed toward evaluating the quality of life as an outcome of controlled clinical trials.

References

1. Wagner JS, Adson MA, van Heerden JA, Adson MH, Ilstrup DM: The natural history of hepatic metastases from colorectal cancer. A comparison with resective treatment. Ann Surg 199: 502-508, 1984.
2. Cady B, McDermott WV: Major hepatic resection for metachronous metastases from colon cancer. Ann Surg 201: 204-209, 1985.
3. Balch CM, Urist MM, Soony S-J, McGregor ML: A prospective phase II clinical trial of continuous FUDR regional chemotherapy for colorectal metastases to the liver using a totally implantable drug infusion pump. Ann Surg 198: 567-573, 1983.
4. Barofsky I, Sugarbaker PH: Health status indexes: Disease specific vs. general population measures. Proceedings of Public Health Conference on Records and Statistics. June, 1978, Washington, D.C., Department of Health, Education and Welfare (PHS) 79-1214: 263-269, 1979.
5. Karnofsky DA, Abelman WH, Craver LF, Burchenal JH:: The use of the nitrogen mustards in the palliative treatment of carcinoma. Cancer 1: 634-656, 1948.
6. Spitzer WO, Dobson AJ, Hall J, Chesterman E, Levi J, Shephard R, Battista RN, Catchlove BR: Measuring the quality of life of cancer patients. J Chron Dis 34: 585-597, 1981.
7. Schipper H, Clinch J, McMurray A, Levitt M: Measuring the quality of life of cancer patients: The functional living index-cancer: Development and validation. J Clin Oncol 2: 472-483, 1984.
8. Sugarbaker PH, Barofsky I, Rosenberg SA, Gianola FJ: Quality of life assessment of patients in extremity sarcoma clinical trials. Surgery 91: 17-23, 1982.

SECTION III.

THE PREVENTION AND LOCAL TREATMENT OF COLORECTAL METASTASIS

9

REGIONAL INFUSION CHEMOTHERAPY FOR COLORECTAL HEPATIC METASTASES

John M. Daly and Nancy Kemeny

SUMMARY

Large bowel cancer is the second most common malignancy with the liver being the predominate site of distant metastases. Prospective studies evaluating the natural history of advanced disease suggest a median survival of five to six months, however, there is a wide range depending upon the extent of hepatic involvement. Disappointment with systemic chemotherapy has led to increased investigations regarding regional therapy directed at the liver. In the past, improved response rates have been noted with hepatic arterial infusion chemotherapy, however, complications of the technique have not led to widespread acceptance. Use of an implantable pump has decreased technical and infectious complications associated with this method of treatment. A phase II trial at Memorial Sloan-Kettering Cancer Center showed that previously untreated patients had a response rate of 50% while in previously treated patients the response rate was 31%. Toxicity involved the gastrointestinal tract with chemical hepatitis and gastritis being the predominate manifestations. Further, prospective clinical trials of intra-arterial chemotherapy for colorectal hepatic metastases are indicated to provide definitive conclusions regarding tumor response rates, length of patient survival, cost, morbidity, and quality of life during treatment.

INTRODUCTION

More than 130,000 new cases of colorectal cancer are diagnosed in the United States each year, with more than 50,000 deaths occurring as a result of metastatic disease. Forty to 70% of patients with colorectal cancer who develop metastatic disease have liver involvement. The liver is the sole initial site of recurrent disease in 30% of patients. Thus, approximately 12,000 patients per year are candidates for therapy directed specifically to hepatic metastases, and successful drug treatment would provide major palliation for many patients. Most clinicians choose either systemic or regional chemotherapy for treatment. Choice of treatment methods should depend on a knowledge of the natural history of the disease and on knowledge of the progression of colorectal cancers that have metastasized to the liver.

NATURAL HISTORY OF HEPATIC METASTASES

Retrospective studies have delineated the natural history of patients with hepatic metastases from colorectal cancer (1,2). In the past, liver metastases were usually discovered either at laparotomy performed for other reasons, or they were found when symptoms such as fever, fatigue, abdominal pain, anorexia, and weight loss occurred. Thus, hepatic metastases were often comparatively advanced at the time of their discovery. The single most important determinant of patient survival is the extent of hepatic involvement by tumor. In a study of 113 patients by Wood et al., the mean survival time for all patients was 6.6 months (3). For 87 patients with widespread liver metastases, the mean survival time was 3.1 months, with a one-year survival rate of 5.7%. For the 11 patients with localized liver metastases, the mean survival time was 10.6 months with a one-year survival rate of 27%. For the 15 patients with solitary liver metastases, the mean survival time was 16.7 months, and the one-year survival rate was 60%. The overall survival time for patients in this series is similar to the results of Jaffe et al., who noted a median survival time of 146 days in patients with colorectal hepatic metastases (2). Wagner et al. studied 252 patients with colorectal hepatic metastases retrospectively and demonstrated one-year survival rates of 40%, 60%, and 67% respectively in patients with "widespread," "multiple unilateral," and "solitary" disease (4). Similar results have been noted by other investigators who have studied length of survival and correlated it with extent of hepatic involvement (5). Clinical and laboratory indices such as weight loss, jaundice, performance status, hepatomegaly, and serum levels of albumin, bilirubin, alkaline phosphatase, lactic dehydrogenase, and carcinoembryonic antigen (CEA) correlated with length of survival (5). These data indicate the critical importance of accurate staging prior to advocating a specific therapy, since patient outcome differs depending upon the extent of involvement with tumor.

SYSTEMIC CHEMOTHERAPY

Systemic chemotherapy using 5-fluorouracil (5-FU) in bolus form results in an average tumor response rate of 15% when the measurement of tumor response is clearly defined. The mean response rate for hepatic metastases in several series is approximately 23% (Table 1) (6). Combination chemotherapy using 5-FU and methyl chloroethyl cyclohexyl nitrosourea (CCNU) with or without vincristine resulted in average response rates of 23%. The use of streptozotocin in addition to these three drugs increased responses in hepatic metastases to 30%. Sequential methotrexate and 5-FU treatment resulted in a 30% average response rate. Thus, conventional systemic chemotherapy in patients with metastatic colorectal cancer results in meaningful tumor responses in approximately 20% of patients.

Table 1. Response of Liver Metastases to 5-FU Treatment for Metastatic Colorectal Carcinoma*

Investigator	Total Population		No. With Liver Metastases	No. of Responders with Liver Metastases (%)
Moertel	144		118	28 (24)
Baker	42		11	- (0)
Seifert	36	bolus	5	1 (20)
Seifert	34	infusion	6	4 (67)
Moertel	23		-	- (0)
Moore	80		-	- (0)
Brennen	45		-	- (0)
Grage	31		31	7 (23)
Total	257 †		171	40 (23)

*   Adapted from Kemeny N, (6).

†   Total number does not include 144 patients (7) in whom the response was not clearly defined or 34 patients receiving infusion therapy.

REGIONAL THERAPY FOR HEPATIC METASTASES

Disappointment with results of systemic chemotherapy led several investigators to evaluate other modes of treatment, such as direct regional chemotherapeutic infusion (8-10). Controversy exists as to the best route for infusing the liver. Hepatic arterial infusion, hepatic artery ligation with arterial or portal vein infusion, and portal vein infusion have all been used.

In 1962, Clarkson et al. reported the method of chemotherapy by continuous hepatic arterial infusion using a catheter inserted via the brachial artery in 13 patients with advanced metastatic colorectal cancer (11). Duration of tumor response in five patients was short, two weeks to two months. Sullivan et al. noted significant objective tumor regression in 13 of 16 patients with metastatic colorectal cancer that was treated with hepatic arterial infusion chemotherapy (12). Clinical benefit was achieved in 10 of these patients. Other investigators who used hepatic arterial chemotherapy have reported tumor response rates of 55-73% with median patient survivals of 9 to 12 months (8-10). Unfortunately, use of external catheters placed either at operation or by the Seldinger technique has resulted in high complication rates, including catheter displacement, sepsis, and gastrointestinal hemorrhage (12,13). Reed et al. reported a 76% tumor response rate in 88 patients with metastatic colorectal cancer, with a median response duration of 12 months (14). However, complications in this series were frequent; there was an operative mortality of 12% and catheter-related morbidity of 24%. Thus, even though direct hepatic arterial infusion has improved response rates compared with systemic therapy, operative- and treatment-related complications have prevented widespread use of infusion chemotherapy.

In 1980, Buchwald et al. reported the use of an implantable infusion pump for regional hepatic arterial chemotherapy in five patients (15). Initial reports using this device noted tumor response rates of 29-83% with minimal catheter-related complications (16-19). Use of an implantable pump delivery system offers several potential advantages, such as reduction in catheter-related sepsis, ease of drug administration, and greater patient acceptance, without a bulky external device. Direct placement of the catheter eliminates the problem of catheter displacement and allows better determination of the presence of intra-abdominal extrahepatic disease. Cohen et al., for example, reported that 7 of 38 patients who underwent placement of a transaxillary catheter that was connected to an implantable pump experienced withdrawal of the catheter that necessitated catheter replacement (20).

ANATOMIC ANOMALIES AND HEPATIC ARTERIAL CHEMOTHERAPY

The technique of continuous hepatic arterial chemotherapy requires precise knowledge of hepatic arterial anatomic anomalies (21). A retrospective review of 200 cases of celiac and superior mesenteric arteriograms at Memorial Sloan-Kettering Hospital was done to specifically define the relationship of the gastroduodenal artery to the hepatic artery distribution. In 70% of these cases, Type IA anatomy was observed allowing complete infusion of both hepatic lobes using the gastroduodenal artery (Table 2). Patients demonstrating Type IB, II, Type IVB, and Type VB and some "others" required retrograde splenic artery catheterization with ligation of the left and right

104

gastric arteries and the gastroduodenal arteries. In 6% of 200 cases reviewed, the major blood supply to the right hepatic lobe arises from the superior mesenteric artery, while the left hepatic artery arises from the celiac artery. This situation requires either placement of two catheters separately or perhaps anastomosis of the right hepatic artery to the left hepatic artery in order to infuse both hepatic lobes. Because of the reported success of other investigators using the implantable pump system, a phase II study was designed at Memorial Sloan-Kettering Hospital to evaluate the feasibility, operative morbidity, toxicity, and efficacy of continuous hepatic infusion chemotherapy in patients with hepatic metastases from colorectal cancer (7).

Table 2. Hepatic Arterial Anatomy (n=200)

Type[*]	A[†]		B[‡]
I	70%		6%
II		4%	
III		6%	
IV	3%		0.5%
V	2.5%		1.5%
VI	1.5%		0.5%
other		4.5%	

[*] as described in Michels (21)

[†] gastroduodenal artery proximal to bifurcation

[‡] gastroduodenal artery distal to bifurcation

Patients

Forty adult patients with histologically proven, measurable colorectal cancer that metastasized to the liver were included in the trial. All patients underwent preoperative evaluations including chest roentgenogram, complete blood counts, SMA 100 blood chemistry analysis, plasma CEA, prothrombin time and partial thromboplastin time, electrocardiogram, radionuclide liver and spleen scan, and an abdominal computed tomographic (CT) scan. The hepatic arterial blood supply was defined by a preoperative contrast angiogram prior to laparotomy for catheter and pump placement.

Selected patients underwent complete colonoscopy or air-contrast barium enema to ascertain the presence of primary or recurrent malignancies. Three patients had primary colonic carcinomas in the transverse and sigmoid colon and the rectum. With the exception of these three patients, no patient had preoperative evidence of extrahepatic metastatic disease. Patients were excluded from the study if they had isolated hepatic metastasis amenable to resection, if they had known extrahepatic metastatic disease, if their performance status was less than 60, or if they had evidence of hepatic failure (e.g., serum bilirubin > 4 mg/dl). Patients were not excluded from the study based on volume of hepatic involvement or failure of previous chemotherapy.

Operative Technique

The operative procedure consisted of an exploratory celiotomy with visual and manual assessment of the entire abdomen for the presence of visceral and parietal metastatic disease. Particular attempts were made to ascertain lymphatic involvement of the inferior and superior mesenteric vessels, celiac and hepatic arteries, and portal vein. The diagnosis of hepatic metastases was confirmed by open biopsy. Determination of the volume of hepatic involvement was performed by manual and visual assessment during surgical exploration.

Hepatic pumps and catheters were placed in 34 patients. Resections of periaortic, celiac, and periportal lymph nodes plus pump and catheter placement were performed in three patients. Two patients underwent transverse and sigmoid colon resection, and one patient underwent fulguration of a rectal cancer, in addition to pump and catheter placement.

Preoperative arteriograms were reviewed and correlated with operative assessment of the hepatic arterial blood suppy. The right gastric artery and small branches to the duodenal bulb were ligated and divided in all patients. In 28 patients, catheterization of the gastroduodenal artery was performed after ligation of the right gastric artery and dissection of the common hepatic, proper hepatic, and gastroduodenal arteries. Particular care was exercised to ligate all branches of the gastroduodenal artery, such as the supraduodenal artery, which arose within 2 cm from its origin from the common hepatic artery. The gastroduodenal artery was ligated distally and temporally and occluded proximally while a transverse arteriotomy was done. The beaded silastic catheter was inserted retrograde so that its tip lay at the junction of the common hepatic and gastroduodenal arteries. The catheter was then secured with three 2-0 silk ligatures.

In 10 patients, retrograde catheterization of the splenic artery was performed after proximal ligation of the right gastric and gastroduodenal arteries and distal (distal to the split of the left hepatic artery) ligation of the left gastric artery. The splenic artery was temporally occluded while a transverse arteriotomy was done. The beaded silastic catheter was inserted so that its tip lay within the celiac artery. In two patients, the gastroduodenal artery was catheterized to allow infusion of the left hepatic artery while the replaced right hepatic artery was cannulated directly using a tapered catheter. This allowed continued blood flow through the nonoccluded right hepatic artery.

After catheterization, 2.0 ml of a fluorescein solution was injected into the pump's sideport, while the abdominal contents were exposed under an ultraviolet light to establish homogeneous uptake in the liver and absence of infusion of the stomach and duodenum. The implantable pumps were placed into the left or right lower quadrant subcutaneous pockets below the belt line, for patient comfort.

Cephalosporin antibiotics were administered preoperatively and for 72 hours postoperatively in all patients. Within five days of the operation, a hepatic perfusion scan was done using ^{99}technetium macroaggregated albumin to confirm that the catheter was infusing both lobes of the liver.

Hepatic arterial chemotherapy was initiated 7 to 14 days after operation. All patients were begun on treatment using floxuridine (FUdR) at a dose of 0.3 mg/kg/day for a 14 day cycle, followed by two weeks of continuous saline infusion. Heparin (10,000 units) was placed in the 50 ml pump reservoir with each refill of drug or saline. Patients with hepatic or extrahepatic disease progression were begun on mitomycin C at a dose of 15 mg/m^2 as a two-hour infusion into the side port every six weeks. Patients entered on the trial during the first 12 months were administered cimetidine orally (300 mg) four times a day and antacids prophylactically; later, patients received Carafate (sucralfate) orally (1 g) four times a day without cimetidine or antacids.

Patients were examined serially at two week intervals with particular attention to known side effects of infusional treatment, such as hepatitis and gastrointestinal ulcerations. Complete blood counts and serum liver function tests (bilirubin, SGOT, SGPT) were determined at these intervals. Plasma CEA levels were determined at least monthly. A radionuclide liver and spleen scan, an abdominal CT scan, or both were done after two months and thereafter as indicated. An upper gastrointestinal endoscopy was performed on patients who developed any symptoms of epigastric pain, fullness, or vomiting; four asymptomatic patients also underwent endoscopy to establish the incidence of gastroduodenal complications and to permit early reduction of the chemotherapeutic dosage.

Results of Therapy

During the 18-month study period, 40 patients underwent placement of the implantable pumps. Twenty-five patients were male; 15 patients were female. Their ages ranged from 33 to 79 years (median age = 59). The patients' performance status (Karnofsky index) ranged from 60 to 90 (median = 80); all patients had an anticipated two-month survival time (7). Twenty-one patients were previously untreated; 19 patients had failed previous chemotherapy, usually with 5-FU or 5-FU as part of a multidrug chemotherapeutic protocol. Hepatic involvement by operative staging ranged from 15-85% (median = 50%). Preoperative plasma CEA levels ranged from 1 to 3900 ng/ml, serum alkaline phosphatase levels ranged from 78 to 1359 IU/ml, and serum lactic dehydrogenase levels ranged from 179 to 2300 IU/ml.

Chemotherapeutic Response

Partial tumor response was strictly defined as a 50% or greater reduction in the sum of the products of the largest perpendicular diameters of measurable lesions by the liver or CT scan, no increase in any other indicator lesion, and no new area of malignant disease in the liver. If hepatomegaly was used as the primary indicator, there had to be a reduction in the sum of the measurements below the costal margin at the xiphoid process and four intervals (5 cm) lateral to the xiphoid process by at least 50%. A minor response occurred if there was a 25-49% reduction in measurable lesions. The patient was considered to have stable disease if there were minimal responses for at least two months, but insufficient regression to meet the above criteria. Progression was defined as an increase in any measurable lesion of more than 25% or the appearance of new areas of metastatic disease. Duration of response was defined as the time interval (months) from determination of partial or minor response to determination of progression of disease either by increase in size of hepatic metastases or by appearance of extrahepatic metastases.

Of the 21 previously untreated patients, three patients were unevaluable, including one patient in whom it was too early to determine response, one patient in whom the pump malfunctioned, and one patient who developed hepatic arterial thrombosis. Eighteen patients were evaluable (Table 3). Nine patients had partial tumor responses, one patient had a minor response, two patients remained stable for a minimum of two months, and six patients had tumor progression. The median duration of response was greater than eight months (range = 2 to more than 17 months).

Of the 19 previously treated patients, three patients were unevaluable, including one patient in whom it was too early to determine response and two patients who were lost to follow-up at our institution. Thus, 16 patients were evaluable (Table 3); five patients had partial tumor response; one patient had a minor response, three patients had disease, and seven patients had tumor progression. The median duration of response was four months (range = two to eight months).

108

Table 3. Chemotherapeutic Treatment Results

<u>Previously Untreated Patients</u> (n=21)

Evaluable Patients (n=18)[*]

Partial Response	9/18	(50%)
Minor Response	1/18	(6%)
Stable Disease	2/18	(11%)
Disease Progression	6/18	(33%)

<u>Previously Treated Patients</u> (n=19)

Evaluable Patients (n=16)[†]

Partial Response	5/16[‡]	(31%)
Minor Response	1/16	(6%)
Stable Disease	3/16	(19%)
Disease Progression	7/16	(44%)

[*] 1 too early for evaluation, 1 pump failure, 1 hepatic artery thrombosis

[†] 1 too early for evaluation, 2 lost to follow-up

[‡] 3 responded to FUdR above; 2 responded to FUdR plus mitomycin C

Chemotherapy Toxicity

Toxicity related to continuous FUdR infusion was associated primarily with the gastrointestinal tract. Twelve patients had ulcer disease documented by endoscopy; seven patients had documented gastritis or duodenitis without discrete ulceration. Thus, gastroduodenal inflammation or ulceration was noted in 48% of these patients.

Narset et al. described gastric ulceration in eight patients during intrahepatic arterial infusion with 5-FU (22). In all cases, the catheter tip was dislodged and was proximal to its correct position, allowing the stomach to be directly infused with 5-FU. Crowley reported one case of duodenal ulceration with erosion around the silastic catheter from an implantable pump in a patient receiving continuous hepatic arterial chemotherapy with FUdR (12). Ensminger et al. reported gastritis in 60% and ulcers in 8% of 60 patients receiving continuous hepatic arterial chemotherapy (13). The etiology of gastroduodenal ulceration and inflammation in our patients is uncertain; catheter placement and drug dosage schedules may be important determinants.

The direct arterial supply to the stomach and duodenum (right gastric and gastroduodenal arteries) was ligated proximally in all patients. In addition, ligation of the supraduodenal artery and small branches of the gastroduodenal artery was accomplished.   Celiac angiograms in two of our patients who developed ulcers demonstrated small collateral vessels from the common hepatic artery months after retrograde catheter placement in the splenic artery.   Prophylaxis with cimetidine and antacids did not seem to benefit patients, and recently, we have placed patients on 1 g Carafate four times a day.   The incidence of gastritis or ulcerations in patients during the past year has decreased substantially.   However, early reduction of drug dosages resulting from increased physician awareness has probably been the major factor in reducing this problem.

Hepatic toxicity was documented by elevation of serum bilirubin above 3 mg/dl in nine patients.   Serum levels returned to normal in five patients after drug cessation. Elevation of serum SGOT was noted in 65% of the patients; 19 patients had tripling of baseline values.   In all patients, serum SGOT elevations returned to normal by decreasing or stopping chemotherapy.   Two patients developed extrahepatic bile duct strictures that were proven to be unrelated to tumor progression.   They required external biliary drainage.   Ensminger et al. likewise noted a high incidence of hepatitis (46%) (19).   Early recognition of hepatitis and reduction in drug dosage are important in controlling this complication.

Results of this trial demonstrated minimal operative morbidity, but substantial chemotherapy-related complications.   Partial tumor response that was strictly defined occurred in 9 of 18 previously untreated and 5 of 16 previously treated patients.   This tumor response rate is similar to results obtained in most studies of continuous hepatic arterial chemotherapy and seems higher than results obtained in studies of systemic chemotherapy.   However, patient performance status and degree of hepatic involvement are important variables in all of these studies.   Grage et al. reported equivalent tumor response and survival rates in patients who received systemic 5-FU compared with those who received intrahepatic 5-FU (3 weeks) and subsequent 5-FU systemically (23).   A prospective randomized trial comparing intrahepatic arterial and systemic intravenous chemotherapy was designed to determine the relative treatment morbidity, drug toxicity, tumor response, patient survival, and quality of life during treatment.

COMPARISON OF REGIONAL VERSUS SYSTEMIC CHEMOTHERAPY

Patients with measurable colorectal carcinoma metastatic to the liver and without extrahepatic disease were eligible for the protocol.   Patients with a Karnofsky performance status less than 60 and bilirubin measurement greater than 4 mg/ml were excluded.

All patients were randomized to systemic or regional therapy prior to surgery and after stratification by lactic dehydrogenase level (< 300 U/L versus $\geq$ 300 U/L) and

110

percentage of liver involvement (< 50% versus ≥ 50%). The assessment of liver involvement was done medically by evaluation of CT and radionuclide liver scans. The information was placed in a sealed envelope on the patient's chart. The surgeon did not open the envelope until he assessed the extent of the liver involvement. If he disagreed with the preoperative assessment, the patient was randomized again.

All patients had exploratory laparotomy not only for placement of the hepatic catheter and an Infusaid pump (Intermedics Infusaid Corporation, Norwood, Massachusetts), but also to insure that the two arms of the study were comparable by accurately defining the extent of disease in the liver and assuring that there was no disease outside the liver.

Patients with extrahepatic disease or resectable hepatic disease discovered at exploratory surgery were ineligible for the protocol. The remaining eligible patients were randomized between intrahepatic arterial therapy or systemic intravenous therapy with FUdR. The method of administration by continuous infusion for 14 days via the Infusaid pump was the same for both groups. The dose, however, was initially lower in the systemic group (0.15 mg/kg/day versus 0.3 mg/kg/day for the intrahepatic group).

Patients in the intrahepatic group had the hepatic catheter connected to the pump. In the systemic group, the hepatic catheter was connected to an Infus-a-port (Intermedics Infusaid Corporation, Norwood, Massachusetts), and the pump was connected to a catheter placed in the cephalic vein (Figure 1). If a patient in the systemic group experienced tumor progression, a minor surgical procedure allowed a switch from systemic to hepatic arterial therapy, thereby allowing further evaluation of the efficacy of regional delivery (Figure 2).

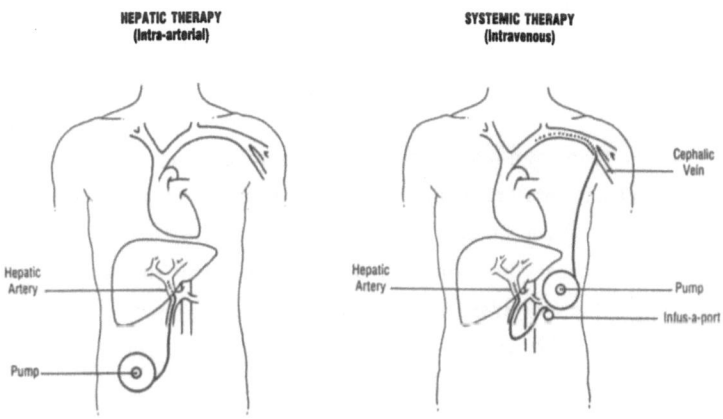

FIGURE 1. Diagrammatic representation of pump and catheter placement in hepatic arterial and systemic intravenous treatment study arms.

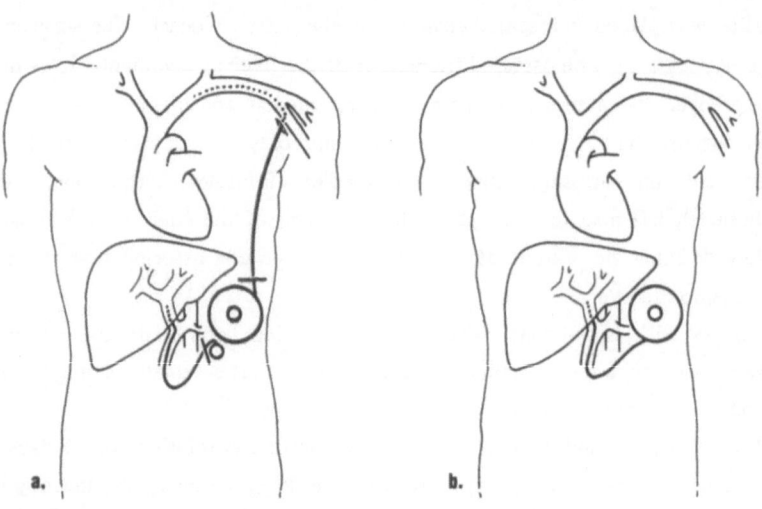

FIGURE 2. Crossover to the arterial arm was done in systemic treatment group patients with progressive disease using a minor surgical procedure.

Sixty-five patients have been referred for entry into the study. Four of the patients refused randomization and three patients were unable to enter because of an anomalous arterial blood supply, i.e. more than three vessels perfused the liver. Therefore, 58 patients were randomized. At surgical exploration, 16 patients were excluded from the study; in 8 patients, the disease was resectable; in 7 patients, extrahepatic disease existed, and in one patient, an intra-abdominal infection was present. Forty-two patients, therefore, received implantable pumps. They were well matched with respect to the percentage of liver involvement, initial laboratory values, performance status, time from liver metastases to protocol entry, and age (Table 4).

At present, 14 patients are evaluable in each group. Two patients had inadequate trials, one in the intrahepatic group because of incorrect catheter placement, and one in the systemic group because the patient died four weeks after surgery and three weeks after starting chemotherapy from very rapidly advancing disease. It is too early to evaluate the remaining 12 patients (4 on the intrahepatic and 8 on the systemic chemotherapy).

Table 4. Patient Characteristics

	Chemotherapy	
	Intrahepatic N=19	Systemic N=23
Median age	62*	62
Percent female	11	48
Performance status	80	80
Initial serum alkaline phosphatase (IU/ml)	213	213
Initial serum lactic dehydrogenase (IU/ml)	398	449
Initial serum carcinoembryonic antigen (ng/ml)	73	178
Initial serum albumin (g/dl)	4.0	4.0

* All numbers represent medians, except percent female.

There were 6 of 14 partial responders in the intrahepatic group, and there were 5 of 14 partial responders in the systemic group. The median duration of response was six months for the intrahepatic group and five months for the systemic group. There was one minor response in each group. In the systemic group there were two patients who had stable disease for more than 12 and more than 3 months. Eight of 16 patients in the intrahepatic group and 6 of 17 patients in the systemic group had a greater than 50% reduction in plasma CEA.

Those patients who did not respond to the systemic treatment had the opportunity to crossover to intrahepatic treatment. Five patients changed groups. One of the five patients experienced a very transient improvement in liver function tests, but this was followed by a thrombosis of the hepatic artery and further progression of disease. Three patients failed to respond to intrahepatic therapy with FUdR and have gone on to receive mitomycin C via the sideport of the pump; one patient responded.

Although the initial dose for the intrahepatic therapy was twice as high as for systemic therapy, the doses in both arms of the study were quite similar after the third cycle of treatment. Five patients required reduction in dosage after their initial treatment with intrahepatic therapy, six patients after the second, and four after the third treatment. The median dose after the third treatment was 0.2 mg/kg/day. In the

113

systemic arm, the original dose in nine patients was 0.15 mg/kg/day. Five of these patients required a reduction in their dose to 0.125 mg/kg/day for 14 days. Two patients developed severe diarrhea at the higher dose, and so after the first nine patients were treated, all patients subsequently were started on a dose of 0.125 mg/kg/day. Fourteen patients have been entered on this dose and seven have already tolerated an increase to 0.15 mg/kg/day. Three of the patients have not been given their second dose. Therefore, the median dose at the present time for the systemic chemotherapy group is 0.15 mg/kg/day.

The toxicity was quite different in the two groups. In the intrahepatic group, the toxicity was mainly gastrointestinal and hepatic. Four of the 14 patients (29%) developed significant gastrointestinal ulcers documented by endoscopy, and a fifth patient had severe gastritis. Seven of 14 (50%) patients developed SGOT elevations greater than 100% over baseline values, and two developed significant bilirubin elevations (9 and 10 mg/ml). In the systemic group, the major toxicity was diarrhea seen in 9 of 14 (64%) adequately treated patients. In two patients sigmoidoscopy revealed severe sigmoid ulcerations suggestive of colitis. Both of these patients required hospitalization for intravenous hydration.

It is too early to draw definite conclusions regarding the results of this randomized trial of continuous intra-arterial versus intravenous chemotherapy. However, it appears that response rates are similar between the two study arms, and gastrointestinal toxicity is common with both types of infusion. Further patient accrural and time are required to fully evaluate these methods of treatment. Other randomized, prospective, clinical trials of intra-arterial chemotherapy for colorectal hepatic metastases are underway and should provide definitive conclusions regarding tumor response rates, length of patient survival, cost, morbidity, and quality of life during treatment.

References

1. Foster JH, Lungy J: Liver metastases. Curr Prob Surg 18: 160-195, 1983.
2. Jaffe BM, Donegan WL, Watson F, Spratt JS: Factors influencing survival in patients with untreated hepatic metastases. Surg Gynecol Obstet 127: 1-11, 1968.
3. Wood CB, Gillis CR, Blumgart LH: A retrospective study of the natural history of patients with liver metastases from colorectal cancer. Clin Oncol 2: 285-288, 1976.
4. Wagner JS, Adson MA, Van heerden JA, Adson MH, Ilstrup DM: The natural history of hepatic metastases from colorectal cancer. Ann Surg 199: 502-508, 1984.
5. Kemeny N, Braun DW: Prognostic factors in advanced colorectal carcinoma: Importance of lactic dehydrogenase, performance status and white blood cell count. Amer J Med 74: 786-797, 1983.
6. Kemeny N: Systemic chemotherapy of hepatic metastases. Semin Oncol 10: 148-158, 1983.

7. Daly JM, Kemeny N, Oderman P, Botet J: Chronic hepatic arterial infusion chemotherapy: Anatomical considerations, operative management and treatment morbidity. Arch Surg 119: 936-941, 1984.

8. Ansfield FJ, Ramirez G, Davis HL, Wirtanen GW, Johnson RO, Bryan GT, Manalo FB, Borden EC, Davis TE, Esmaili M: Further clinical studies with intrahepatic arterial infusion with 5-fluorouracil. Cancer 36: 2413-2417, 1975.

9. Dahl EP, Fredlund PE, Tylen U, Bengmark S: Transient hepatic dearterialization followed by regional intra-arterial 5-fluorouracil infusion as treatment for liver tumors. Ann Surg 193: 82-88, 1981.

10. Fortner JG, Mulcare RJ, Solis A, Watson RC, Golbey RB: Treatment of primary and secondary liver cancer by hepatic artery ligation and infusion chemotherapy. Ann Surg 178: 162-172, 1973.

11. Clarkson B, Young C, Dierick W, Kuehn P, Kim M, Berrett A, Clapp P, Lawrence W: Effects of continuous hepatic artery infusion of antimetabolites on primary and metastatic cancer of the liver. Cancer 15: 472-488, 1962.

12. Sullivan RD, Norcross JW, Watkins E: Chemotherapy of metastatic liver cancer by prolonged hepatic-artery infusion. N Engl J Med 270: 321-327, 1964.

13. Crowley ML: Penetrating duodenal ulcer associated with an operatively implanted arterial chemotherapy infusion catheter. Gastroenterology 83: 118-120, 1982.

14. Reed ML, Vaitkevicius VK, Al-Sarraf M, Vaugn CB, Singhakowinta A, Sexon-Porte M, Izbicki R, Baker L, Straatsma GW: The practicality of chronic hepatic artery infusion therapy of primary and metastatic hepatic malignancies: Ten-year results of 124 patients in a prospective protocol. Cancer 47: 402-409, 1981.

15. Buchwald H, Grage TB, Vassilopoulos PP, Rhode TD, Varco RL, Blackshear PJ: Intraarterial infusion chemotherapy for hepatic carcinoma using a totally implantable infusion pump. Cancer 45: 866-869, 1980.

16. Balch CM, Urist MM, McGregor ML: Continuous regional chemotherapy for metastatic colorectal cancer using a totally implantable infusion pump. Am J Surg 145: 285-290, 1983.

17. Balch CM, Urist MM, Soong SJ, McGregor M: A prospective phase II clinical trial of continuous FUDR regional chemotherapy for colorectal metastases to the liver using a totally implantable drug infusion pump. Ann Surg 198: 567-573, 1983.

18. Ensminger W, Niederhuber J, Dakhil S, Thrail J, Wheeler R: Totally implantated drug delivery system for hepatic arterial chemotherapy. Cancer Treat Rep 5: 393-400, 1981.

19. Ensminger W, Niederhuber J, Gyves J, Thrall J, Cozzi E, Doan K: Effective control of liver metastases from colon cancer with an implanted system for hepatic arterial chemotherapy. (Abstract) Proc Am Soc Clin Oncol 1: 94, 1982.

20. Cohen AM, Kaufman SD, Wood WC, Greenfield AJ: Regional hepatic chemotherapy using an implantable drug infusion pump. Am J Surg 145: 529-533, 1983.

21. Michels NA: Blood supply and anatomy of upper abdominal organs with descriptive atlas. JB Lippincott Co, Philadelphia, 1955, pp. 581.

22. Narsete T, Ansfield F, Wirtanen G, Ramirez G, Wolberg W, Jarrett F: Gastric ulceration in patients receiving intrahepatic infusion of 5-fluorouracil. Ann Surg 186: 734-736, 1977.

23. Grage TB, Vassilopoulos PP, Shingleton WW, Jubert AV, Elias EG, Aust JB, Moss SE: Results of a prospective randomized study of hepatic artery infusion with 5-fluorouracil versus intravenous 5-fluorouracil in patients with hepatic metastases from colorectal cancer: A central oncology group study. Surgery 86: 550-555, 1979.

10

LOCAL SURGICAL TREATMENT OF HEPATIC METASTASES FROM COLORECTAL CARCINOMA: SURVIVAL TIMES AND SITES OF RECURRENCE

Nicholas J. Petrelli, Lemuel Herrera, and Arnold Mittelman

SUMMARY

This chapter summarizes the experience at Roswell Park Memorial Institute with resectable liver metastases and with hepatic artery ligation for unresectable metastases from colorectal carcinoma. Survival times and patterns of recurrence were noted in 36 patients with documented colorectal adenocarcinoma metastatic to the liver who underwent resection. The overall median survival time following liver resection was 22 months. Survival was not influenced by the type of surgical resection performed. Survival time following resection of solitary lesions was 28 months and following resection of multiple lesions, 21 months. The difference between survival times of patients with synchronous metastases (25 months) and patients with metachronous metastases (16 months) from the time of liver resection was not statistically significant. Patterns of recurrence revealed that 11 of 17 patients experienced recurrences in the liver and in extrahepatic sites. Only two patients died with recurrent metastasis only in the liver.

From April 1975 to January 1982, 97 patients underwent hepatic artery ligation for biopsy-proven metastatic adenocarcinoma of the colon and rectum. All patients undergoing ligation had 50% or more of their liver involved with metastases. The overall median survival time was 10 months. The survival rate was determined in relation to performance status, preoperative alkaline phosphatase and total bilirubin levels, and the presence of extrahepatic intra-abdominal disease. We cannot conclude that hepatic artery ligation is an effective means of treating unresectable liver metastases from this retrospective study. What can be concluded is that important patient stratifications in predicting survival time must be taken into consideration for evaluating any form of treatment for unresectable liver metastases. The median survival time for patients with 0-1 performance status was 12 months. Patients with preoperative alkaline phosphatase levels less than two times normal also had a median survival time of 12 months. For patients with total bilirubin levels of less than two times normal the median survival time was four months.

INTRODUCTION

Approximately 138,000 new cases of colorectal carcinoma will occur in the United States this year, and about 27,000 of these patients will develop hepatic metastases (1). The majority of the liver metastases will be unresectable, however, approximately 5% of patients will be candidates for some form of surgical resection (2). The literature contains many reports on the treatment of hepatic metastases. Treatments include hepatic resection (3,4), hepatic artery ligation (5-8), hepatic dearterialization (9-14), hepatic infusion chemotherapy with implantable or external pumps (15-19), portal vein infusion (20), systemic chemotherapy (21,22), and radiation therapy (23,24). Unfortunately, no prospective randomized trials exist for comparing these treatments, and several reports contain small patient populations with varying criteria for success.

For resectable hepatic metastasis some authors (25-27) have reported five-year survival rates from 20-30%, with an overall median survival time of 27 months. For unresectable liver metastases from colorectal carcinoma the survival time has ranged from 6-9 months (28-31).

This chapter summarizes the experience at Roswell Park Memorial Institute with resectable liver metastases and with hepatic artery ligation for unresectable metastases from colorectal carcinoma.

MATERIALS AND METHODS

Resectable Liver Metastasis

This retrospective study involves 36 patients with documented colorectal adenocarcinoma metastatic to the liver who underwent resection at Roswell Park Memorial Institute from January 1972 to September 1983. There were 24 males and 12 females, with a median age of 56 years. The primary colorectal tumor was located in the cecum in 5 patients; in the ascending colon in 2 patients; in the transverse colon in 4 patients; in the descending colon in 2 patients; in the sigmoid colon in 14 patients; in the rectosigmoid colon in 2 patients; and in the rectum in 7 patients. Twenty-three patients (64%) had the sigmoid colon, rectosigmoid colon, and rectum as the primary tumor location.

There were 21 patients (58%) who presented with synchronous liver metastases. Solitary hepatic metastasis was documented in 22 patients, and 9 patients were found to have multiple lesions.

A right lobectomy was performed on 11 patients, a left lobectomy on 2, a wedge resection on 17, and a segmentectomy on 6. Of the six patients who had segmentectomies, there were four who underwent a right trisegmentectomy.

118

From April 1975 to January 1982 there were 97 patients who underwent hepatic artery ligation for biopsy-proven metastatic adenocarcinoma of the colon or rectum involving 50% or more of the estimated liver volume. There were 31 patients who received previous systemic chemotherapy and 66 patients who had no prior treatment. Preoperative celiac and superior mesenteric angiograms were used to identify the hepatic blood supply and to evalute the venous phase for portal vein obstruction or reversal of portal flow, which were contraindications for ligation. During hepatic artery ligation no attempts were made at dearterialization by interrupting the hepatic triangular ligaments. However, any accessory hepatic arteries identified by preoperative angiography were ligated.

Patients were stratified into subgroups for which median survival times were determined.   The first stratification was synchronous extrahepatic intra-abdominal disease with hepatic metastases versus hepatic metastases only.   The second stratification evaluated preoperative serum alkaline phosphatase and total bilirubin levels. The last stratification was patient performance status (Table 1).

Statistical comparisons of survival distributions were performed using the logrank test. The survival curves were calculated using the Kaplan and Meier method for both resectable and unresectable liver metastases (32). Comparison of survival rates between groups was evaluated with the Mantle-Cox test (33).

Table 1. Definition of Patient Performance Status

Classification	Definition	Status
0	Normal performance	Normal
1	Symptoms of metastases but ambulatory	Normal
2	Spends <50% of time in bed	Ambulatory
3	Spends >50% of time in bed	Ambulatory
4	Spends 100% of time in bed	Bedridden

RESULTS

Resectable Liver Metastasis

The overall median survival time following hepatic resection in the 36 patients was 22 months. Postoperative mortality, defined as death within 30 days of resection, was

119

documented in 5 of the 36 patients (14%). Three of the five patients who died postoperatively had undergone right trisegmentectomy and died of hepatic failure. Of the remaining two patients, one died from a pulmonary embolus and one from cardiopulmonary failure.

The medain survival time from the time of liver resection in patients with metachronous metastases was 16 months, in patients with synchronous lesions, 25 months. These survival-time differences were not statistically significant ($\underline{P}$=.75). Also, when survival times were classified by the type of surgical resection performed, no statistically significant difference among them was found; that is, the median survival time following lobectomy was 21 months; following segmentectomy, 22 months; and following wedge resection, 16 months ($\underline{P}$=.61).

Survival times from the time of liver resection was also compared between patients with solitary and patients with multiple liver metastases. The median survival time for patients with solitary lesions was 28 months and for patients with multiple lesions, 21 months. No statistically significant difference in survival times was noted ($\underline{P}$=.24).

The two-year survival rate following hepatic resection was 45%. However, of the 36 patients reviewed, 25 (69%) died. Postoperative mortality was seen in five patients, as previously noted; a sixth patient died of complications from a perforated duodenal ulcer; and an additional patient died at home from unknown causes. There have been 18 patients who have died secondary to recurrent tumor.

Eleven of the 36 patients (30%) are presently alive. Eight of these patients remain free of any cancer recurrence. The remaining three patients have histologic proof of tumor recurrence; one in the liver only, one in the liver and the lung, and one in the left axillary lymph nodes with abdominal wall involvement.

In this review, no one has survived five years. The longest-living survivor is a patient who in the fall of 1980 underwent a left colectomy and a subsequent right lobectomy for a synchronous solitary hepatic metastasis.

Clinical and Autopsy Data of Tumor Recurrence at Time of Death

To evaluate patterns of recurrence, either clinically determined patterns of failure or autopsy information can be reviewed. The former method has limitations because of the sensitivity and specificity of clinical tests, which vary at different organ sites in the body. On the other hand, the latter information very often represents end-stage, widespread, disseminated disease, which limits the value of assessing patterns of early spread. Despite these shortcomings, 23 patients were studied at the times of their deaths for site of tumor recurrence. Ten patients underwent autopsies , but six were not evaluable for patterns of recurrence because five patients succumbed to postoperative mortality and the sixth died of a perforated duodenal ulcer. Therefore, four patients were evaluable for patterns of failure. Two of these four patients were documented to have lung, liver and other intra-abdominal metastases, the third had liver and brain metastases, and the fourth patient had extrahepatic intra-abdominal carcinomatosis.

Clinically determined patterns of failure were evaluated in 13 patients who died and did not have an autopsy performed. Only two patients died with the liver as the only site of recurrence, whereas five of 13 patients (39%) died with liver and other intra-abdominal metastases. Table 2 illustrates the sites of recurrence that could best be determined by clinical evaluation (including nuclear scans and roentgenograms) in these 13 patients.

Table 2. Recurrence Sites Determined by Clinical Evaluation

Recurrence Site	Patients
Liver and extrahepatic intra-abdominal	5
Liver only	2
Abdominal wall	1
Liver and pelvis	1
Liver and pulmonary	1
Lung and liver	1
Extrahepatic intra-abdominal only	1
Lung only	1

Unresectable Liver Metastases

At Roswell Park Memorial Institute, one of the methods for treating unresectable liver metastases has been hepatic artery ligation. It should be emphasized that only those patients with 50% or more of the liver involved with metastases, determined by the surgeon at the time of exploration, were candidates for ligation. The overall median survival time of these 97 patients was 10 months.

In this review, median survival times are reported in three categories. The first category compares survival times in patients with simultaneous intra-abdominal metastases and hepatic metastases versus hepatic metastases only. In the 51 patients who were documented to have hepatic metastases and other intra-abdominal sites of tumor involvement, the median survival time was 7 months, whereas the median survival of the 46 patients with liver metastases only was 10 months ($P < .01$).

The second category evaluated survival times in relation to preoperative liver function tests, specifically alkaline phosphatase and total bilirubin levels. The alkaline phosphatase levels were divided into three ranges: less than two times normal, between two and four times normal, and greater than four times normal. There were 43 patients whose preoperative alkaline phosphatase levels were less than two times normal, and their median survival time was 12 months. In the 29 patients whose preoperative alkaline phosphatase levels were between two and four times normal, the median survival time was seven months. In the 25 patients whose alkaline phosphatase levels were greater than four times normal, the median survival time was also seven months. The difference between the survival times was statistically significant ($\underline{P}$= <.01).

Preoperative levels of total bilirubin were also evaluated. An elevation of the preoperative total bilirubin level to twice the upper limit of normal in patients undergoing hepatic artery ligation had no impact on survival time. In the 62 patients with normal preoperative total bilirubin levels, the median survival time was nine months, and in the 21 patients with total bilirubin levels two times normal, the median survival time was also nine months. However, when the bilirubin level rose to greater than two times normal, the median survival time was 4 months ($\underline{P}$= < .01).

The last category to be discussed is performance status. Normal performance status (0-1) was seen in 12 patients, who had a median survival time of 12 months following hepatic artery ligation. There were 76 patients considered to have ambulatory performance status (2-3) whose median survival time was eight months. In the last group of patients considered to be performance status 4 (100% bedridden), the median survival time was three months. Again, the differences in survival times were statistically significant ($\underline{P}$= <.01).

There were nine patients who developed right pleural effusions, none requiring thoracocentesis. There was one postoperative wound infection and no instances of intrahepatic abscesses requiring reexploration. This results in a morbidity rate of 10%. There were two deaths in this series. One patient succumbed to hepatic failure and the other to respiratory failure, for a mortality rate of 2%.

DISCUSSION

In this review we attempt to identify certain prognostic factors in patients with resectable and unresectable liver metastases from colorectal carcinoma. We also evaluate sites of recurrence for resectable liver metastasis from clinical and autopsy data. The prognostic factors and sites of recurrence are important data necessary to make intelligent treatment decisions on an individual-patient basis. These factors become even more significant when taken in the context of the report by Adson and associates (26), in which the natural history of unresected hepatic metastases that could have been removed shows clearly that survival rates of treated patients should be interpreted very critically. As stated by these authors, surgeons should not take credit for what the natural course of the disease might have been. Unfortunately there is no decisive way of knowing whether survival rates two or three years after liver resection for colorectal metastasis can be attributed to the surgical removal of the lesions or to the natural history of the disease.

Our overall median survival time following for the 36 patients was 22 months. Also, survival time was not influenced by type of resection performed, as noted in a previous series (25). The difference between survival times of patients with solitary (median 28 months) and patients with multiple (median 21 months) metastases was not statistically significant. It is interesting to note that contrary to an earlier report by Wilson and Adson (34), the overall survival time of patients with resectable multiple liver metastases did not differ from that of patients with solitary lesions resected in a more recent study by some of the same authors. In the latter study by Adson and associates (26) it was shown that survival time after resection of multiple hepatic metastases may be determined by the size of the metastases and the time of detection and their surgical removal.

In this series of 36 patients there are as yet no five-year survivors, but this may change with continued follow-up of the remaining 11 patients. Two years after hepatic resection, 45% of the patients in this report were alive. This percentage is similar to that in other reported series (25,35).

The difference between the survival times of patients with synchronous metastases and patients with metachronous metastases from the time of liver resection was not statistically significant. It is important to emphasize that survival time was determined from the time of liver resection and not from the time of diagnosis of the primary colorectal tumor. We feel that the former time period is more significant because one can never know how long the liver metastases coexisted with the primary colorectal tumor.

The surgical mortality rate for liver resection for colorectal metastases ranges from 2-9% (2,34-36). In this series, surgical mortality was seen in five patients (14%). At the time of autopsy there were no technical surgical errors noted in the procedures used on these patients, all of whom died from hepatic failure. Because of the difficulty in determining liver reserve in the lateral segment of the left lobe after right trisegmentectomy, the policy at Roswell Park Memorial Institute has been to abandon right trisegmentectomy for liver metastases from colorectal carcinoma. This has not been the case in other series (27,37).

Seventeen patients were evaluated for sites of recurrence after liver resection. In 11 of these patients (65%) tumor recurrence was found in the liver and other extrahepatic sites. There were only two patients who died with the liver as the single site of recurrence. Steele and associates (38) have also noted that tumor recurrence tends to appear in extrahepatic sites after liver resection. In a series of 30 patients evaluated after liver resection for colorectal metastases, 50% of successfully resected patients still relapsed with most recurrences documented outside the liver parenchyma. These data call for the evaluation of adjuvant chemotherapy following liver resection from colorectal metastases once chemotherapeutic drugs effective against this cancer become available.

Of the 20,000 patients who will develop hepatic metastasis from colorectal carcinoma this year, the majority of these patients will have surgically unresectable disease. There are basically three approaches to treating unresectable liver metastases. The first consists of systemic chemotherapy (22), and the second is hepatic artery infusion, either percutaneously or with a portable or an implantable pump (15-19). The third category consists of hepatic artery ligation with or without dearterialization, hyperthermia, or concomitant chemotherapy infusion (6-14). These three treatment modes basically tell investigators that the most efficient means of treating unresectable liver metastases from colorectal carcinoma has not been identified. No prospective randomized trials of the above-stated techniques have been reported and no large series exist for some of these forms of treatment. In studies that have been done, patient stratifications and response criteria have varied to the point that treatment groups are not comparable. This is illustrated most clearly in series utilizing intra-arterial chemotherapy via an implantable pump (15-19). The response rates in these series range from 29-88%, with a median duration of response from 6-13 months. There are several reasons for this variability in response rates. One of the most critical is that total liver perfusion has not been adequately documented in many reports. Another is that the small size of some series does not allow clinical experience for early detection of local regional toxicity. Modification in the regimens can also be expected to alter response rates. Lastly, the above-described series have a mixed population of previously treated and previously untreated patient groups.

In this series of 97 patients undergoing hepatic artery ligation with 50% or more liver involvement, the overall median survival time was 10 months with minimal morbidity and mortality. Because this study is retrospective and uses historical controls for comparison of survival rates, we cannot conclude that hepatic artery ligation is an effective means of treating unresectable liver metastases. A prospective randomized study is needed to compare this form of treatment to the others mentioned above. What can be concluded is that important patient stratifications in predicting survival times must be taken into consideration for evaluating any form of treatment for unresectable liver metastases. In a report by Petrelli and associates on hepatic artery ligation (5), median survival times were determined in relation to six categories. However, in this study only three categories have been emphasized. It is apparent that preoperative levels of alkaline phosphatase and total bilirubin have an impact on survival. These two liver function tests have also been noted in other series (17-19) to be important prognostic determinants. The presence of extrahepatic intra-abdominal disease in this series of patients was another important prognostic determinant. This factor is notable, because to analyze comparable studies, intra-abdominal extrahepatic metastases must be ruled out. The last category that was analyzed as a prognostic determinant was the performance status of the patient. Those patients whose performance status was normal or who had symtpoms but were ambulatory were shown to have a median survival time of 12 months as opposed to patients with a performance status of 4, who had a median survival time of 3 months. Thus performance status, alkaline phosphatase level, total bilirubin levels, and the presence of extrahepatic intra-abdominal metastases are important prognostic determinants. These factors have also been emphasized by Goslin and associates (39) to be important determinants of survival irrespective of the form of treatment patients underwent for liver metastases from colorectal carcinoma. We feel that these prognostic determinants are important enough to be adopted in a proposed liver-disease classification system (40).

The bottom line is that a group of patients with good prognostic factors who undergo placement of implantable pumps for intra-arterial chemotherapy cannot be compared with a group of patients who undergo hepatic artery ligation with poor prognostic determinants. Although the survival time of patients with implantable pumps may be 24 months and the survival time of patients undergoing hepatic artery ligation may be 10 months, the groups are not comparable. The important question is whether the patient with good prognostic determinants would survive 24 months without any form of treatment. Thus, we concur with Goslin and associates (39), that prospectively controlled trials with matched untreated controls using survival time as the measure of response are necessary.

Our knowledge concerning the management of liver cancer is mostly derived from series of patients with metastatic disease, especially those of colorectal origin. It has been noted retrospectively that as we gain better control of liver metastases, extrahepatic disease has become an important factor in determining survival rates. This once again emphasizes the systemic nature of colorectal carcinoma and the need for the multimodality treatment.

References

1. Silverberg E: Cancer Statistics, 1985. CA 35: 19-35, 1985.
2. Wanebo J, Semoglou C, Attiyeh F, Stearns M: Surgical management of patients with primary operable colorectal cancer and synchronous liver metastases. Am J Surg 135: 81-85, 1978.
3. Foster JH, Berman MM: Solid liver tumors. WB Saunders, Philadelphia, 1977.
4. Logan SE, Meier SJ, Ramming KP: Hepatic resection of metastatic colorectal carcinoma. Arch Surg 117: 25-28, 1982.
5. Petrelli NJ, Barcewicz PA, Evans JT, Ledesma EJ, Lawrence DD, Mittelman A: Hepatic artery ligation for liver metastasis in colorectal carcinoma. Cancer 53: 1347-1353, 1984.
6. Larmi TKI, Karkola P, Klintrup H, Heikkinen E: Treatment of patients with hepatic tumors and jaundice by ligation of the hepatic artery. Arch Surg 108: 178-183, 1974.
7. Fortner JG, Mulcare RJ, Solis A, Watson RC, Golbey RB: Treatment of primary and secondary liver cancer by hepatic artery ligation and infusion chemotherapy. Ann Surg 178: 162-172, 1973.
8. Sparks FC, Mosher MB, Wolfgang G, Hallaver WC, Silverstein MJ, Rangel D, Passaro E Jr, Morton DL: Hepatic artery ligation and postoperative chemotherapy for hepatic metastases: Clinical and pathologic results. Cancer 35: 1074-1082, 1975.
9. Gulesserian HP, Lawton RL, Condon RE: Hepatic artery ligation and cytotoxic infusion in treatment of liver metastasis. Arch Surg 105: 280-295, 1972.
10. Cady B, Oberfield RA: Regional infusion chemotherapy of hepatic metastases from carcinoma of the colon. Am J Surg 127: 220-227, 1974.
11. Ramming KP, Sparks FC, Eilber FR, Holmes EC, Morton DL: Hepatic artery ligation and 5-fluorouracil infusion for metastatic colon carcinoma and primary hepatoma. Am J Surg 132: 236-242, 1976.
12. Grage TB, Vassilopoules PP, Shingleton WW, Jubert AV, Elias EG, Aust JB, Moss SE: Results of a prospective randomized study of hepatic artery infusion with 5-fluorouracil versus intravenous 5-fluorouracil in patients with hepatic metastases from colorectal cancer: A Central Oncology Group Study. Surgery 86: 550-555, 1979.
13. Lise M, Cagol PP, Nitti I, Feltrin G, Fosser V, Cecchetto A, Rubaltelli L, Pucciarelli S: Temporary occlusion of the hepatic artery plus infusion and systemic chemotherapy for inoperable cancer of the liver. Int Surg 65: 315-323, 1980.
14. Dahl EP, Fredlung PE, Tylen U, Bengmark S: Transient hepatic dearterialization followed by regional intraarterial 5-fluorouracil infusion as treatment for liver tumors. Ann Surg 193: 82-88, 1981.
15. Grage TB, Shingleton WW, Jubert AV, Elias EG, Aust JB, Moss SE: Results of a prospective randomized study of hepatic artery infusion with 5-fluorouracil versus intravenous 5-fluorouracil in patients with hepatic metastases from colorectal cancer. Front Gastrointest Res 5: 116-129, 1979.
16. Balch CM, Urist MM, Soong SJ, McGregor M: A prospective phase II clinical trial of continuous FUdR regional chemotherapy for colorectal metastases to the liver using a totally implantable drug infusion pump. Ann Surg 198: 567-573, 1983.
17. Kemeny N, Daly JM, Oderman P, Schike M: Hepatic infusion chemotherapy for metastatic colorectal carcinoma, results and complications (Abstract). Proc Am Soc Clin Oncol 2: 123, 1983.

18. Weiss GR, Garnick MB, Osteen RT, Steele GD Jr, Wilson RE, Shade D, Kaplan W, Boxt L, Kandarpa K, Mayer R, Frei ET III: Long-term hepatic arterial infusion of 5-fluorodeoxyuridine for liver metastases using an implantable infusion pump. J Clin Oncol 1: 337-344, 1983.
19. Niederhuber JE, Ensminger W, Gyves J, Thrall J, Walker S, Cozzi E: Regional chemotherapy of colorectal cancer metastatic to the liver. Cancer 53: 1336-1343, 1984.
20. Taylor I: Cytotoxic perfusion for colorectal liver metastases. Br J Surg 65: 109-114, 1978.
21. Douglass HO Jr, Lavin PT, Woll J, Conroy JF, Carbone P: Chemotherapy of advanced measurable colon and rectal carcinoma with oral 5-fluorouracil, alone or in combination with cyclophosphamide or 6-thioguanine, with intravenous 5-fluorouracil or beta-2'-deoxythioguanosine or with oral 3(4-methyl-cyclohexyl)-1(2-chloroethyl)-1-nitrosourea. A phase II-III study of the Eastern Cooperative Oncology Group (EST 4273). Cancer 42: 2538-2545, 1978.
22. Petrelli NJ, Mittelman A: An analysis of chemotherapy for colorectal carcinoma. J Surg Oncol 25: 201-206, 1984.
23. Borgelt BB, Gelber R, Brady LW, Griffin T, Hendrickson FR: The palliation of hepatic metastases: Results of the Radiation Therapy Oncology Group Pilot Study. Int J Radiat Oncol Biol Phys 7: 587-591, 1981.
24. Barone RM, Byfield JE, Goldfarb PB, Frankel S, Ginn C, Greer S: Intra-arterial chemotherapy using an implantable infusion pump and liver irradiation for the treatment of hepatic metastases. Cancer 50: 850-862, 1982.
25. Logan S, Meier S, Ramming K, Morton D, Longmire W: Hepatic resection of metastatic colorectal carcinoma. Arch Surg 117: 25-28, 1982.
26. Adson MA, van Heerden JA, Adson MH, Wagner JS, Ilstrup DM: Resection of hepatic metastases from colorectal cancer. Arch Surg 119: 647-651, 1984.
27. Iwatsuki S, Shaw BW, Starzl TE: Experience with 150 liver resections. Ann Surg 197: 247-253, 1983.
28. Flanagan K Jr, Foster JH: Hepatic resection for metastatic cancer. Am J Surg 113: 551-557, 1967.
29. Cady B, Monson DO, Swinton NW: Survival of patients after colonic resection for carcinoma with simultaneous liver metastases. Surg Gynecol Obstet 131: 697-700, 1970.
30. Bengmark S, Hafstrom L: The natural history of primary and secondary malignant tumors of the liver. I. The prognosis for patients with hepatic metastases from colonic and rectal carcinoma by laparotomy. Cancer 23: 198-202, 1969.
31. Jaffe BM, Donegan WL, Watson F, Spratt J: Factors influencing survival in patients with untreated hepatic metastases. Surg Gynecol Obstet 127: 1-11, 1968.
32. Kaplan E, Meier P: Nonparametric estimation from incomplete observations. J Amer Stat Assoc 53: 457-481, 1958.
33. Engelman L, Frame JW, Jennrick RI: BMDP Biomedical Computer Programs, P-series. In: Dixon WJ, Brown MB (eds), Publications in Automatic Computation. University of California Press, Los Angeles 1979, pp 880.
34. Wilson SM, Adson MA: Surgical treatment of hepatic metastases from colorectal cancers. Arch Surg 111: 330-334, 1976.
35. Foster J: Survival after liver resection for secondary tumors. Am J Surg 135: 389-394, 1978.
36. Adson M, van Heerden J: Major hepatic resections for metastatic colorectal cancer. Ann Surg 191: 576-583, 1980.
37. Starzl TE, Koep LJ, Weil R, Lilly JR, Putnam CW, Aldreter JA: Right trisegmentectomy for hepatic neoplasms. Surg Gynecol Obstet 150: 208-213, 1980.

38. Steele G, Osteen RT, Wilson RE, Brooks DC, Mayer RJ, Zamcheck N, Ravikumar TS: Patterns of failure after surgical cure of large liver tumors: A change in the proximate cause of death and a need for effective systemic adjuvant therapy. Am J Surg 147: 554-559, 1984.
39. Goslin R, Steele G, Zamcheck N, Mayer R, MacIntyre J: Factors influencing survival in patients with hepatic metastases from adenocarcinoma of the colon or rectum. Dis Colon Rectum 25: 749-754, 1982.
40. Petrelli NJ, Bonnheim DC, Herrera LO, Mittelman A: A proposed classification system for liver metastasis from colorectal carcinoma. Dis Colon Rectum 27: 249-252, 1984.

11

ENDOSCOPIC LASER SURGERY FOR COLONIC NEOPLASIA

John H. Bowers, Randall W. Burt, and John A. Dixon

SUMMARY

The potential role of endoscopically directed light amplification by stimulated emission of radiation (LASER) surgery for the palliative treatment of colorectal neoplasms and adenomas in selected patients is reviewed. This technique relies on the precise thermal destruction of exposed tissue. The depth of penetration is determined by the wavelength of the incident laser source, most commonly the argon laser or the neodymium YAG laser. In selected patients, because of the size configuration or location of a lesion, laser surgery appears to be a safe alternative to endoscopic diathermic removal or incisional surgery. This procedure has been well tolerated without complications. Nevertheless, the encouraging preliminary experience reported here is best regarded as palliative treatment.

INTRODUCTION

Laser energy delivered via a flexible waveguide makes possible thermal destruction of neoplastic tissue within the bowel. The depth of the injury to the tissue is predictable and largely depends on the wavelength of the laser light (1,2), a fact that makes it possible to photocoagulate the neoplastic tissue selectively, while preserving the bowel wall integrity. On the other hand, the depth of tissue necrosis after monopolar electrocautery is unpredictable (3), thus limiting the usefulness of that treatment modality. It is the precision of the laser and tissue interaction that enables the laser to be used for the local treatment of colonic neoplasms. For this reason, we examined the potential role of endoscopically directed laser energy in the treatment of selected patients with benign and malignant colonic neoplasms.

Laser energy is absorbed by biologic tissues. The energy is converted to heat, which leads to coagulation or vaporization of tissue. The depth of the injury to the tissue is mainly determined by the wavelength of the incident laser light. With the argon laser, the depth of the injury is approximately 1 mm so that the integrity of the muscularis and the serosa is preserved (1). After the application of argon laser light to a normal colonic surface, the mucosal layer sloughs after four days, leaving an acute ulceration (4). These laser-induced ulcerations heal completely and leave a normal-appearing mucosal surface within 12 days (4). The neodymium YAG (Nd:YAG) laser leads to greater depth of tissue damage and frequently causes full-thickness injury to normal bowel tissue in experimental animals (2,5,6). This situation is worsened because the gas-distended colonic wall is perhaps only 1-2 mm thick. This makes the risk of perforation higher with the Nd:YAG compared to the argon laser. However, the serosa is believed to be relatively transparent to the Nd:YAG laser, a fact that should help preserve the integrity of the bowel wall, even in the face of a near full-thickness injury. In addition, areas of tumor involvement are usually thicker than the surrounding tissue in a normal colon. The greater depth of tissue injury associated with Nd:YAG laser makes possible the more rapid photocoagulation of a given volume of neoplastic tissue. Nonetheless, the choice of laser and the ultimate role for laser therapy in the management of colonic neoplasms remain to be established.

Some patients with colonic cancer may require therapy for the local complications of their disease, even though the tumor is unresectable or metastatic. Additionally, because of the size, configuration, or location, some benign colonic polyps do not readily lend themselves to endoscopic diathermic removal or incisional surgery. Safe alternative treatments are therefore needed for these patients.

METHODS

Twelve patients with Gardner's syndrome, four with other benign colonic adenomas, and nine with colonic adenocarcinoma were selected for laser photocoagulation therapy. The choice of argon or Nd:YAG laser was determined by the location, size, and configuration of each lesion to be treated and by its benign or malignant nature. The argon laser was generally used in patients with small benign sessile polyps. The Nd:YAG laser was used for the treatment of large benign polyps and of frankly malignant lesions. All patients with Gardner's syndrome had had subtotal colectomies.

Access to tumor areas was normally gained by flexible fiberoptic endoscopy; two-channel therapeutic endoscopes were preferred to facilitate gas removal. Laser energy was delivered via flexible fiberoptic waveguide with coaxial CO_2 gas. Treatment distances were in the range of 0.5 to 3.0 cm. For the argon laser, the energy was applied in the continuous wave mode, with pulse durations up to 10 seconds, at a power setting of 4-6 six watts. A typical 5 mm sessile polyp required only a few seconds for coagulation.

130

For Nd:YAG laser, the maximal pulse duration was limited to 2.0 seconds, at a power setting of approximately 60 watts. The total time required for treatment depended on the size, configuration, and location of the polyp. Total energy per Nd:YAG laser treatment session was in the range of 1,000-5,000 joules. Laser treatment variables are summarized in Table 1.

Table 1. Laser Treatment Variables

	Argon	Nd:YAG
Power (watts)	4-6	30-70
Maximum pulse duration (sec)	continuous	2.0
Treatment distance (cm)	0.5-2.0	0.5-3.0
Total energy per treatment session (Joules)	NA	1,000-5,000

Laser treatments were performed at two- to four-day intervals, often on an outpatient basis, until the desired mucosal effect was observed. Subsequent examinations and treatments were normally scheduled at two- to six-month intervals, according to the patient's individual circumstances.

RESULTS

Twelve Gardner's syndrome patients underwent outpatient argon laser photocoagulation for rectal polyposis. Acute and chronic studies were performed. One of these patients had been scheduled for proctectomy because of an inability to control polyp regrowth with monopolar electrocautery. Four days prior to surgery, 15 rectal polyps were photocoagulated with the argon laser. Pathologic examination of the rectum after removal showed that the polyps had been ablated and that there was thrombosis of the submucosal vessels. The depth of the tissue injury was limited to the submucosa. The remaining 11 Gardner's syndrome patients had 211 rectal polyps photocoagulated with argon laser. Follow-up endoscopic examinations after four days showed that the polyps were gone and small superficial ulcers were present. After 12 days, the mucosal surface had healed and polyps were no longer evident. These same patients have returned at three- to six-month intervals for photocoagulation of new polyps; more than

131

500 polyps have been removed, in total. Treatments have been well tolerated and no significant complications have occurred.

Four patients with 27 sessile adenomatous colonic polyps underwent outpatient argon laser photocoagulation of the lesions. Polyps selected for laser therapy met three criteria: they were sessile, were more than 5 mm in transverse diameter, and were not easily removed by standard endoscopic techniques. Subsequent endoscopic examination after four months demonstrated complete healing and the absence of polyps. However, one large (20 mm) tubular adenoma recurred 13 months after the completion of the argon laser photocoagulation treatment. Additional treatment with Nd:YAG laser was required. The polyp did not recur during the next 18 months of follow-up.

Nine additional patients with biopsy-proven adenocarcinomas of the rectosigmoid colon have received Nd:YAG laser photocoagulation therapy. In three patients with large nonobstructive tumors, the size of the lesion could be reduced with the Nd:YAG laser, but it could not be eradicated. Mean survival for these patients was 5.5 months. It was not apparent from this experience that reduction of the tumor was beneficial. It must be noted that these individuals had end-stage disseminated cancer at the time of the laser treatment and that they had had other treatments previously. One patient with imminent obstruction of the sigmoid colon from cancer was maintained in an asymptomatic state for 15 months with interval Nd:YAG laser treatments until his death from cardiovascular disease. Three patients with early rectosigmoid cancers were considered to have had their tumors completely removed with Nd:YAG laser. Two of these patients died within 4 months from cardiovascular disease, but without any evidence of recurrence of the tumor; the third patient is alive and free of clinically evident disease after 23 months. One patient with disseminated cancer who was treated for intractable bleeding remained free of hemorrhage until his death three months later from renal failure that was the result of bilateral ureteral obstruction by tumor. No complications of the laser therapy were observed.

DISCUSSION

Laser photocoagulation offers the capacity to destroy and remove neoplastic tissue via the transluminal route without the necessity for incisional surgery. This capability is an important factor in patients whose life expectancies may be limited. The extent of the tissue injury is more predictable with laser than with electrocautery. Our previous studies had shown the safety of the argon laser in the normal canine colon (4). The duration of argon irradiation required for perforation was well beyond pulse durations that are expected to be used clinically. The Nd:YAG laser causes a greater depth of

132

tissue injury (5), and the risk of perforation would seem to be higher; however, the argon laser was not effective for the treatment of the larger malignant lesions. For that reason, the Nd:YAG laser is now used exclusively for the treatment of cancers. To date, there have been no perforations. It should be noted that treatments are begun centrally, and care is taken to avoid the irradiation of normal-appearing areas in the colon. In other studies, complications have included perforation (7), hemorrhage (7), rectal stenosis (8), and late recurrence (9). Fever, proctalgia, and minor bleeding may occur, but are usually inconsequential.

Persons affected by familial polyposis and Gardner's syndrome are highly prone to develop colon cancer at an early age (10). Prior to the appearance of the cancer, these patients have numerous adenomatous polyps, which are considered premalignant. Total colectomy is the most reliable method for preventing death from colon cancer (10); however, many of our patients had elected to undergo subtotal colectomy combined with interval removal of rectal polyps by diathermic means. It was this group of patients who were considered for argon laser photocoagulation. In this study, we found that the argon laser was effective and well tolerated when performed at regular intervals on outpatients with Gardner's syndrome. Spinelli et al. have used a similar approach with the Nd:YAG laser for the treatment of the rectal remnant after colectomy in patients with familial polyposis (11). The long-term utility of laser treatment in polyposis patients remains to be determined.

The preferred treatment for benign colonic adenomas is endoscopic removal. Most of these polyps are easily removed with a monopolar electrocautery snare device (12) or with hot biopsy forceps (13). However, large sessile polyps may be difficult to remove safely by standard endoscopic diathermic techniques. Surgical excision has been the standard treatment for this type of lesion (12). In circumstances where surgical excision is considered undesirable or unsafe, laser photocoagulation may play a role. Small polyps can be easily treated with the argon laser. Larger polyps may require the application of the Nd:YAG laser. Large villous adenomas occurring in elderly patients may be especially suitable for treatment with the Nd:YAG laser. Other investigators have reported the complete healing of benign and malignant rectal villous adenomas after Nd:YAG laser photocoagulation (7,8,9). When used as definitive therapy for colonic cancer, laser therapy must be reserved for those patients who are unable to have surgery. Persons with inoperable colonic cancer may develop local complications, such as obstruction or bleeding, which have required surgical treatment in the past. Endoscopically directed laser treatment offers an alternative that does not require incisional surgery. This approach may be of particular value in those patients with limited life expectancies.

In our experience, tumor size was reduced with laser photocoagulation. In addition, the Nd:YAG laser has been effective in the palliation of obstructing esophageal (14,15) and gastric (15) cancers. It should be possible to prevent the progression of colonic cancer to complete obstruction by the technique of intermittent endoscopic laser removal of the intraluminal portion of the tumor. This goal is accomplished more readily if treatments are performed prior to the development of complete obstruction. Once complete obstruction has occurred, it may be difficult to ascertain the exact location of the bowel lumen. Following the initial treatment series, outpatient intermittent treatments may be undertaken as necessary, usually at three- to six-month intervals.

It was not clear in this study that the reduction of tumor volume, per se, was necessarily beneficial. Unless one is able to remove the entire tumor, the underlying tissue would not be expected to heal. However, three patients with early rectal cancers were treated with Nd:YAG laser because of their inability to tolerate proctectomy. In all three, the tumor was completely eradicated. Unfortunately, two of these patients died of causes unrelated to their cancers. The third patient has remained free of recurrence 23 months after the completion of laser therapy. Lambert et al. (7) and Harada et al. (16) have reported cure in patients with early rectal cancers after treatment with the Nd:YAG laser. The criterion of cure in these patients was the simple demonstration that the tumor site had healed completely following laser treatment. Long-term results are not available. It must be recognized that some of these patients may have had regional lymph node metastases that might have been surgically removed had surgery been considered feasible. Some patients may, therefore, develop clinically evident metastases. For that reason, the use of the laser should be regarded as strictly palliative in patients with colonic carcinoma.

In summary, promising short-term results for the maintenance of luminal patency, for control of hemorrhage, and for probable cure of villous adenomas and early cancers have been obtained in selected patients wth colonic neoplasms. The major advantages for transluminal laser therapy include absent or minimal morbidity and outpatient treatment status. Nevertheless, laser treatment for colonic cancer is best regarded as palliative because the detection and removal of regional lymph node metastases are not possible by endoscopic means alone.

References

1. Kelly DF, Bown SG, Salmon PR, Calder BM, Pearson H, Weaver BMQ: The nature and extent of biological changes induced by argon laser photocoagulation in canine gastric mucosa. Gut 22: 1047-1055, 1980.

2.   Bown SG, Salmon PR, Storey DW, Calder BM, Kelly DF, Adams N, Pearson H, Weaver BMQ: Nd:YAG laser photocoagulation in the dog stomach. Gut 21: 818-825, 1980.
3.   Piercey JRA, Auth DC, Silverstein FE, Willard HR, Dennis MB, Ellefson DM, Davis DM, Protell RL, Rubin CE: Electrosurgical treatment of experimental bleeding canine gastric ulcers: Development and testing of a computer control and a better electrode. Gastroenterology 74: 527-534, 1978.
4.   Dixon JA, Burt RW, Rotering RH, McCloskey DW: Endoscopic argon laser photocoagulation of sessile colonic polyps. Gastrointest Endosc 28: 162-165, 1982.
5.   Protell RL, Silverstein FE, Auth DL, Dennis MB, Gilbert DA, Rubin CE: The Nd:YAG is dangerous for photocoagulation of experimental bleeding gastric ulcers when compared with the argon laser (Abstract). Gastroenterology 74: 1080, 1978.
6.   Dixon JA, Berenson MM, McCloskey DW: Neodymium-YAG laser treatment of experimental canine gastric bleeding. Acute and chronic studies of photocoagulation, penetration and perforation. Gastroenterology 77: 647-751, 1979.
7.   Lambert R, Sabben G: Laser therapy in colorectal tumors: Early results (Abstract). Gastroenterology 84: 1223, 1983.
8.   Brunetaud JM, Mosquet L, Bourez J, Triboulet JP, Delmotte JS, Cortot A: Laser applications in nonhemorrhagic digestive lesions. In K Atsumi (ed), New Frontiers in Laser Medicine and Surgery. Excerpta Medica, Amsterdam, 1983, pp 455-461.
9.   Kiefhaber P, Kiefhaber K: Present endoscopic laser therapy in the gastrointestinal tract. In K Atsumi (ed), New Frontiers in Laser Medicine and Surgery. Excerpta Medica, Amsterdam, 1983, pp 439-446.
10.   Erbe RW: Inherited gastrointestinal polyposis syndromes. N Engl J Med 294: 1101-1106, 1976.
11.   Spinelli P, Pizzetti P, Mirabile V, Marchesini R, Andreola S, Fava G, Emanuelli H: Neodymium-YAG laser treatment of the rectal remnant after colectomy for familial polyposis. In: K Atsumi and N Nimsakul (eds), Laser-Tokyo '81, Japan Society for Laser Medicine, Tokyo, 1981, pp 23-49 -- 23-50.
12.   Wolff WI, Shinya H: Endoscopic polypectomy. Cancer 36: 683-690, 1975.
13.   Schrock TR: Management of the discovered colon lesion. Gastrointest Endosc 26 (Suppl): 365-375, 1980.
14.   Fleischer DE, Kessler F, Haye O: Endoscopic laser therapy for carcinoma of the esophagus: A new palliative approach. Am J Surg 143: 280-283, 1982.
15.   Bown SG, Swain CP, Edwards DAW, Salmon PR: Palliative relief of malignant upper gastrointestinal obstruction by endoscopic laser therapy (Abstract). Gut 23: A918, 1982.
16.   Harada K, Mizushima K, Namiki M, Kasai S, Mito M: Endoscopic YAG laser treatment of lesions in the distal colon with experimental studies (Abstract). In: K Atsumi and N Nimsakul (eds), Laser-Tokyo '81, Tokyo. Japan Society for Laser Medicine, 1981, pp 20-32.

12

PHARMACOKINETICS OF HEPATIC ARTERIAL CHEMOTHERAPY

William D. Ensminger and John W. Gyves

SUMMARY

The pharmacokinetic objective of hepatic arterial chemotherapy (HAC) is to generate increased drug exposure in the tumor-bearing liver relative to that generated by standard intravenous administration. The pertinent pharmacokinetic principles have been defined. The increased exposure potentially achievable is directly proportional to the total body clearance (Cl_{TB}) of the drug in question, thus making it essential that a drug used for HAC has a relatively high Cl_{TB}. Exposure is inversely proportional to hepatic arterial blood flow. Thus, the ratio of a drug's Cl_{TB} to the hepatic arterial blood flow is a relative measure of the potential exposure increase.

The amount of drug extracted by passage through the hepatic vasculature is also important in that drugs with higher hepatic extraction (E_H) generate higher hepatic exposure per given degree of systemic exposure. The increased exposure achievable with HAC in a given patient may be limited by the degree of arterial to venous shunting present. Dose rate is also important in that drugs may display nonlinear pharmacokinetics showing decreased Cl_{TB} and E_H with increasing dose rates, thus leading to a decreased exposure advantage at high dose rates.

Recent studies have indicated that tumors within the liver are often hypervascular at the microcirculatory level. This increased microvascular density provides a mechanism for selective treatment using microsphere therapy either with starch microspheres plus drug or with radiotherapeutic yttrium-90 (^{90}Y) microspheres. Phase I studies of starch microspheres have been completed. Studies examining the toxicity of ^{90}Y microspheres alone and with the radiosensitizer, 5-bromodeoxyuridine (BUdR), are currently underway in dogs. The pharmacokinetics of BUdR in dogs indicates that it is a rational drug for HAC, at appropriate dose rates, owing to nonlinear pharmacokinetics.

INTRODUCTION

There has been a recent increase of interest in hepatic arterial chemotherapy (HAC) based on a number of developments. Despite a great deal of effort, no new systemic (intravenous) agents with efficacies approaching the low 20% efficacy of fluorouracil have been developed. Meanwhile, the technology of HAC has progressed. Nuclear medicine techniques have been developed to monitor drug distribution within the liver. Implantable devices and catheters have been tested and found to be reliable and convenient in the delivery of HAC. Essentially all phase II studies conducted with HAC have demonstrated higher response rates than would be expected with intravenous chemotherapy administration. HAC has primarily used the fluorinated pyrimidines, 5-fluorouracil (5-FU) or 5-fluorodeoxyuridine (FUdR, floxuridine). In the past several years, the pharmacokinetic principles relevant to HAC and intra-arterial chemotherapy in general have been delineated (1,2). This chapter will describe the practical pharmacokinetic factors that are relevant to HAC and will briefly review some of the ongoing research at the University of Michigan aimed at the development of new, more selective therapies using the hepatic arterial route of delivery.

GENERAL PRINCIPLES

From a pharmacokinetic standpoint, the major aim of direct hepatic arterial drug infusion is achieving higher drug exposures within the hepatic arterial distribution, i.e., within the tumor-bearing liver. If a given agent has no potential for increased exposure with direct hepatic arterial infusion or if such exposure is compromised by the dose rate of administration, there will be little advantage when compared to direct intravenous infusion. Other relevant aspects of HAC, such as the necessity for complete drug infusion to the entire tumor-bearing liver and the primary dependency of the hepatic tumor on hepatic arterial blood for nutrition, have been reviewed elsewhere (3) and will not be covered here. Based on mass balance considerations (1,2), the exposure (advantage) generated by direct hepatic arterial infusion compared to intravenous infusion is directly proportional to the total body clearance (Cl_{TB}) of the agent in question and inversely proportional to the hepatic arterial blood flow times the quantity, 1-hepatic extraction (E_H). This means that for marked increased exposure with hepatic arterial infusion, a drug should have a high Cl_{TB} relative to hepatic arterial blood flow. Although not essential, a high E_H, i.e., the fraction of drug removed by passage through the liver, will further increase the exposure advantage. As an example, FUdR has a Cl_{TB} of 10-15 ℓ (4). This compares with the usual hepatic arterial blood flow of

138

0.25-.5 ℓ/min. Hence, the high Cl_{TB} of FUdR generates by itself about a 20- to 60-fold exposure advantage. However, some 90-95% of the FUdR is extracted by the liver (E_H = 0.90-0.95) (4). Hence, the high hepatic extraction of FUdR increases the relative exposure advantage by 10-20 times, thus potentially generating a 200- to 1200-fold advantage on a theoretic basis. The average advantage determined by direct drug measurements at calculated dose rates and blood flows is about 400-fold for FUdR (3,4).

A major limitation, which has recently been identified, to the potential increased drug exposure with hepatic arterial infusion is the hepatic arterial to hepatic venous shunting that occurs in patients with hepatic tumors (5). One mechanism for defining the shunting that occurs has been the hepatic arterial administration of technetium macroaggregated albumin (Tc-MAA) and the determination of the amount of this microparticulate substance (of 30μ diameter) lodging in the lung compared to the total of lung and liver entrapment. This value defines a percent lung shunt index and ranged from 5.8-26% in 18 patients with hepatic metastases, primarily from colorectal cancer (5). The mean percent shunt index in these patients was 12.6%. The E_H of a drug in a given patient will be limited by the degree of arterial-venous shunting in that the drug must pass through small nutrient vessels for extraction to occur. There is some evidence that patients receiving FUdR who have a high degree of arterial-venous shunting to the lung determined by Tc-MAA technique have more systemic toxicity. This would be expected from the generation of higher systemic levels because of a diminished E_H.

A second major element, not often considered, that may limit the usefulness of a particular drug in hepatic arterial infusion is nonlinear pharmacokinetics. 5-FU provides an excellent example of this phenomenon. The initial studies of the E_H and the regional exposure advantage of 5-FU achieved with hepatic arterial infusion utilized short, high-dose infusions because of the relative insensitivity of the assay techniques employed (4). At high doses, such as would be achieved by bolus or short-term infusion into the hepatic artery, the Cl_{TB} and E_H are markedly diminished owing to saturation of the clearance mechanisms (6,7). The relative exposure advantage can fall as much as twofold for HAC with 5-FU. However, at doses of 15-30 mg/kg/d of 5-FU (as are usually employed), the Cl_{TB} of 5-FU appears to be approximately 2 ℓ/min with an E_H of approximately .80 (6). Thus, HAC with 5-FU at appropriate dose rates can achieve a 50- to 100-fold advantage. It should be noted that at doses from 30 to 90 mg/kg/d, significant systemic (intravenous) levels of 5-FU within the micromolar range are maintained, thus providing a potential systemic therapeutic effect. It is significant that, at high-dosage rates of infusion, FUdR appears to maintain its linearity of clearance and E_H (4). Thus, it appears essential that drugs considered for hepatic arterial infusion be administered at dosage rates that have been studied and are within the linear range. The relative roles of

139

hepatic dysfunction and the proportion of liver replaced by tumor on the pharmacokinetics of drugs has not been investigated and is probably also an important factor for those agents in which linearity is not demonstrated.

MICROCIRCULATION DIFFERENCES BETWEEN TUMOR AND NORMAL LIVER

Hepatic arterial injection of Tc-MAA has been developed and widely applied as a mechanism for defining the distribution of drug flow in HAC (8, 9). In the process of such hepatic arterial nuclide angiography, it became evident to us that most tumors had at least some regions that appeared to entrap more of the Tc-MAA than did normal liver (3,10). The distribution on a nuclide scan of Tc-MAA, which is homogenously mixed with a hepatic arterial blood and flows to small nutrient vessels, should directly reflect the microcirculatory blood flow at the time of the injection. The technique of single photon emission computed tomography allows the examination of cross-sections taken through tumor nodules in patients undergoing scan (3,10). Our examination of patients with colorectal cancer liver metastases using the Tc-MAA injection with tomographic scanning indicates that tumor nodules smaller than 8 or 9 cm in diameter are generally hypervascular, with 2.5 times or more greater entrapment of Tc-MAA compared to normal liver. Tumor nodules greater than 9 cm in diameter appear to have a hypervascular rim, 3-3.5 cm thick, and a hypovascular core. Because of this hypovascular core, integration of the relative blood flow throughout the liver will lead to the faulty conclusion that a tumor is hypovascular. The finding that the pertinent growing regions of tumors within the liver entrap more microparticulate and have a greater microcirculatory density provides a mechanism for selective therapy using therapuetic microspheres of similar size distribution to the radiolabeled tracer Tc-MAA. Two forms of therapeutic microspheres have been investigated, starch microspheres (Spherex, Pharmacia, Uppsala, Sweden) and yttrium-90 (^{90}Y) radiotherapeutic resin microspheres.

STARCH MICROSPHERES

Starch microspheres that have a mean diameter of 40 μ and a half-life of 10-15 min because of dissolution by serum amylase have been developed for therapeutic use (11,12). When these starch microspheres are suspended in a drug solution of high concentration and injected into the hepatic artery, they produce blockage of blood flow in the microcirculation and generate a semistatic blood column containing a high

140

concentration of drug within the microcirculation. This high intravascular drug concentration provides a gradient for movement of drug into the surrounding tissue. It has been shown for bis-chloroethyl nitrosourea (BCNU) and mitomycin C that coadministration of starch microspheres with these drugs can lead to greater deposition of the drug within the liver and decreased flow of the drug into the systemic circulation (11,12).

Recently, we conducted phase I studies in an attempt to determine an appropriate dose of microspheres to be used in subsequent therapeutic trials. There are some six million starch microspheres per milliliter of the standard formulation. Escalating doses of microspheres were administered with a set dose of mitomycin C, and the effect of given microsphere dose on the systemic mitomycin exposure (area under concentration multiplied by the time curve) was determined. Toxicity as related to the dose administered was also measured. Those studies indicated that six milliliters (or 36 million) of microspheres achieved most of the effect of higher doses in terms of increasing the deposition of mitomycin within the liver and diminishing systemic exposure without the acute side effects found at higher dose rates. Recently, a phase II study of hepatic arterial mitomycin C with starch microspheres using the six milliliter dose has been initiated. Toxicities have been tolerable with this regimen, and 5 of the first 11 patients have responded.

BROMODEOXYURIDINE AND YTTRIUM-90 MICROSPHERES IN A DOG MODEL

Bromodeoxyuridine (BUdR) is an analogue of thymidine and is incorporated into double-stranded deoxyribonucleic acid (DNA) in place of thymidine in cells exposed to the drug. BUdR is a potent and selective sensitizer. Radiosensitization is a direct function of the amount of BUdR incorporated into the DNA of cells undergoing DNA synthesis (13,14). In humans, BUdR has a Cl_{TB} that exceeds 3 ℓ/min (15). In preparation for clinical trials, we have studied both the pharmacokinetics of hepatic arterial infusion of BUdR and the effect of BUdR on the toxicity of hepatic arterially administered ^{90}Y microspheres using a dog model. Although the BUdR pharmacokinetic studies are incomplete, intravenous bolus administration of varying doses indicates that the pharmacokinetics are nonlinear and that at low dose rates, Cl_{TB} can be as high as 10 ℓ/min. Dose rates of 5 mg/kg/hr and 50 mg/kg/hr have been administered both by the intravenous and by the hepatic arterial route to two dogs. The pharmacokinetics are nonlinear in that a dosage increase from 5 mg/kg/hr to 50 mg/kg/hr results in a 25- to 100-fold increase in the systemic levels achieved. Whereas, the E_H is 60-80% at

5 mg/kg/hr, the E_H falls to approximately 8-10% at 50 mg/kg/hr. The high Cl_{TB} and the relatively high E_H seen at appropriate dosage levels indicates that BUdR will be an appropriate agent for hepatic arterial administration, and clinical studies are projected for the future.

Based on the microcirculatory studies described above, we have been interested in the potential therapeutic use of ^{90}Y microspheres on liver metastases. At present, there is no active investigational new drug (IND) for these microspheres, although in the past, they have been used and have shown a degree of activity (16,17). Currently, we are conducting studies examining the toxicity of hepatic arterial microspheres alone and preceeded by an HAC infusion of BUdR in dogs. Standard clinical Infusaid pumps (Intermedics Infusaid Corporation, Norwood, Massachusetts) were implanted in 10 dogs so as to infuse the majority of the liver. Half of the dogs received BUdR at 10 mg/kg/d for a four-week infusion, and the other half received four weeks of saline alone. All dogs were then treated with an injection of ^{90}Y microspheres given through the hepatic arterial catheter via the side port of the Infusaid pump. Blood counts, liver function tests, and serum amylase were measured throughout the experiment and animals were sacrificed for pathologic examination eight weeks after ^{90}Y microsphere administration. There were no effects of treatment on blood counts or serum amylase either with BUdR or with ^{90}Y microspheres alone or with BUdR plus ^{90}Y microspheres. The administration of ^{90}Y microspheres alone had no effect on serum glutamate-pyruvate transaminase levels or on serum alkaline phosphatase. BUdR treatment alone produced a rise in serum glutamate-pyruvate transaminase levels, which initially fell after ^{90}Y microsphere treatment, rose again, and then ultimately fell back to control levels by eight weeks after ^{90}Y microsphere administration. Serum alkaline phosphatase levels began to rise three weeks into the BUdR infusion and continued to rise once the BUdR was stopped and ^{90}Y microspheres were administered in dogs treated with both agents. Elevated serum alkaline phosphatase levels then generally began to fall four weeks after ^{90}Y microsphere administration in the BUdR-treated animals and were back to the baseline levels by eight weeks, when the dogs were sacrificed. Although the microscopic examination is as yet incomplete, at autopsy, little hepatic toxicity was noted macroscopically and other organs appeared to be normal in all dogs. The effect of varying the schedule of BUdR administration relative to initiation of ^{90}Y microsphere treatment will be examined in future sets of dogs. Hopefully, an IND for the clinical study of ^{90}Y microspheres alone will be obtained in the near future, and subsequently, the effect of BUdR with ^{90}Y microspheres may be investigated in later clinical trials.

CONCLUSIONS

As described, regional (hepatic) drug exposure was increased when there was a high Cl_{TB} of the agent in question relative to the hepatic blood flow. When there is a high degree of E_H by the agent, regional selectivity is further increased. For FUdR, an agent with a 10 to 15 ℓ/min Cl_{TB} and an E_H of 90-95%, the regional exposure advantage achieved may range from 200- to 1200-fold over that achieved with intravenous administration. Although there has been little investigation of the phenomena, it is highly likely that hepatic arterial-venous shunting, as noted with the flow of hepatic arterially injected Tc-MAA to the lungs, can limit E_H of the drug. With lowered E_H, not only does the regional exposure decrease, but the potential for systemic toxicity may also increase. As shown through the example of 5-FU and BUdR, increasing dosage rates, when there are nonlinear pharmacokinetics, can decrease the regional advantage through the generation of a lower Cl_{TB} for the agent and lowered E_H at the higher dosage rates. It is essential that new agents considered for hepatic arterial infusion be studied pharmacokinetically.

Recent investigations using nuclear angiography coupled with nuclear tomography have indicated that the pertinent regions of hepatic tumors are generally hypervascular at the microcirculatory level. This hypervascularity may provide a selective mechanism for the delivery of therapy. Phase I studies have been concluded and phase II studies are under way, using starch microspheres (Spherex) with BCNU and mitomycin. There have been responses in the phase II study to the combination of starch microspheres and mitomycin. Investigations are under way that examine, in a dog model, the toxicity of hepatic arterial ^{90}Y microspheres as a radiotherapeutic modality. The pharmacokinetics of BUdR, a potent radiosensitizer, have been studied in the dog and suggest that hepatic arterial infusion is an extremely rational mechanism for achieving a selective regional exposure advantage. A toxicity study of ^{90}Y microspheres alone and with hepatic arterial BUdR in dogs is under way. Results to date suggest that such therapy may be clinically useful in the future.

ACKNOWLEDGMENT

Supported in part by Public Health Service grants CA-28478, CA-28490, and CA-33825 (National Cancer Institute), and M01-RR-00042 (Division of Research Resources), National Institutes of Health, Department of Health and Human Services, and by the Burroughs Wellcome Fund.

References

1. Collins JM, Dedrick RL: Pharmacokinetics of anticancer drugs. In: B Chabner (ed). Pharmacologic Principles of Cancer Treatment. WB Saunders, Philadelphia, 1982, pp 77-99.
2. Chen H-SG, Gross JF: Intra-arterial infusion of anticancer drugs: Theoretic aspects of drug delivery and review of responses. Cancer Treat Rep 64: 31-40, 1980.
3. Ensminger W, Gyves J: Regional cancer chemotherapy. Cancer Treat Rep 68: 101-115, 1984.
4. Ensminger WD, Rosowsky A, Raso V, Levin DC, Glode M, Come S, Steele G, Frei E III: A clinical pharmacologic evaluation of hepatic arterial infusions of 5-fluoro-2'-deoxyuridine and 5-fluorouracil. Cancer Res 38: 3784-3792, 1978.
5. Ziessman H, Thrall J, Gyves J, Ensminger W, Niederhuber J, Tuscon M, Walker S: Quantitative hepatic arterial perfusion scintigraphy and starch microspheres in cancer chemotherapy. J Nucl Med 24: 871-875, 1983.
6. Ensminger W, Stetson P, Gyves J, Walker S, Janis M, Zlotecki R, Meyer M, Brady T, Niederhuber J: Dependence of hepatic arterial fluorouracil pharmacokinetics on dose rate and the duration of infusion (Abstract). Proc Am Soc Clin Oncol 2: C-98, 1983.
7. Collins JM, Dedrick RL, King FG, Speyer JL, Myers CE: Nonlinear pharmacokinetic models for 5-fluorouracil in man: intravenous and intraperitoneal routes. Clin Pharmacol Ther 28: 235-246, 1980.
8. Kaplan WD, D'Orsi CJ, Ensminger WD, Smith EH, Levin DC: Intra-arterial radionuclide infusion: a new technique to assess chemotherapy perfusion patterns. Cancer Treat Rep 62: 699-703, 1978.
9. Kaplan WD, Ensminger WD, Come SE, Smith EH, D'Orsi CJ, Levin DC, Takvorian RW, Steele GD Jr: Radionuclide angiography to predict patient response to hepatic artery chemotherapy. Cancer Treat Rep 64: 1217-1222, 1980.
10. Gyves J, Ensminger W, Thrall J, Ziessman H, Niederhuber J, Keyes J, Walker S: Definition of hepatic tumor microcirculation by single-photon emission computed tomography (SPECT). J Nucl Med 25: 972-977, 1984.
11. Dakhil S, Ensminger W, Cho K, Niederhuber J, Doan K, Wheeler R: Improved regional selectivity of hepatic arterial BCNU with degradable microspheres. Cancer 50: 631-635, 1982.
12. Gyves J, Ensminger W, VanHarken D, Niederhuber J, Stetson P, Walker S: Improved regional selectivity of hepatic arterial mitomycin by starch microspheres. Clin Pharmacol Ther 34: 259-265, 1983.
13. Djordjevic B, Szybalski W: Genetics of human cell lines. III. Incorporation of 5-bromo- and 5-iododeoxyuridine into the deoxyribonucleic acid of human cells and its effect on radiation sensitivity. J Exp Med 112: 509-531, 1960.
14. Schindler R, Ramseier L, Grieder A: Increased sensitivity of mammalian cell cultures to radiomimetic alkylating agents following incorporation of 5-bromodeoxyuridine into cellular DNA. Biochem Pharmacol 15: 2013-2023, 1966.
15. Russo A, Gianni L, Kinsella T, Klecker RW Jr., Jenkins J, Rowland J, Glatstein E, Mitchell JB, Collins J, Myers C: Pharmacological evaluation of intravenous delivery of 5-bromodeoxyuridine to patients with brain tumors. Cancer Res 44: 1702-1705, 1984.
16. Ariel IM: Treatment of inoperable primary pancreatic and liver cancer by the intra-arterial administration of radioactive isotopes (Y^{99} radiating microspheres). Ann Surg 162: 267-278, 1965.
17. Grady E: Internal radiation therapy of hepatic cancer. Dis Colon Rectum 22: 371-375, 1979.

13

ADJUVANT RADIATION THERAPY FOR COLORECTAL CANCER

Tyvin A. Rich

SUMMARY

The use of adjuvant radiation therapy (XRT) after potentially curative surgery for colorectal cancer has decreased the incidence of local and regional failure more than in historical surgical controls. When radiation is most suitable for the patient with rectal cancer is unclear, since studies employing either pre- or postoperative XRT have demonstrated that both are beneficial. The patients with the highest risk of relapsing can be well defined by an assessment of the clinical description and the pathologic stage of the tumor. Compared with surgery alone, postoperative radiation treatment, with strict attention to treatment planning and localization to avoid excessive radiation doses in the small intestine, has been successful in reducing local recurrence to 10% or less without an increased complications rate. The continued use of adjuvant XRT (either pre- or postoperatively) in combination with systemic therapy is indicated if survival rates are to be improved.

INTRODUCTION

The use of adjuvant radiation therapy (XRT) for colorectal cancer has become increasingly popular because of the need to improve local control rates after potentially curative surgery. Identification of the anatomic and pathologic risk factors associated with local treatment failure has made it possible to select those patients with the highest risk of local disease relapse. The differences between the risk of local recurrence for rectal cancer and the risk of local recurrence from colon cancer after surgical treatment only are believed to reflect the anatomic constraints associated with tumor removal in the low pelvis versus the less difficult tumor surgery in the abdomen. In either anatomic location, however, a higher tumor stage (e.g., degree of transmural tumor extension) is directly associated with an increasing risk of local relapse.

There are now several retrospective analyses of the incidence of local and regional failure in patients treated only by surgery for rectal cancer (1-5). In these studies, the scope of local and regional failure includes any recurrence in the pelvis, regardless of the presence of distant metastasis. By defining local failure in this way, the importance of local recurrence either alone or as a component of local failure is emphasized. The aim of radiation therapy is twofold: to decrease the amount of symptomatic local recurrence in the pelvis and, for a smaller subpopulation (not yet clearly identifiable) who will ultimately relapse only in the pelvis, to prevent a fatal relapse and by doing so improve the survival rate.

The risk for local failure is related to the stage of disease. Although the Dukes' staging system is useful in assigning an overall prognosis, radiation therapists have found that assessment of local failure can be refined by a careful examination of the degree of extramural tumor extension (Table 1) (5). For lesions confined to the bowel wall, the risk of local failure is small (8-15%). Even patients having lymph nodes positive for disease, but with lesions still confined to the bowel wall, have a low risk of local recurrence (~20%). With extension beyond the bowel wall, the rate of pelvic failure increases to 27-35% for lesions without lymph node involvement (stages B_2 and B_3), and to 50-67% for lesions with lymph node involvement (stages C_2 and C_3) (Table 2). In one study from the Massachusetts General Hospital (MGH), these differences, based on the degree of extramural extension within the lymph nodes, were significant (4). The highest incidence of local pelvic failure was found in cases in which tumors involved adjacent organs or structures, whether clinically or pathologically (stages B_3 and C_3) (Table 3). In a similar type of analysis, Withers and Romsdahl also found a high pelvic recurrence rate for patients with tumors that were described as "difficult to resect" or with adherence to or proven pathologic involvement of adjacent pelvic organs (2).

Other factors in addition to pathologic stage seem to influence local failure after potentially curative surgery. The location of the tumor is important, particularly if it is below the peritoneal flexure or on the posterior wall, where operative removal may be limited because of proximity to the sacrum. Blood vessel invasion is associated with both increased local failure and poorer survival rates, and it appears to be independent of lymph node status or pathologic stage (4). Some investigators have found a higher incidence of pelvic recurrence in patients with high-grade tumors, even though recurrence is usually correlated with pathologic stage (1,4). In assessing any patient for risk of local failure, these additional factors are sometimes useful to radiation therapists in making decisions about dose and volume of irradiation.

Table 1. Staging Systems for Colorectal Carcinoma: Comparison of Dukes' Scheme with TNM and a Modification of the Astler-Coller System by Gunderson and Sosin[*]

Staging System			Description
Dukes'	Modified Astler-Coller	TNM[†]	
A	A	T_1N_0	Nodes negative; lesion limited to mucosa
	B_1	T_2N_0	Nodes negative; extension of lesion through mucosa, but still within bowel wall
B	B_2[‡]	T_3N_0	Nodes negative; extension through entire bowel wall, including serosa if present
C	C_1	T_2N_1	Nodes positive; lesions limited to bowel wall
	C_2[‡]	T_3N_1	Nodes positive; extension of lesion through entire bowel wall, including serosa

[*] Modified from Gunderson, (5).

[†] By definition M_0 equals no evidence of metastasis.

[‡] A separate notation is made regarding the degree of extension through the bowel wall: microscopic only -- m; gross extension confirmed by microscopy -- m + g; adherence to or invasion of surrounding organs or structures -- $B_3 + C_3$ (TNM system -- T_5).

For optimal treatment of patients with rectal cancer, a close collaboration between the surgeon and radiation therapist is essential. For most lesions, radiation is not the treatment method of choice, but it should be considered a useful tool for achieving local disease control when it is combined with potentially curative surgery. Surgical extirpation remains the treatment of choice for nearly all mobile lesions, and for patients with this type of disease, it provides an excellent chance for cure. The choice of operation for rectal cancer is either combined abdominoperineal resection (CAPR) or low anterior resection (LAR), depending on tumor site and stage, sex of the patient, and the surgeon's training and preference. Whenever adjuvant irradiation is a possibility, consideration should be given to certain maneuvers aimed at improving the therapeutic ratio of tumor control: complications. After CAPR, the pelvic floor should be reconstructed whenever feasible to minimize the volume of small intestine in the true pelvis. The placement of omentum beside a difficult operative area will sometimes minimize the chance of a "stuck" loop of small bowel in an area requiring high-dose radiation. Some investigators advocate the placement of a foreign body (silastic-rubber implant) in the true pelvis, thereby preventing the chance of postoperative adherence of

Table 2. Extent of Disease Compared with Later Local Recurrence (Minimum 2-Year Follow-up Time)[*]

Series[†]	Reference	Tumor Site	Modified Astler-Coller Stage[*]					
			Within Wall			Through Wall		
			A	B_1	C_1	$B_2(\pm B_3)$	$C_2(\pm C_3)$	B_3+C_3
UFL	(1)	Colorectum	0/30	3/20 (15%)	4/19 (21%)	29/106 (27%)	33/64 (52%)	--
MDAH	(2)	Rectum and rectosigmoid	--	13/92 (14%)	1/8 (12%)	16/90 (18%)	18/52 (35%)	8/14 (57%)
ME	(3)	Rectum and rectosigmoid	0/1	6/42 (11%)	1/5 (20%)	13/37 (35%)	24/37 (65%)	--
MGH	(4)	Rectum and rectosigmoid	0/3	3/36 (8%)	2/4 (50%)	18-59 (30%)	20/40 (50%)	(53-67%)
UMN	(5)	Rectum and rectosigmoid	--	--	4/7 (57%)	--	28/40 (70%)	--

[*] Modified from Gunderson et al., (17).

[†] UFL - University of Florida, Gainesville, Florida; MDAH - M. D. Anderson Hospital, Houston, Texas; ME - Maine Medical Center, Portland, Maine; MGH - Massachusetts General Hospital, Boston, Massachusetts; UMN - University of Minnesota, Rochester, Minnesota.

the small bowel (6). Primary or partial closure should be considered to speed healing and to decrease the interval between surgery and irradiation. The surgeon should accurately describe the location of the primary bowel tumor and mark any areas of residual disease with radio-opaque clips so the radiotherapist can precisely aim the boost irradiation. There is less concern for small bowel injury after LAR because the chance of adherent small bowel is reduced. Postoperative radiation is also simpler; since the entire perineum does not require treatment, therapy can start sooner.

Table 3. Extent of Rectal or Rectosigmoid Cancer and Percent of Local Recurrence after Potentially Curative Surgery[*]

Tumor Stage	Local Recurrence	%
Nodes negative for disease		
A	0/3	0
B_1	3/36	8
B_2 micro [†]	2/12	17
B_2 macro [†]	8/32	25
B_3 Adherent or adjacent involvement	8/15	53
Nodes positive for disease		
C_1/C_2 micro [†]	4/11	36
C_2 macro [†]	14/27	52
C_3 Adherent or adjacent involvement	4/6	67
Total	43/142	30

[*]   Modified from Rich et al., (4).

[†]   Micro and macro refer to microscopic or macroscopic transmural tumor invasion.

ADJUVANT IRRADIATION: TREATMENT TECHNIQUES

There are three sequence options for adjuvant XRT for the patient with rectal cancer. The first is preoperative irradiation, which can contribute to reducing the disease stage (fewer stage C tumors than before treatment) and improving local disease control and survival rates in both randomized and nonrandomized trials (7-13). The doses used have ranged from single fractions of 500 centigray (cGy) given immediately after surgery to doses of 1000-2500 cGy administered over 1-3 weeks. Moderate doses of 3450-4500 cGy have sometimes been used, especially for patients with large or immobile tumors. In cases where tumor fixation is found on palpation, high doses of 5000-6000 cGy can be used in order to convert the mass to a potentially resectable tumor. The preoperative radiation studies have demonstrated slight survival rate advantages for most patients treated, particularly patients with tumor fixation or patients with Stage C tumors below the peritoneal reflection (Table 4). The disadvantages of preoperative XRT for all patients with rectal cancer are the potentially unnecessary treatment of 10-30% of those with mobile lesions who are highly curable with surgery alone and the irradiation of those patients with occult metastasis. The identification of such patients may be easier with the better diagnostic techniques available now. Continued study of preoperative XRT is indicated.

Table 4. Preoperative Irradiation

Series/ Reference[*]	Randomized	Preoperative Dose (cGy)	Five-Year Survival Rate (%)	
			XRT + Surgery	Surgery
Toronto (7)	yes	500	37	19
Medical Research Council (8)	yes	500-2000	40	38
Veterans Administration Hospitals (9)	yes	2000-2500	47	34
Memorial (10)	no	2000-2500	35	41
	yes	2000-2500	ND[†]	ND[†]
Yale (11)	yes	4500	41	25
Holland (12)	yes	3450	58	32
Oregon (13)	no	5000-6000	53	38

[*] Ontario Cancer Institute, Toronto, Ontario, Canada; Medical Research Council, London, England; Veterans Administration Hospital - includes all Veterans Administration Hospitals in USA; Memorial - Memorial Sloan-Kettering Hospital, New York, New York; Yale - Yale University, New Haven, Connecticut; Holland - Rottedamsch Radio-Theraputisch Institute (RRTI), Rotterdam, The Netherlands; Oregon - University of Oregon, Portland, Oregon.

[†] ND - no difference.

Another treatment approach is the use of postoperative XRT based on the pathologic stage of disease. There are now several nonrandomized studies reported that demonstrate the utility of 4500-5000 cGy given postoperatively for patients with stage B_2, B_3, C_2, or C_3 disease (2,5,14,15). A comparison of the rates of local control for patients treated with or without postoperative XRT is shown in Table 5. The local recurrence rate for equivalent groups (stage B_2, B_3, C_2 or C_3) ranges from 35-50% for operation alone and is reduced to 6-8% by adjuvant XRT. These studies are not randomized, but may be interpreted to show that the natural history of rectal cancer after potentially curative surgery can be altered, especially regarding local recurrence. These pilot studies have demonstrated several other important points regarding radiation treatment. There is sufficient evidence to support a dose-response relationship for local control and that doses of no less than 4500-5000 cGy (tumor minimum) are necessary for tumor sterilization (16). Radiation treatment should involve multiple fields and a small bowel series so as to avoid unnecessarily high doses of radiation to the small intestine (17).

Another postoperative adjuvant study is the Gastrointestinal Tumor Study Group's randomized prospective trial, in which patients were assigned to a control arm of surgery alone or to one of three adjuvant treatment groups. The adjuvant treatment consisted of chemotherapy (5-fluorouracil plus methyl chloroethyl cyclohexyl nitrosourea; CCNU), pelvic XRT, or a combination of chemotherapy plus XRT (18). The preliminary results show a superior disease-free survival rate in all three treatment arms compared with the survival rate after surgery alone at follow-up intervals of 130-150 weeks. The difference between the chemotherapy plus XRT versus surgery alone is statistically significant (P < .03). Local recurrence rate (analyzed as the first site of failure) ranges from 19% for surgery alone to less than 10% for combination treatment. In the radiation-alone treatment arm, however, the minimum local recurrence rate is 15%, which is high compared with an overall 6-8% rate in the nonrandomized studies. This difference is possibly a result of lower radiation doses in the randomized trial, in which doses ranged from 4000-4800 cGy, than in the nonrandomized studies.

As a third alternative for adjuvant XRT for rectal cancer, some investigators have advocated the use of the "sandwich" technique, employing a low-dose (500 cGy in one fraction or 1000 cGy in five sessions), preoperative course of radiation combined with postoperative XRT for those patients with "high-risk" tumors (19,20). In the two studies that have now been reported, the local failure rate varies from 6-20%. Since this combined approach offers potential advantages over either pre- or postoperative treatment alone, particularly for resectable lesions, further investigation is warranted. For the patient with an unresectable lesion, however, higher doses of preoperative XRT are preferred in conjunction with CAPR.

Table 5. Postoperative Adjuvant Radiation Therapy for Colorectal Cancer

Extent of Disease	After Operation Alone	After Postoperative Adjuvant Radiation Therapy — Recurrences				Total No. with Recurrence/Total No. Treated
		MDAH(2)	LDSH(14)	MGH(15)	MH(16)	
Confined to wall Nodes positive (C_1)	20-30%	0/3	0/2	1/9	--	1/14 (7%)
Through wall Nodes negative (B_2)	25-35%	1/18	0/10	2/29	0/10	3/67 (4%)
Through wall Nodes positive (C_2)	45-70%	3/33	2/16	5/49	4/28	14/127 (11%)
Adherent or invasive Nodes negative or positive (B_3, C_3)	50-75%	1/8	--	2/17	1/13	4/38 (11%)
Total						22/246 (9%)

* MDAH - M. D. Anderson Hospital, Houston, Texas; LDSH - Latter Day Saints Hospital, Salt Lake City, Utah; MGH - Massachusetts General Hospital, Boston, Massachusetts; MH - Memorial Hospital/University of Miami, Hollywood, Florida.

152

In the patient with residual, recurrent, or unresectable disease, the task of achieving local control by surgical or radiotherapeutic means is more difficult because radiation dose levels greater than 6000 cGy are required for permanent tumor control. The data in support of this are derived from patients treated for advanced disease with preoperative radiation in doses of 4500-5000 cGy and who have a local failure rate of 35-45% (21). Similarly, patients with microscopic or gross residual disease who receive postoperative XRT still have a 15-54% local failure rate (16). Since high dosage levels are required in these clinical situations, a new technique employing intraoperative radiation therapy is being developed in order to safely deliver very high radiation doses (>6000 cGy) to the tumor, while maximally sparing normal tissues (22). Pilot studies indicate this method may be useful in advanced disease, but the role for this type of treatment as adjuvant therapy has not yet been determined.

COLON CANCER

The problem of local and regional recurrence after curative resection of colon cancer (all sites proximal to the sigmoid colon segment) can be substantial. Summaries of studies from the University of Minnesota (23), from the University of Washington (24), and from MGH (25) describing the patterns of failure are shown in Table 6. There is an increased risk of local and regional failure associated with tumor extension through the full thickness of the bowel wall, but the single most important factor predicting the risk of local failure of colon cancer is advanced pathologic stage. For tumors confined to the bowel wall, the risk of local relapse is 2%, but it increases to 11-19% with full-thickness involvement. Of patients with tumors adherent to or invading adjacent organs or structures, 35-37% will have recurrence later in the local area. Fixed anatomic locations (splenic or hepatic flexure versus transverse or sigmoid colon) were indicated by one study (24) to have a slightly higher incidence of local and regional failure than the mobile colon location (21% versus 5%). In this study from the University of Washington (24), however, no differences were found regarding fixed or mobile portions of the colon. Disease-positive lymph nodes are associated with a slightly higher incidence of local and regional failure (32-49%) compared with disease-negative lymph nodes (2-30%). In the MGH study (25), an increasing number of lymph nodes (>5) was related to a higher local failure rate (13-50%). Two other pathologic factors found in the MGH study were associated with a higher local recurrence rate. Twenty-eight percent of patients with colloid tumors relapsed versus 15-18% with noncolloid tumors, regardless of the histologic grade. The other finding was the relation of tumor size to risk of local

153

Table 6. Colon Cancer: Patterns of Recurrence*

| Series† | Number of Cases | | | | No. with recurrence / Total No. Cases |
	Local/Regional	Abdominal/Peritoneal Seeding	Liver	Extra Abdominal	
UMN (23)					
Location:					
Transverse	38	13	--	25	3/8 (38%)
Cecum	49	16	--	27	26/37 (70%)
Ascending/descending and flexures	50	30	--	37	29/46 (63%)
UWA (24)					
Extent of tumor penetration:					
Confined (A, B_1, C_1)	2 (16%)	4 (42%)	4 (39%)	3 (27%)	19/184 (11%)
Full thickness (B_2, C_2)	11 (27%)	16 (38%)	18 (43%)	11 (27%)	138/326 (42%)
Adherent/invasive (B_3, C_3)	35 (49%)	33 (45%)	20 (28%)	13 (17%)	29/40 (72%)
MGH (25)		Distant Metastasis‡			
Extent of tumor penetration:					
Confined (A, B_1, C_1)	2 (21%)	9 (93%)		14/138 (10%)	
Full thickness (B_2, C_2)	19 (56%)	28 (82%)		90/263 (34%)	
Adherent/invasive (B_3, C_3)	37 (83%)	33 (75%)		59/132 (45%)	

* Autopsy series, Gunderson LL, Sosin H, unpublished data.
Recurrence determined at reoperation in 12% (UWA) and 25% (MGH).

† UMN – University of Minnesota, Rochester, Minnesota; UWA – University of Washington, Seattle, Washington; MGH – Massachusetts General Hospital, Boston, Massachusetts.

‡ "Distant Metastasis" included any patient with abdominal or extra-abdominal failure. The first number is the total group at risk; the percentage is the percent of the group that relapsed.

154

failure. Patients with tumors more than 5 cm in diameter had nearly double the risk of patients with smaller tumors (25% versus 13%), and the risk appeared to be independent of tumor stage.

The importance of local and regional failure in colon cancer should not be underestimated, because up to 30% of patients who relapse do so only in the original tumor site. The recurrence patterns of colon cancer are more complex, however, than those of rectal cancer because of their location within the abdominal cavity and the possibility of early dissemination via direct peritoneal spread. Diffuse peritoneal seeding and liver metastasis occur frequently, and overall, up to 70% of patients will experience recurrence with a component of disease at a site below the diaphragm.

XRT has been used less often for primary colon tumors than for rectal cancer, partly because of the lack of good data regarding the patterns of relapse. These are now sufficient data available to identify subgroups of patients at risk for local and regional relapse, but because of the complex failure pattern for colon cancer patients, local therapy alone may have only a small impact on the ultimate outcome of this disease. The types of adjuvant-therapy studies can be separated into local-regional treatment or whole abdominal treatment.

In a study from MGH, 49 patients with locally advanced tumors (stages B_2, B_3, C_2, and C_3) were treated with localized fields of radiation to the tumor bed in doses of 4500–5500 cGy after curative surgery (26). The follow-up results of treatment for all patients seen for a minimum of 18 months showed a 94–95% local failure-free survival rate for patients with stage B_2 or B_3 disease. In 39 patients with tumors and disease-positive nodes, the local failure-free survival rate ranged from 75% (stage C_2 disease) to 57% (stage C_3 disease). Serious morbidity occurred in two patients who required small bowel resection for radiation injury. Adjuvant radiation in this setting appears to have acceptable toxicity as long as diligent efforts are made to localize the small intestine during treatment planning and to avoid excessive radiation doses by employing precise radiation techniques. Prospective and randomized studies to investigate the combination of postoperative local XRT with or without whole abdominal radiation are underway.

In another approach, investigators have used whole abdominal XRT for patients with colonic primary tumors after complete or incomplete resection (26). Forty-seven patients with stage B_2, B_3, C_1, and C_2 tumors of the proximal colon were treated with postoperative whole abdominal (including the liver) XRT by a strip technique delivering 2100 cGy over eight days. Nine patients with residual disease received additional doses of 1000-1500 cGy to reduced fields. Sixty percent of patients (28/47) were alive and free of disease after a minimum follow-up time of 12 months. Complications were encountered in three patients (6%), including one death from radiation enteritis. This report is encouraging, compared with historical data, but the results need to be confirmed in prospective randomized trials.

ACKNOWLEDGEMENT

This work supported in part by grants CA06294 and CA16672 awarded by the Department of Health and Human Services, National Institutes of Health, through the National Cancer Institute.

References

1. Cass AW, Million RR, Pfaff WW: Patterns of recurrence following surgery alone for adenocarcinoma of colon and rectum. Cancer 37: 2861-2865, 1976.
2. Withers HR, Romsdahl MN, Barkely HT Jr, Saxton J, McBride C, McMurtrey M: Postoperative radiotherapy for rectal cancer. In: SE Jones and SE Salmon (eds), Adjuvant therapy of cancer II. Grune and Stratton, New York, 1979, pp 621-628.
3. Gilbert SG: Symptomatic local tumor failure following abdomino-perineal resection. Int J Radiat Oncol Biol Phys 4: 801-807, 1978.
4. Rich TA, Gunderson LL, Lew R, Galdibini JJ, Cohen AM, Donaldson G: Patterns of recurrence of rectal cancer after potentially curative surgery. Cancer 52: 1317-1329, 1983.
5. Gunderson LL: Combined irradiation and surgery for rectal and sigmoid cancer: Emerging roles of radiotherapy in four selected areas. Curr Prob Cancer 1: 40-53, 1976.
6. Sugarbaker PH: Intrapelvic prosthesis to prevent injury of the small intestine with high dosage pelvic irradiation. Surg Gynecol Obstet 157: 269-271, 1983.
7. Rider WD: Is the Miles operation really necessary for the treatment of rectal cancer? J Cancer Assoc Radiol 26: 167-175, 1975.
8. Smith AN, MRC Working Party: The evaluation of low dose preoperative x-ray therapy in the management of operable rectal cancer: Results of a randomly controlled trial. Br J Surg 71: 21-25, 1984.
9. Roswit B, Higgins GA, Keeham RS: A controlled study of preoperative irradiation in cancer of sigmoid colon and rectum. Radiology 97: 133-140. 1970.
10. Stevens KR, Allen CV, Fletcher WS: Preoperative radiotherapy for adenocarcinoma of the rectosigmoid. Cancer 37: 2866-2874, 1976.
11. Kligerman MM, Urdanetta N, Knowlton A: Preoperative irradiation of rectosigmoid carcinoma including its regional lymph nodes. Am J Roentgenol 114: 498-503, 1972.
12. Wassif SB, Langenhorst BG, Hop WCJ: The contribution of preoperative radiotherapy in the management of borderline operability rectal cancer. In: SE Jones and SE Salmon (eds), Adjuvant therapy of cancer II. Grune and Stratton, New York, 1979, pp 613-620.
13. Stevens RK, Fletcher WS, Allen CV: Anterior resection and primary anastomosis following high dose preoperative irradiation for adenocarcinoma of the rectosigmoid. Cancer 41: 2065-2071, 1978.

14. Hoskins RB, Gunderson LL, Dosoretz DE, Rich TA, Galdibini JJ, Donaldson GA, Cohen AM: Adjuvant postoperative radiotherapy in carcinoma of the rectum and rectosigmoid carcinoma including its regional lymph nodes. Cancer 55: 61-71, 1985.

15. Brizel HE, Tepperman BS: Postoperative adjuvant irradiation for adenocarcinoma of the rectum and sigmoid. Am J Clin Oncol, 1985, in press.

16. Allee PE, Gunderson LL, Munzenrider JE: Postoperative radiation therapy for residual colorectal carcinoma. Int J Radiat Oncol Biol Phys 7: 1208, 1981.

17. Gunderson LL, Meyer JE, Sheedy P, Munzenrider JE: Radiation oncology, part XVIII. In: AR Margolis and JH Buzhenne (eds), Alimentary Tract Radiology (3rd edition). CV Mosby, St. Louis, 1983, pp 2409-2446.

18. Moertel CG: Surgical adjuvant therapy of GI cancer. In: SE Jones and SE Salmon (eds), Adjuvant therapy of Cancer II. Grune and Stratton, New York, 1980, pp 573-580.

19. Gunderson LL, Dosoretz DE, Hedberg SE, Blitzer PH, Rodkey G, Hoskins B, Shipley WU, Cohen AM: Low-dose preoperative irradiation, surgery, and elective postoperative radiation therapy for resectable rectum and rectosigmoid carcinoma. Cancer 52: 446-451, 1983.

20. Mohiuddin M, Marks G, Kramer S, Pajale T: Adjuvant radiation therapy for rectal cancer. Int J Ratiat Oncol Biol Phys 10: 977-980, 1984.

21. Dosoretz DE, Gunderson LL, Hoskins B: Preoperative irradiation for localized carcinoma of the rectum and rectosigmoid: Patterns of failure, survival, and future treatment strategies. Cancer 52: 814-818, 1983.

22. Gunderson LL, Tepper JE, Biggs PJ, Goldson A, Martin JK, McCullough EC, Rich TA, Shipley WU, Sindelar WF, Wood WL: Intraoperative external beam irradiation. Curr Prob Cancer 7: 1-69, 1983.

23. Russell AH, Tong D, Dawson LE, Wisbeck W: Adenocarcinoma of the proximal colon: Sites of initial dissemination and patterns of recurrence following surgery alone. Cancer 53: 360-367, 1984.

24. Willett C, Tepper JE, Cohen AM, Orlow E, Weld C, Donaldson G: Local failure following curative resection of colonic adenocarcinoma. Int J Radiat Oncol Biol Phys 10: 645-651, 1984.

25. Duttenhaver J, Hoskins B, Gunderson LL, Tepper J, Willett C: Adjuvant postoperative radiation therapy in cancer of the colon above the peritoneal reflection (Abstract). Int J Radiat Oncol Biol Phys 9 (Supp 1): 101, 1983.

26. Ghossein NA, Samala EC, Alpert S, DeLuca FR, Ragins H, Turner SS, Stacey P, Flax H: Elective postoperative radiotherapy after incomplete resection of colorectal cancer. Dis Colon Rectum 24: 252-256, 1981.

14

HEPATIC RESECTION FOR COLORECTAL CARCINOMA METASTASES: PRESENT STATUS AND FUTURE PROSPECTS

Kevin S. Hughes, David A. August, Reyer T. Ottow, Paul H. Sugarbaker

SUMMARY

In reviewing the literature and in updating the experience at the National Cancer Institute, two conclusions become apparent: 1) liver resection offers the only significant chance of cure in patients with colorectal cancer metastases, and 2) 60-80% of patients who undergo liver resection are not cured. The multifactorial nature of the problem makes it difficult to define specific prognostic groups when dealing with small individual series. Therefore, to encourage future collaborative efforts, a discussion of the staging of hepatic metastases and a protocol matrix for uniform data collection and reporting are proposed. If all data can be synthesized into a central data base, it should be possible to define a group of patients who will benefit from surgery alone, a group who will benefit from surgery plus adjuvant treatments, and a group who will not benefit from surgery. This will allow more knowledgeable patient selection for this major surgical procedure.

INTRODUCTION

Liver resection is the only treatment available for colorectal metastases that has a significant chance of curing the patient. Five-year survival rates varying from 23% (1) to 55% (2) have been reported, with the majority of series finding less than 40% surviving five years (3-9). This means that 45-77% of patients undergo a major operative resection without being cured, though a prolongation of life has been suggested in some reports. In order to increase the benefit of resection, we need to select which patients will be cured by this procedure and which patients will relapse. If groups that have high recurrence rates can be defined, we can develop therapies adjuvant to resection that will improve the prognosis of these patients.

In this paper, we report the National Institutes of Health (NIH) experience with liver resection for colorectal metastases and with adjuvant intraperitoneal 5-fluorouracil (5-FU). In updating this experience (10) and in reviewing the literature, we have found that the prognostic significance of various factors is difficult to evaluate with a single-institution series. Therefore, to encourage future collaborative efforts, a discussion of staging systems for hepatic metastases is presented and a protocol matrix for uniform data collection and reporting are proposed.

NATIONAL INSTITUTES OF HEALTH EXPERIENCE WITH HEPATIC RESECTION FOR COLORECTAL CANCER METASTASES

Seventy-seven patients with suspected liver metastases from colorectal cancer were seen at the Surgery Branch of the National Cancer Institute (NCI) between January 1980 and January 1983. Forty-seven of these patients had disease thought to be resectable after preoperative assessment, and 46 patients underwent laparotomies. One patient refused surgery. Thirty patients had disease confined to their livers which were resected of all gross disease. Three had simultaneous resections of second sites of metastasis (two in the lung, one in a lymph node) and were excluded from this analysis. Of the remaining 13 patients, resection was not performed because of unresectable liver involvement in seven patients, the presence of extrahepatic metastases in one patient, and the presence of metastases in lymph nodes draining the liver in five patients. The following discussion deals with the 30 patients undergoing resection for liver metastases only, plus three patients who underwent hepatic resection at the NCI between 1976 and 1979.

Twenty-three men and 10 women ranging in age from 17-74 years were evaluated. All patients had primary adenocarcinomas of the colon or rectum. Primary tumors were classified according to the Astler-Coller modification of Dukes' staging system (11). Fifteen patients had synchronous hepatic metastases, and 18 had disease-free intervals ranging from 2-90 months.

Twenty patients underwent resection of metastases, 11 of which involved both lobes of the liver. Twelve patients underwent lobectomy, four of whom also had resection of metastases of the contralateral lobe. One patient underwent a trisegmentectomy with a wedge resection of a left lateral segment metastasis.

Twenty-one patients received intraperitoneal chemotherapy following hepatic resection, in a pilot protocol. Twelve patients did not receive this treatment for various

160

reasons, five had resections prior to initiation of this protocol, three refused chemotherapy, two had infectious complications that contraindicated chemotherapy, and two had medical contraindications. Chemotherapy was administered via a Tenckhoff catheter implanted at the time of resection.

Chemotherapy was initiated at a median of 34 days after surgery and was given on days 1-5 of a 28-day cycle. The initial cycle used 1040 mg of 5-FU given daily in two liters of Inpersol (Abbott Park, N. Chicago, Illinois), with subsequent cycles escalating the daily dose to 1820 mg or until limited by toxicity. Treatment was continued for 12 cycles unless toxicity or tumor recurrence indicated earlier cessation.

Time until recurrence and survival data were estimated and plotted using the Kaplan-Meier product-limit method (12). The Mantel-Haenszel test (13) was used to compare outcomes between different groups of patients. All probability values cited are two-tailed.

For all patients, the two- and three-year survival rates were 78% and 48%, respectively. An estimated five-year survival rate was 26%, but only two patients were actually available for analysis after five years. For all patients, the two- and three-year disease-free survival rates were 35% and 18%, respectively. In the 22 patients who developed recurrent disease, the liver was the site of initial recurrence in 11 (50%), the lung was the site of initial recurrence in 7 (32%), and more than one organ was involved at first evidence of recurrence in the remaining 4 patients (18%).

When the patients were grouped by factors that had prognostic significance, certain trends became apparent. However, because of the small numbers, these trends should be interpreted carefully.

The most significant prognostic factor was the number of metastases resected. Patients with one to three metastases resected had two- and three-year survival rates of 84% and 53% and two- and three-year disease-free survival rates of 47% and 23%, respectively. Patients with four or more metastases had two- and three-year survival rates of 20% and 10% (Figure 1A,B). In comparing survival rates, a P value of .006 was found.

The distribution of metastases (unilobar versus bilobar) was also predictive of disease-free survival, with unilobar metastases indicating an increased survival time. This difference in survival rates based on metastases distribution was not stastistically significant when solitary metastases were excluded from the analysis, but the number of cases of multiple metastasis is too small and the follow-up times are too short to draw conclusions (Figure 2A). Patients with multiple unilobar metastases (n = 7) had a two-year disease-free survival rate of 28%, and patients with multiple bilobar metastases (n = 15) had a two-year disease-free survival rate of 13% (Figure 2B).

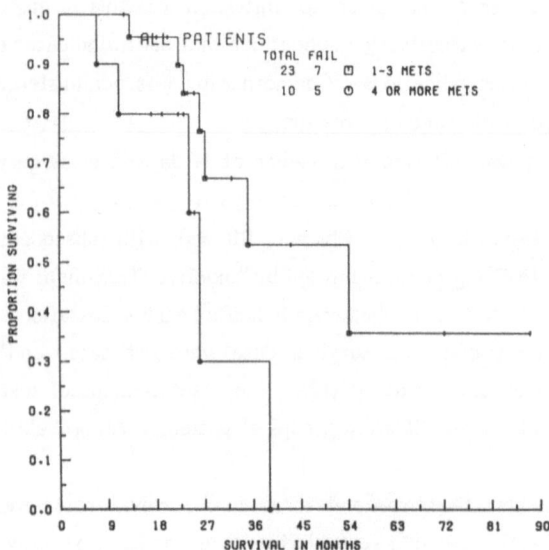

FIGURE 1A. Survival rates of all patients, based on the number of metastases resected.

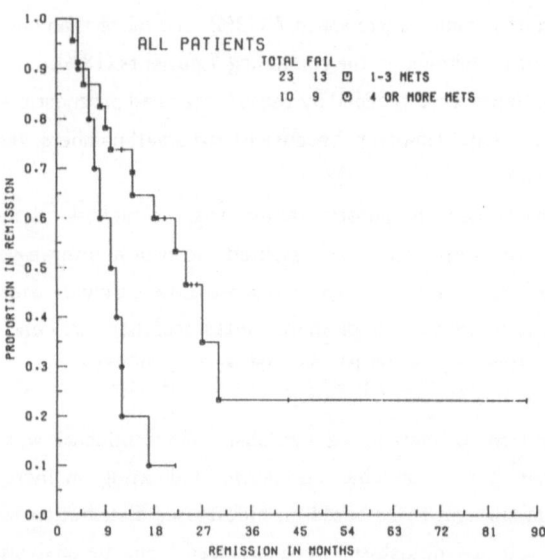

FIGURE 1B. Disease-free survival rates of all patients, based on the number of metastases resected.

162

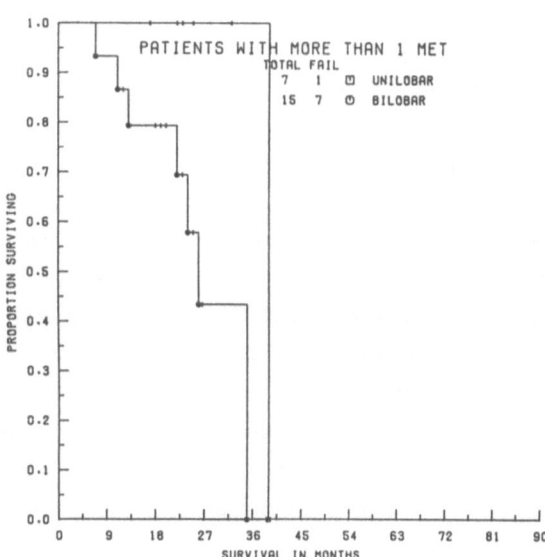

FIGURE 2A.   Survival rates of patients with more than one metastasis, based on metastases distribution.

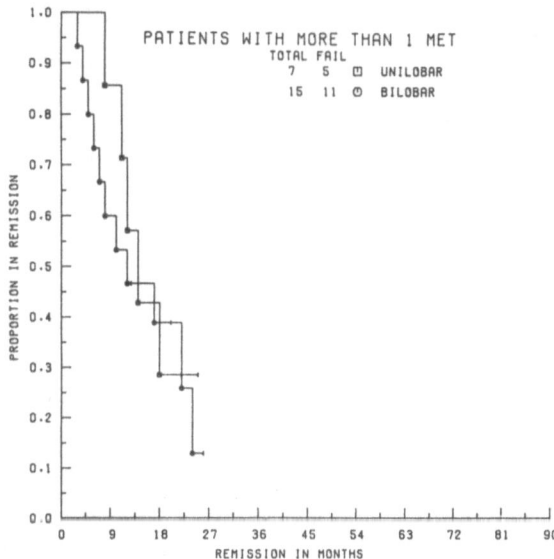

FIGURE 2B.   Disease-free survival rates of patients with more than one metastasis, based on metastases distribution.

All four patients with microscopic disease in the surgical margins developed clinically apparent recurrent disease within one year, but all survived beyond two years.

Sex, the Dukes' stage of the primary lesion, the location of the primary tumor (colon versus rectum), the interval between bowel resection and detection of hepatic metastases (disease-free interval), the preoperative carcinoembryonic antigen (CEA) level, the method of detection of hepatic metastasis, and the type of operation (lobectomy versus wedge resection) were not found to significantly affect survival rates; but again, the number of cases is small and the follow-up time is short.

Twenty-one patients underwent intraperitoneal 5-FU treatment as part of a pilot study. There was no significant increase in survival time among patients treated with intraperitoneal 5-FU. However, patients receiving 5-FU had an average of 3.7 metastases versus an average of 2.2 metastases among the untreated group. Among patients with one to three metastases, there is a trend toward an increased survival time in the treated group, but follow-up time is short, and the differences are not statistically significant (Figure 3A,B).

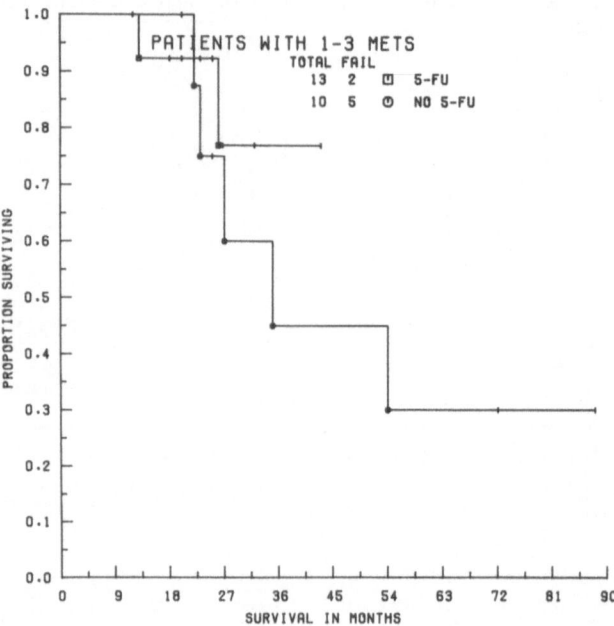

FIGURE 3A. Survival rates of patients with one to three metastases, based on treatment regimen.

164

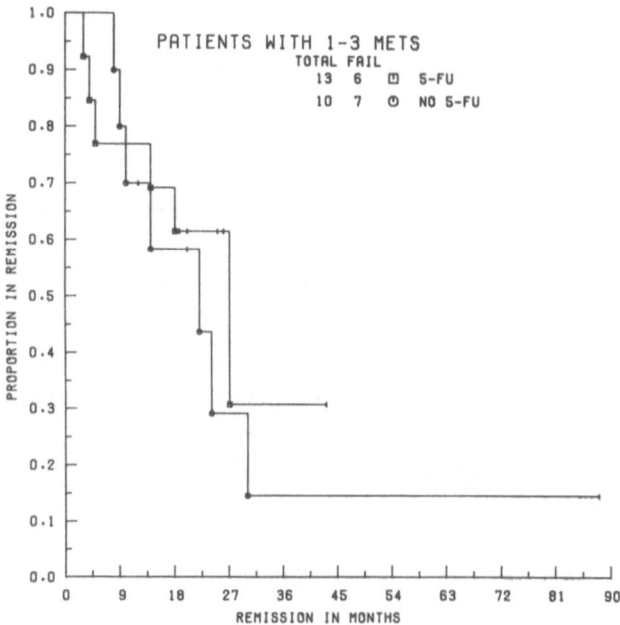

FIGURE 3B. Disease-free survival rates of patients with one to three metastases, based on treatment regimen.

A prospective, randomized trial comparing intraperitoneal 5-FU versus no further treatment is now being conducted at the NCI.

SURVEY OF THE LITERATURE

Liver resection is the only treatment option currently available that can lead to the cure of metastatic colorectal cancer. This procedure must be considered, therefore, for any patient with liver metastases. But the question remains, how do we determine who will benefit from liver resection?

The literature is replete with operative series of resected colorectal metastases, and all series come to similar general conclusions . The reported five-year survival rates range from 23% (1) to 55% (2), with a mixture of actual and actuarial survival, but with the majority sharing a less-than-40% five-year survival rate (3-9). This means, according

165

to the majority of the reports, that more than 60% of patients underwent liver resection without being cured.

Improved techniques and experience have resulted in decreased mortality rates to less than 10%, and this has encouraged surgeons to extend the indications for this operation. However, the incidence of complications is still 20-40%, and about six weeks are required before the patient can resume his normal activities. The surgical treatment of this disease would be improved if we could determine who would benefit from resection and whose prognosis would not be changed. We would then be able to define a group of patients who needed adjuvant treatment and begin clinical trials.

Factors that may have prognostic significance are listed in Table 1. According to this list, we find 12 preoperative factors, 8 operative factors, and 4 postoperative factors. After resection, the parameters that need to be followed include survival time, disease-free survival time, site of initial recurrence, other sites of recurrence, and future liver involvement. With such a large number of prognostic factors, a large number of patients is obviously required to perform significant multifactorial analysis.

Table 1. Factors that may have prognostic significance

Type	Factor
Preoperative	Sex of patient, site of primary tumor, Dukes' stage of primary tumor, histologic type, grade of primary tumor, how metastases were detected, presence or absence of symptoms, time of detection of liver metastases, time from detection to resection, liver function (Child's), extrahepatic disease, CEA* level
Operative	Presence and type of extrahepatic disease, number of nodules involved, lobes of the liver involved, size of nodules, histologic type, grade of metastasis, type of resection, margin of resection
Postoperative	Whether chemotherapy administered, type of chemotherapy, route of administration, CEA level

*   CEA: carcinoembryonic antigen

The literature comprises 16 series (1-10, 14-19) whose patient populations appear to be mutually exclusive. These series contain from 5-231 patients; only two of these series have greater than 70 patients (1,5). There are few patients reported who have been followed longer than five years in any series, as shown in Table 2.

Table 2 Sixteen Series Collected from the Surgical Literature

Report	Year	No. of Patients	No. of patients Followed longer than 5 years
(Series that include only colorectal metastases to the liver)			
Adson et al. (5,20-23)	1984	141	< 31(?)
August et al. (10)	1984	33	2
Cady and McDermott (6)	1984	23	< 5(?)
Nims (19)	1984	9	0
Fortner et al. (4)	1984	65	13
Kambouris (14)	1983	5	0
Lim and McPherson (18)	1983	7	0
Bengmark et al. (15)	1982	39	3
Rajpal et al. (16)	1982	34	0
Foster and Lundy (1,24-26)	1981	231	53
Attiyeh et al. (3)	1978	25	8
(Series that include noncolorectal metastases and primary liver tumors)			
Kortz et al. (8)	1984	16	(?)
Steele et al. (17)	1984	30	1
Iwatsuki et al. (2)	1983	24	(?)
Morrow et al. (9)	1983	29	3
Thompson et al. (7)	1983	22	3

Among the 16 reports found in the literature (1-10, 14-19) those factors which have been suggested to correlate with survival time include sex (5), site of primary tumor (9), stage of primary tumor (3-5), the detection of synchronous versus metachronous metastases (3,5), the presence of extrahepatic disease of indistinguishable type (5), size of nodules (5), number of nodules (1,5,6,10), pathology at the margin of resection (6,10,16), the unilobar versus bilobar distribution of metastases (10), and the type of liver resection (5). There is an equal number of series that deny the correlation of one or

167

more of these factors with survival (1,4-10,15) and a number of series that can not make any serious comment about any of the factors because of failure to report on the factor, small numbers of patients, or short follow-up (2,14,17-19). These observations are summarized in Table 3.

Table 3. Suggested Prognostic Factors in Hepatic Resection

Factor	References 1	2	3	4	5	6	7	8	9	10	14	15	16	17	18	19
Sex	0	0	0	-	+	-	0	0	0	0	0	0	0	0	0	0
Site of primary tumor	0	0	0	-	-	-	0	0	0	+	0	0	0	0	0	0
Stage of primary tumor	-	0	+	+	+	-	-	0	-	-	0	0	0	0	0	0
Disease-free interval	-	0	+	-	+	0	0	-	0	-	0	-	0	0	0	0
Extrahepatic disease	0	0	0	0	+	0	0	0	0	0	0	0	0	0	0	0
Size of metastases	+	0	0	0	+	-	0	0	0	0	0	0	0	0	0	0
Number of metastases	+	0	0	-	+	+	0	0	0	+	0	0	0	0	0	0
Margin of resection	-	0	0	-	0	+	0	0	0	+	0	0	+	0	0	0
Preresection CEA*	0	0	0	-	0	0	0	0	0	-	0	0	0	0	0	0
Type of resection	-	0	0	-	+	0	0	0	0	-	0	0	0	0	0	0
Distribution of metastases (unilobar vs. bilobar)	0	0	0	0	0	0	0	0	0	+	0	0	0	0	0	0

There is no information available regarding the effect of delaying hepatic resection after hepatic metastases are detected. Divergent opinions are expressed by Cady and McDermott (6) and August et al. (27). Cady suggests that delaying resection several months will help avoid unnecessary surgery by allowing other subclinical hepatic or extrahepatic metastases to become clinically detectable. Our opinion, as expressed by August et al. (27), is that metastases metastasize and that the longer a hepatic metastasis is in place, the more chance it has to shed viable cancer cells. In our series of 46 laparotomies for apparently resectable metastatic lesions, five patients were found to have unresectable disease after metastatic deposits were discovered in lymph nodes draining the liver at laparotomy. The most likely source of these metastases was the hepatic lesion. The proper surgical strategy regarding early versus delayed operation cannot be ascertained from the available data.

Why is it that prognostic factors have not yet been better defined? The main problems are the large number of prognostic factors, the small size of the single-institution experience, and the relatively short time that liver resection has been popular. In putting together the 16 major series we found 733 colon resections reported, but only a small fraction of these have follow-up reports beyond five years. Each series uses a different method of reporting degree of liver involvement and a different method of reporting follow-up data. Because of those differences, the data reported so far cannot be synthesized into a single data base, and many answerable questions remain unanswered.

The major factors believed to influence prognosis are disease-free interval, or the time of detection of liver metastases (synchronous, early and late metachronous), number of metastases, (1,2-3, >3), size of metastases, (small, medium, large), and presence or absence of preoperative symptoms. In evaluating these four factors, we find 11 subgroups. If each factor is considered an independent variable, there are 54 possible combinations. It is not possible to evaluate 54 separate combinations when most series have fewer than 50 patients. The difficulty is emphasized by Adson et al. (5), who have the largest single-institution series with 141 patients. They state that when studying time of detection of liver metastasis (synchronous versus metachronous), size of metastasis (small versus large), and number of metastases (single versus multiple), eight combinations are created. In that study, "small sample size precluded some comparisons and eroded statistical analysis." Furthermore, when Wilson and Adson studied 60 patients in 1976 (23), they found that the presence of multiple metastases resulted in an extremely poor prognosis. Yet, in 1984, when the results from this study were combined with the results from a study of 81 other patients, the original analysis was eroded; patients with multiple metastases survived just as well as patients with solitary metastases (20). This example illustrates the fallibility of small series.

Despite the problems encountered selecting patients for surgery, currently, hepatic resection is the only hope for cure in metastatic colorectal cancer. After reviewing the natural history of hepatic colorectal metastases, Wagner et al. (21) note that almost all unresected patients are dead within five years. There is a definite difference between three-year survival rates of patients with single metastases (21%), multiple unilobar metastases (6%), and widespread bilobar disease (4%). More specific observations on unresected metastases again are hindered by small numbers of cases, but in solitary unresected metastases, less well differentiated tumors have a poorer prognosis and patients with Dukes' C stage primary tumors have a poorer prognosis than those with B stage primary tumors. These observations were not found to be statistically significant when dealing with multiple metastases.

Even the natural history of hepatic metastases is not completely clear. One of the patients reported by Attiyeh et al. (3) had multiple bilobar metastases 5 and 10 years after a biopsy of her tumor. The patient survived 11 years and died of her disease. A patient reported by Levine et al. (28) lived 14 years treated with chemotherapy despite documented bilobar metastases, although all other patients on the same regimen died within 3 years.

STAGING OF HEPATIC METASTASES FROM COLORECTAL CANCER

Uniform staging of hepatic metastases would be of help in comparing the treatment results from different institutions. Many staging systems have been proposed in an attempt to separate patients into specific prognostic groups. In 1982, Gennari (29) reviewed eight classification systems for colorectal cancer metastases to the liver and proposed a ninth. In 1984, Petrelli (30) proposed a tenth classification system. Several prognostic factors are considered important for stratifying patients. Degree of hepatic involvement is probably the main factor; it is measured by estimating the percentage of hepatic replacement, the size of the liver, general liver function test values including alkaline phosphatase level or bilirubin level. Other factors considered important include the number of metastases, their distribution (unilobar versus bilobar), their size, their resectability, the disease-free interval (detection of synchronous versus metachronous metastases), absence or presence of extrahepatic disease, type of extrahepatic disease (contiguous versus distant), performance status of the patient, and the presence or absence of symptoms.

In 1984, a group of surgeons with an interest in liver resection met in Leiden, The Netherlands, to consider the staging systems currently in use. They proposed a staging system that included the major prognostic indicators and was simple enough for general use (31). Stratification is based on tumor resectability, extent of hepatic involvement, the presence or absence of symptoms, and the presence or absence of extrahepatic disease.

Extent of hepatic involvement is recorded as percent hepatic replacement (PHR). P1 is less than 25 PHR, P2 is 26-75 PHR, and P3 is greater than 75 PHR. Extrahepatic disease is designated by the letter E, and the presence of symptoms is designated by the letter S. Four stages are defined (Table 4). Stages I, II, and III disease are all unresectable. This is a useful classification for tumors that should be treated by regional or systemic modalities. Stage 0 is obviously a very broad category and needs further definition. However, the data is not yet available to better define this stage. This brings us to the second phase of this project, which is to develop uniform recording and reporting methods in order to define the significant prognostic factors in stage 0 disease.

170

Table 4. Leiden Classification System for Hepatic Metastases

Stage	Description
0	Curatively resected metastases
I	P1 (no E, no S)
II	P2 (no E, no S)
III	P3 (no E, no S) or P1, P2, or P3 with E,S, or both

Uniform Recording and Reporting of Stage 0 Disease

As discussed previously, stage 0 includes a diverse group of patients that cannot be separated into prognostic groups because of insufficient data. Prognostic factors would become apparent if data were recorded in a standardized fashion; therefore, data sheets have been developed at the NCI (Figure 4) that are simple and easily computerized and that contain information on all factors currently considered to have prognostic significance. A separate sheet is used to record the pathology of the disease (Figure 5), and a follow-up sheet (Figure 6) is updated every six months. Follow-up data to be obtained are survival time, disease-free survival time, method of detection of recurrence, site of initial recurrence, and other sites of recurrence.

At the NCI, patients are followed after resection according to the flow sheet shown in Figure 7. The CEA level is checked monthly for two years, a computed tomographic (CT) scan of the abdomen is performed every three months for three years, and frequent physical examinations are performed. The follow-up reports should help determine which tests are valuable in detecting recurrence and whether early detection after hepatic resection allows further effective treatments.

If all surgeons resecting hepatic metastases from colorectal cancer would use these data sheets, a central data base could be formed, and answers to specific questions could be found. All patients who undergo laparotomy for possible resection should also be reported so the preoperative assessment of resectability could be evaluated.

Once it has been determined which patients are likely to relapse, and where the disease is likely to recur, more effective adjuvant therapies can be tested. In the NCI series, disease recurred only in the liver in 52% of the patients, and only in the lungs in 32% of the patients. When these findings are evaluated in a multi-institutional series, adjuvant treatments can be planned in a site-specific manner.

171

RESECTION OF COLORECTAL HEPATIC METASTASES
CLINICAL RECORD

Patient Name:_____ Hospital:_____

Hospital Number:_____ Surgeon:_____

Birthdate:_____

(A) PRIMARY COLON OR RECTAL TUMOR

1. Date of Resection:____/____/____   2. Location: 3. Duke's Stage (Astler-Coller)
                                                Ascending   A   B1   B2   C1   C2
                                                Transverse
                                                Descending
                                                Sigmoid
                                                Rectum

4. Nodes Resected: 5. Contiguous Structures Invaded:
                                        Omentum   Small Bowel
        ____/____   Prostate   Abdominal Wall
      Pos.   Total   Bladder   Pelvic Side Wall
                                        Ovaries   Other_____
                                        Uterus   None

6. Histology: 7. Grade: 8. Other Treatment Prior to
      Adenocarcinoma   Poor   Liver Metastases:
      Signet Ring Adenocarcinoma   Moderate   None
      Carcinoma Simplex   Well   Radiation Therapy
      Mucinous Adenocarcinoma   Chemotherapy
      Scirrhous

(B) PREOPERATIVE TO HEPATIC RESECTION

1. Date of Diagnosis:____/____/____   2. Determined By: 3. Karnofsky Scale:
                                                L/S Scan   Rising CEA   0   1   2   3   4
                                                CT Scan   Ultrasound
                                                Laparotomy   Other

4. Symptoms: 5. Nutrition: 6. Ascites:
      Present   Excellent   None
      Absent   Good   Easily Controlled
                              Poor   Poorly Controlled

7. Bilirubin (mg%):   8. Alkaline Phosphatase: 9. Albumin (g%):
      <2   <2 x Normal   >3.5
      2 - 3   2 - 4 x   3 - 3.5
      >3   >2 x   <3

(C) OPERATION FOR HEPATIC RESECTION

1. Date:____/____/____   2. Number of Metastases Found:_____ _____   3. Wedges:
                                                                                  No. L Lobe____
                                                                                  No. R Lobe____

4. Major Resection: 5. Extrahepatic Disease: 6. Other Organs Resected:
      L Lobe   None   None   Small Bowel
      R Lobe   Nodes   Diaphragm   Abdominal Wall
      L Lat. Seg.   Contiguous   Adrenal   Omentum
      Triseg   Discontinuous   Kidney   Other_____

7. Made NED:
      Yes
      No

(D) POSTOPERATIVE

1. CEA (Nadir):   2. Complications: 3. Chemotherapy and Route:
                              None   None   IV (periph)
      _____ Date:_____   Bleeding   5-FU   Intra-peritoneal
                              Infection-Intraabdominal   FUDR   Intra-arterial
                              Infection-Wound   Other   Intra-portal
                              Other____ _____

FIGURE 4. Data sheet for recording factors with prognostic significance for colorectal hepatic metastases. (Abbreviations: L/S - liver/spleen; CEA - carcinoembryonic antigen; CT - computed tomography.)

172

RESECTION OF COLORECTAL HEPATIC METASTASES
PATHOLOGIC RECORD

Patient Name: _____   Hospital: _____

Hospital Number: _____

(F) GROSS EXAM

1. Total Number of Nodules on the Surface of Specimen: _____

2. Total Number of Nodules Seen Upon Cutting Specimen into 1 cm Slices: _____

3. Location of Individual Metastases:

	1.		2.		3.		4.		5.	
	L	R	L	R	L	R	L	R	L	R
Left/Right:	M	L	M	L	M	L	M	L	M	L
Med./Lat.:	A	P	A	P	A	P	A	P	A	P
Ant./Post.:	U	L	U	L	U	L	U	L	U	L
Upp./Lower:										

5. Extrahepatic Invasion:
    None
    Nodes
    Contiguous
    Discontinuous

4. Closest Margin:
    Gross Inspection: _____
    Microscopic: _____

(G) ANALYSIS OF INDIVIDUAL METASTASES

	#1	#2	#3	#4	#5
1. Size (greatest Diameter)					
2. Grade (1 [poor] to 3 [well])					
3. Histologic Type					
4. Hepatic Venous Invasion (Y/N)					
5. Lymphatic Invasion (Y/N)					
6. Portal Venous Invasion (Y/N)					
7. Inflammatory Response (Y/N)					
8. Tumor Border (1=pushing, 2=infiltrating) . .					
9. Necrosis (0 [least] to 4 [most])					
10. Daughter Metastases (number)					

KEY: 2. 1 = Poor   2 = Moderate   3 = Well

      3. 1 = Adenocarcinoma   2 = Scirrhous   3 = Mucinous   4 = Signet Ring

          5 = Carcinoma Simplex

FIGURE 5. Data sheet for recording pathology of colorectal hepatic metastases.

173

RESECTION OF COLORECTAL HEPATIC METASTASES
FOLLOW-UP RECORD

Patient Name: _____

Hospital Number: _____   Hospital: _____

(E) FOLLOW-UP

1. Date of Follow-Up: ____/____/____

2. Status: 3. Karnofsky Scale:
        ANED   0   1   2   3   4
        DNED
        AWD
        DWD

4. Site of Initial Recurrence: 5. Date of Initial
        Liver   Lung   Recurrence: ____/____/____
        Local/Regional Bone
        Retroperitoneal Other_____

6. Diagnosis By: 7. Hepatic Recurrence: 8. Date of Hepatic
        L/S Scan   Rising CEA   Yes   Recurrence:
        CT Scan   Laparotomy   No   ____/____/____
        Other   Whole Lung Tomograms

9. Other Sites of Recurrence: 10. Made NED After Recurrence:
        Liver   Yes
        Local/Regional   No
        Retroperitoneum
        Lung
        Bone
        Other_____

FIGURE 6. Data sheet for recording follow-up report information on colorectal hepatic metastases. (Abbreviations: CEA - carcinoembryonic antigen; CT - computed tomography; ANED - alive, no evidence of disease; DNED - dead, no evidence of disease; AWD - alive, with disease; DWD - dead, with disease; L/S scan - liver/spleen scan; CT - computed tomography; CEA - carcinoembryonic antigen, NED - no evidence of disease.

174

RESECTION OF COLORECTAL HEPATIC METASTASES
FOLLOW-UP FLOW SHEET

Follow-up Months - From Surgery

Month	1	2	3	4	5	6	7	8	9	10	11	12	13	14	15	16	17	18	19	20	21	22	23	24	27	30	33	36	39	42	45	48	51	54	57	60
Date																																				
CEA	x	x	x	x	x	x	x	x	x	x	x	x	x	x	x	x	x	x	x	x	x	x	x	x	x	x	x	x	x	x	x	x	x	x	x	x
CBC & SMAC	x	x	x	x	x	x			x			x			x			x			x			x		x		x		x		x		x		x
Physical Exam	x		x						x			x			x			x			x			x		x		x		x		x		x		x
CT Abdomen (or Ultrasound, or Liver/Spleen Scan)									x			x			x			x			x			x	x	x	x	x		x		x		x		x
Chest X-ray						x						x						x						x												x
Lung Tomograms						x						x						x						x				x				x				x
Bone Scan												x												x				x				x				x
Barium Enema/ Sigmoidoscopy and IVP												x												x												x

FIGURE 7. Flow sheet of clinical data for follow-up of patients after hepatic resection. (Abbreviations: CEA - carcinoembryonic antigen; CBC - complete blood count; SMAC - sequential multiple analytic computer; CT - computed tomography; IVP - intravenous pyelogram.

ADJUVANT TREATMENTS FOLLOWING HEPATIC RESECTION

There have been no reported prospective, randomized trials of adjuvant therapy after hepatic resection to date, but many ideas have been advanced. Possible adjuvant treatments include intra-arterial 5-FU or fluorodeoxyuridine (FUdR), intraportal 5-FU, or intravenous 5-FU.

The NCI is currently conducting a randomized prospective trial comparing intraperitoneal 5-FU with no further treatment after potentially curative hepatic resection. The rationale behind this therapy is that high local levels of chemotherapy prevent peritoneal carcinomatosis (32), and high portal levels prevent hepatic metastases (33).

Intra-arterial FUdR given after resection has been suggested by Kemeny and co-workers (personal communication, September 1984). This may be an effective adjuvant treatment against hepatic recurrence (the liver was the site of initial recurrence in 50% of the NCI patients). However, the effects of FUdR on hepatic regeneration are not known, and nonhepatic recurrence will most likely remain unaffected.

Intraportal 5-FU has been used after resection by Fortner (4), but because of the small numbers of patients studied, it is not possible to draw conclusions. This mode of treatment has drawbacks similar to those of intra-arterial FUdR, in that the effects on hepatic regeneration or extrahepatic metastases are not known. Fortner did report one death from portal vein thrombosis when using this method (4). Multi-institutional, randomized, prospective trials will give the most extensive information on the effectiveness of these adjuvant treatments.

PREVENTION OF HEPATIC METASTASES

Another approach to hepatic metastases that is only beginning to be explored is prophylaxis. In 1967, Turnbull et al. (34) popularized the no-touch technique, its rationale being that manipulation of the tumor would shower viable cancer cells into the portal vein. He reported decreased liver metastases in patients treated by the no-touch isolation technique. In a randomized prospective trial, (Hans Jeekel, personal communication, 1984) has recently reported the suggestion of a decrease in hepatic metastases when the no-touch technique is used.

Taylor (35) has reported favorable preliminary results of a randomized, prospective trial in which the umbilical vein is catheterized after colon or rectal cancer resection and 5-FU is infused into the portal vein for seven days. The reasoning behind this treatment is that blood-borne metastases in the liver are effectively treated by 5-FU chemotherapy. Decreased hepatic metastases have been noted in treated patients. Further studies are needed to confirm these preliminary results.

Hepatic resection for colorectal carcinoma metastases is a multifactorial problem and requires a cooperative approach to find meaningful answers to the questions surrounding this issue.

References

1. Foster JH, Lundy J: Pathology of liver metastasis. Curr Probl Surg 18: 157-202, 1981.
2. Iwatsuki S, Shaw BW, Starzl TE: Experience with 150 liver resections. Ann Surg 197: 247-253, 1983.
3. Attiyeh FF, Wanebo HJ, Stearns MW: Hepatic resection for metastasis from colorectal cancer. Dis Colon Rectum 21: 160-162, 1978.
4. Fortner JG, Silva JS, Golbey RB, Cox EB, MacLean BJ: Multivariate analysis of a personal series of 247 consecutive patients with liver metastases from colorectal cancer. Ann Surg 199: 306-316, 1984.
5. Adson MA, van Heerden JA, Adson MH, Wagner JS, Ilstrup DM: Resection of hepatic metastases from colorectal cancer. Arch Surg 119: 647-651, 1984.
6. Cady B, McDermott WV: Major hepatic resection for metachronous metastases from colon cancer. Ann Surg 201:204-209, 1985.
7. Thompson HH, Tompkins RK, Longmire WP: Major hepatic resection: A 25-year experience. Ann Surg 197: 375-388, 1983.
8. Kortz WJ, Meyers WC, Hanks JB, Schirmer BD, Jones RS: Hepatic resection for metastatic cancer. Ann Surg 199: 182-186, 1984.
9. Morrow CE, Grage TB, Sutherland DE, Najarian JS: Hepatic resection for secondary neoplasms. Surgery 92: 610-614, 1983.
10. August DA, Sugarbaker PH, Ottow RT, Gianola FJ, Schneider PD: Hepatic resection of colorectal metastases: Influence of clinical factors and adjuvant intraperitoneal 5-FU via Tenckhoff catheter on survival. Ann Surg 201: 210-218, 1985.
11. Astler VB, Coller FA: The prognostic significance of direct extension of carcinoma of the colon and rectum. Ann Surg 139: 846-852, 1954.
12. Kaplan EL, Meier P: Nonparametric estimation from incomplete observations. J Am Stat Assoc 53: 457-481, 1958.
13. Mantel N, Haenszel W: Statistical aspects of the analysis of data from retrospective studies of disease. J Natl Cancer Inst 22: 719-748, 1959.
14. Kambouris AA: The role of major hepatic resections for liver metastases from colorectal cancer. Henry Ford Hosp Med J 31: 25-29, 1983.
15. Bengmark S, Hafstrom L, Jeppsson B, Jonsson P, Ryden S, Sundqvist K: Metastatic disease in the liver from colorectal cancer: An appraisal of liver surgery. World J Surg 6: 61-65, 1982.
16. Rajpal S, Dasmahapatra KS, Ledesma EJ, Mittelman A: Extensive resections of isolated metastases from carcinoma of the colon and rectum. Surg Gynecol Obstet 155: 813-816, 1982.
17. Steele G, Osteen RT, Wilson RE, Brooks DC, Mayer RJ, Zamcheck N, Ravikumar T: Patterns of failure after surgical cure of large liver tumors. Am J Surg 147: 554-559, 1984.
18. Lim CN-H, McPherson TA: Surgery as an alternative to chemotherapy for hepatic metastases from colorectal cancer. Cancer J Surg 26: 458-459, 1983.

19. Nims TA: Resection of the liver for metastatic cancer. Surg Gynecol Obstet 158: 46-48, 1984.
20. Wagner JS, Adson MA, van Heerden JA, Adson MH, Ilstrup DM: The natural history of hepatic metastases from colorectal cancer. Ann Surg 199: 502-508, 1984.
21. Adson MA: Hepatic resection. Dis Colon Rectum 22: 366-370, 1979.
22. Adson MA: Hepatic metastases in perspective. Am J Radiol 140, 695-700, 1983.
23. Wilson SM, Adson MA: Surgical treatment of hepatic metastases from colorectal cancers. Arch Surg 111: 330-334, 1976.
24. Wanebo HJ, Semoglou C, Attiyeh F, Stearns MJ: Surgical management of patients with primary operable colorectal cancer and synchronous liver metastases. Am J Surg 135: 81-85, 1978.
25. Macphee IW: The excision of malignant secondary hepatic deposits. Br J Surg 56: 831-832, 1969.
26. Foster JH: Survival after liver resection for secondary deposits. Br J Surg 135: 389-394, 1978.
27. August DA, Sugarbaker PH, Schneider PD: Lymphatic dissemination of hepatic metastases: Implications for the follow-up and treatment of patients with colorectal cancer. Cancer 1985 (In press).
28. Levine AW, Donegan WL, Irwin M: Adenocarcinoma of the colon with hepatic metastasis, fifteen-year survival. J Am Med Assoc 247: 2809-2810, 1982.
29. Gennari L, Doci R, Bozzetti F, Veronesi U: Proposal for a clinical classification of liver metastases. Tumori 68: 443-449, 1982.
30. Petrelli NJ, Bonnheim DC, Herrera LO, Mittelman A: A proposed classification system for liver metastases from colorectal carcinoma. Dis Colon Rectum 27: 249-252, 1984.
31. Sugarbaker PH, van de Velde C, Veenhof CHN: A matrix for controlled clinical trials for the study of hepatic metastases: Proceedings of a workshop. J Surg Oncol 1985 (In press).
32. Speyer JL: Intraperitoneal chemotherapy . . . a possible role in the treatment of hepatic metastases. In: CJH van de Velde and PH Sugarbaker (eds), Liver metastasis: Basic aspects, detection and management. Martinus Nijhoff Publishers, Dordrecht, The Netherlands, 1984, pp 249.
33. Sugarbaker PH, Speyer JC, Gianola FJ, Meyers CE: Prospective randomized trial of intravenous vs. intraperitoneal 5-FU in patients with advanced primary colon and rectal cancer. Surgery 1985 (In press).
34. Turnbull RB Jr, Kyle K, Watson FR, Spratt J: Cancer of the colon: The Influence of the No-Touch Isolation technique on survival rates. Ann Surg 166: 420-427, 1967.
35. Taylor I, Brooman P, Rowling JT: Adjuvant liver perfusion in colorectal cancer: Initial results of a clinical trial. Br Med J 2: 1320-1325, 1977.

15

NEW DIAGNOSTIC TECHNIQUES IN HEPATIC MASS DETECTION

Michael E. Bernardino

SUMMARY

During the past five years there have been rapid advances in technology and in the development of contrast agents and other techniques used to enhance hepatic imaging capabilities. This chapter briefly summarizes some of these new techniques, including sonography, computed tomography, and magnetic resonance imaging. An overview of the strengths and the limitations of these various techniques, together with their specific applications, is presented.

COMPUTED TOMOGRAPHY AND SONOGRAPHY

Until recently radionuclide imaging, sonography, and computed tomography (CT) have been used in hepatic screening or problem solving. Most of the previous comparative studies dealing with these diagnostic modalities have shown CT to be the most accurate method (1-3). The accuracy varies depending on the institution, quality of equipment, and expertise of the individuals involved. Some authors have stated that the accuracy of CT is not significantly greater than the other diagnostic techniques and does not warrant the added cost (2,3). These data do not take into account the fact that CT and ultrasound image more than the liver (4,5). It is quite possible for a patient with colon carcinoma to have a normal liver and to have disease in the adrenal glands or retroperitoneum. Thus, data comparing the various modalities are somewhat skewed and do not consider the other sites of disease. No other single diagnostic test yields as much information about multiplicity of disease sites at the initial staging procedure.

Previous accuracy figures do not take into account the newer diagnostic techniques of any of the three modalities. Radionuclide imaging can now be obtained with tomographic potential scanning (6). This new technique allows one to detect lesions of roughly 1-2 cm. Few institutions currently have this technique available. However, it has increased the accuracy of routine radionuclide hepatic imaging.

Sonography has not changed significantly over the past four years (7). Advances in real time have not changed the basic resolution of 1-2 cm. New data are being generated with the use of hepatic-specific sonographic agents (8). These agents raise the echogenicity of the normal liver. It is hoped that they will create an echogenic difference between normal and abnormal hepatic parenchyma so that smaller lesions can be detected with greater accuracy and reliability. However, utilization of such materials is at least four to five years away.

CT can be augmented with hepatic-specific contrast agents (9-12). These agents vary from heavy metals to Ethiodol compounds. The most promising agents are the liposomes and emulsions. These materials are taken up by the reticuloendothelial system, much like radionuclide imaging, and transferred to the hepatocytes. They raise the inherent density of normal tissue, depending on the dose. Usually, it is in the range of 30-50 Hounsfield units. The amount of iodine used is less than for routine intravenous pyelography. This is due to the fact that the iodine is aimed at a single organ rather than being dispersed in the extravascular space. The agent that has been used the most is EOE-13, an oily emulsion of Ethiodol. It is excreted almost entirely by the kidneys over 72 hours. It has increased the diagnostic accuracy of routine CT by 42% in one study (Figure 1A & B) (13). In another study dealing with splenic involvement by lymphoma, it increased the diagnostic accuracy ninefold (14). Smaller lesions, some less than .5 cm, are detected with this material. Many of the larger lesions are also more reliably detected owing to the fact that the true edge of the tumor is noted rather than its blending in with the surrounding hepatic parenchyma. In a recent study of 225 examinations using this material, there was less than a 4% complication rate (15). Thus, the agent is relatively safe. At present, the greatest drawback to these materials is their lack of availability. They are still experimental.

Delayed iodine imaging is the most recent advance in CT. Delayed iodine CT scans are performed after administering 60-80 g of iodine, intravenously. The liver naturally excretes 1-2% of the iodine load. Thus, the density of the liver is increased at four hours after the administration of iodine. The relative increase is roughly 22 Hounsfield units. This is a 40% increase over the normal density of the liver. Therefore, the delayed iodine images look very much like the hepatic-specific contrast images (Figure 2A & B). However, because knowledge of this imaging techinique is new, there are no data comparing this type of imaging with routine imaging, angiography, or hepatic-specific agents. Delayed iodine imaging holds the potential for increased accuracy in hepatic CT without the use of more invasive techniques or hepatic-specific agents. Also, the side effects of currently used intravenous urographic agents are well known. Thus, the technique may be applicable at every institution.

180

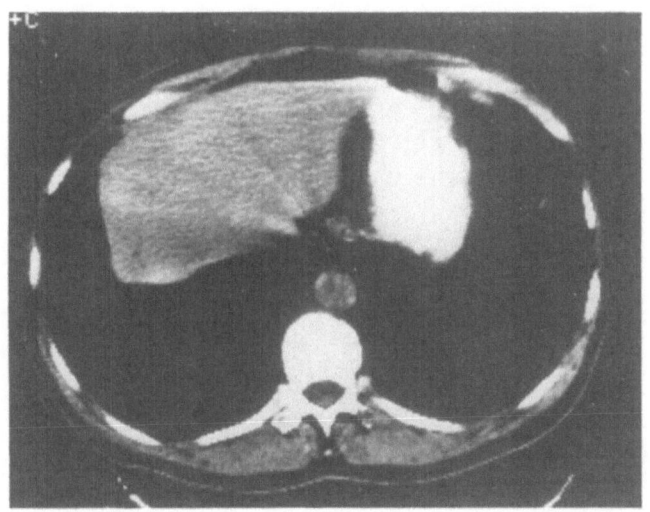

FIGURE 1A. CT scan through the upper portion of the liver demonstrates no focal lesions.

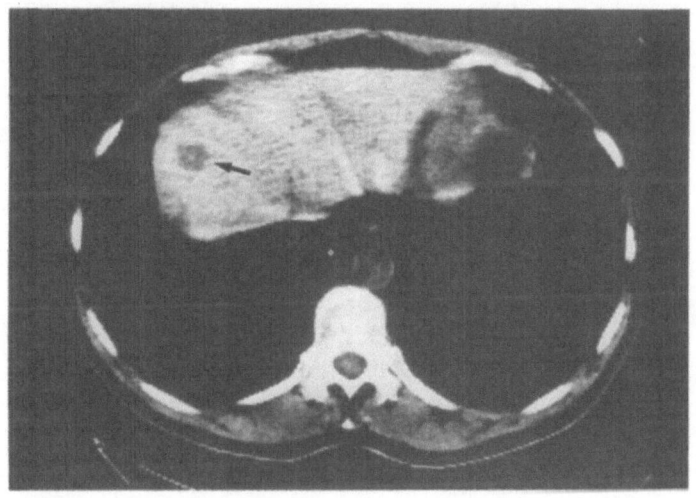

FIGURE 1B. After EOE-13, a single solitary lesion (arrow) is noted.

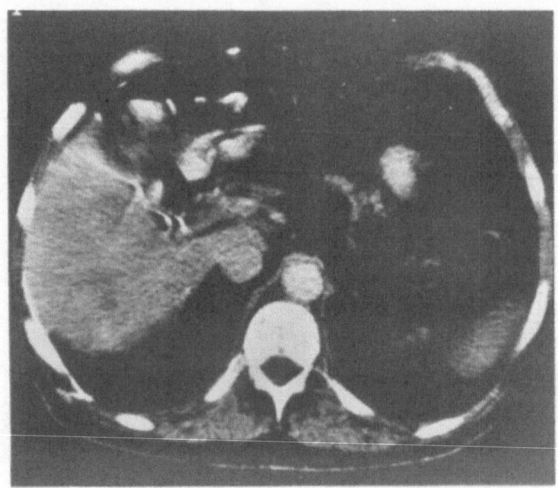

FIGURE 2A. After dynamic sequential CT, some mottled areas are noted in the lower portion of the right hepatic lobe.

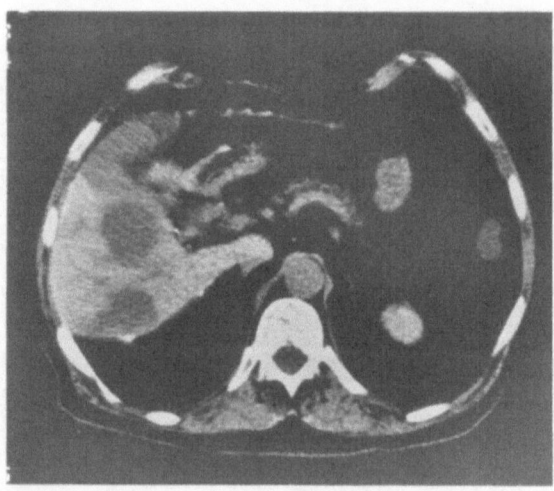

FIGURE 2B. Repeat CT scan four hours later demonstrates multiple large hepatic metastases. The delayed iodine studies are very similar to the EOE-13 studies.

CT angiography combines the two procedures (16). A catheter may be placed in the hepatic artery or celiac axis. A slow infusion of 30% iodine is perfused through the catheter while the CT study is performed. The images are detected because metastases are fed predominantly from the hepatic artery. Therefore, the periphery of the tumors is enhanced. If there is portal venous obstruction, a high-density wedge-shaped defect may be located in the periphery. The high-density wedge is due to arterial portal communication distal to the tumor obstruction (Figure 3). Using this technique, 60% more lesions were detected than by either angiography or CT alone (17). This technique significantly decreased the number of patients who might have been considered for possible partial hepatectomy.

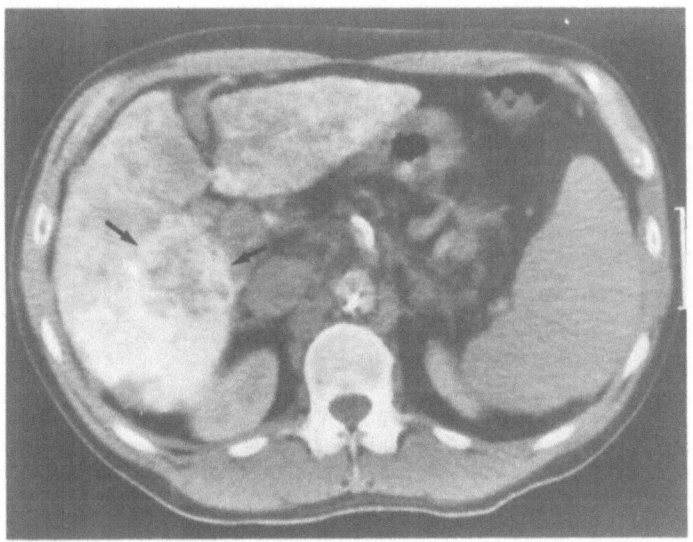

FIGURE 3. A CT angiogram with the catheter placed in the hepatic artery demonstrates a hepatoma in the right hepatic lobe. The periphery (arrows) of the hepatoma is of higher density because of its increased vasculature. The area distal to the hepatoma is almost entirely opacified because of hepatic artery-portal vein shunting resulting from obstruction to the portal vein proximally.

A variation of this technique is injecting contrast material through the superior mesenteric artery. This is the variation favored by the Japanese (18). In this technique, the liver increases in density owing to the return of blood flow from the superior mesenteric vein and portal vein. Since tumors are not fed from the portal system, they appear as low-density defects within a high-density liver (Figure 4). If there is portal-venous obstruction by tumor, a wedge-shaped defect of low density is noted rather than the high density seen in the hepatic artery technique. Again, there is a significant increase in diagnostic accuracy using this technique. However, because CT angiography is invasive, it should be reserved for specially selected cases and patients who are being considered for partial hepatectomies.

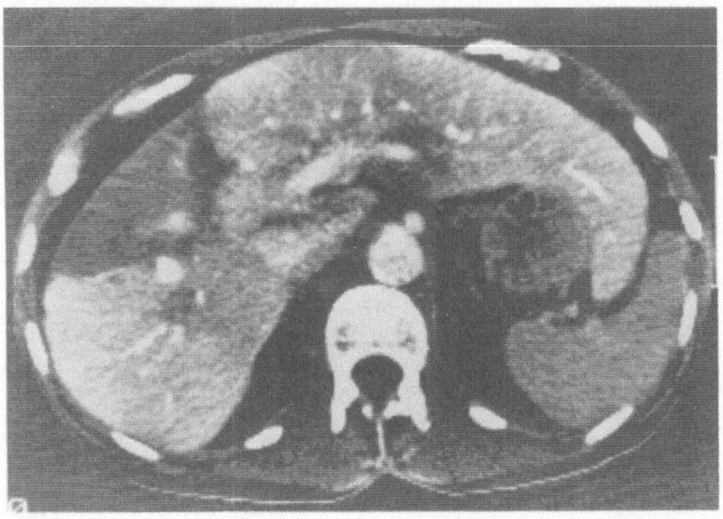

FIGURE 4. A CT angiogram performed with the superior mesenteric artery technique demonstrates enhancement of the normal liver. Most tumors seen on this technique are low density defects demonstrated against the high density surrounding normal hepatic parenchyma.

The problem with such sensitive techniques is that they also detect benign lesions. Autopsy series reveal that roughly 10% of the population has either benign hepatic cysts or small hemangiomas less than 1 cm. Thus, many of the lesions detected by these sophisticated imaging techniques may not represent metastatic disease. Therefore, it is important to perform percutaneous biopsies of these newly detected small lesions before therapy is administered. The accuracy of hepatic biopsies at our institution is greater than 92% (19). Reliable biopsy results can be obtained for lesions between .5 and 1 cm. Our complication rate for the last 151 hepatic biopsies was less than 1.5%.

Despite the many new imaging techniques, small subcapsularly located lesions may be missed. This has always been the greatest limitation of diagnostic imaging and will continue to be so until there are further significant technological advances.

MAGNETIC RESONANCE IMAGING

At present, most data show that magnetic resonance imaging (MRI) offers no significant advantage over CT in the detection of focal lesions (20-22). MRI takes a great deal of time to perform, and multiple scanning sequences are used. On some of the scanning sequences (inversion recovery or spin echo technique), a large lesion (as great as 5 cm) may be missed. Thus, many scanning sequences must be performed before one can feel comfortable with the diagnosis of no focal hepatic masses. In the future, with the use of organ-specific contrast agents the detection of lesions may be easier with MRI. Also, the speed with which MRI examinations can be performed should increase, but this is at least three to five years in the future.

The newer techniques have allowed us to see more hepatic lesions. This has also brought about the problem of determining which lesions are metastatic and which are not. It has also significantly decreased the number of candidates for potential cure, since many patients who were thought to be potentially curable in the past may in actuality have had multiple sites of disease.

References

1. Temple, DF, Parthasarathy KL, Bakshi SP, Mittelman AE: A comparison of isotopic and computerized tomographic scanning in the diagnosis of metastasis to the liver in patients with adenocarcinoma of the colon and rectum. Surg Gynecol Obstet 156: 205-208, 1983.
2. Alderson PO, Adams DF, McNeil BJ, Sanders R, Sieelman SS, Finberg HJ, Hessel SJ, Abrams HL: Computed tomography, ultrasound, and scintigraphy of the liver in patients with colon or breast carcinoma: A prospective comparison. Radiology 149: 225-230, 1983.
3. Smith TJ, Kemeny MM, Sugarbaker PH, Jones, AE, Vermess M, Shawker TH, Edwards BK: A prospective study of hepatic imaging in the detection of metastatic disease. Ann Surg 195: 486-491, 1982.
4. Phillips VM, Knopf DR, Bernardino ME: Percutaneous hepatic biopsy in suspected pancreatic carcinoma. CT. J Comput Tomogr 8: 307-310, 1984.
5. Doiron MJ, Bernardino ME: A comparison of noninvasive imaging modalities in the melanoma patient. Cancer 47: 2581-2584, 1981.
6. Jaszcak RJ, Whitehead FR, Lim CB, Coleman RE: Lesion detection with single-photon emission computed tomography (SPECT) compared with conventional imaging. J Nucl Med 23: 97-102, 1982.
7. Bernardino ME, Thomas JL, Maklad N.: Hepatic sonography: Technical considerations, present applications and possible future. Radiology 142: 249-251, 1982.

185

8. Mattrey RF, Scheible FW, Gosink BB, Leopold GR, Long DM, Higgins CB: Perfluoroctylbromide: A liver/spleen- specific and tumor-imaging ultrasound contrast material. Radiology 145: 759-762, 1982.
9. Seltzer SE, Adams DF, Davis MA, Hessel SJ, Havron A, Judy PF, Paskins-Hurlburt AJ, Holenberg NK: Hepatic contrast agents for computed tomography: High atomic number particulate material. J Comput Assist Tomogr 5: 370-374, 1981.
10. Marincek B, Young SW, Enzmann DR: Time-density evaluation of the liver after iosulamide meglumine: A tissue-specific CT contrast agent. Invest Radiol 17: 90-94, 1982.
11. Vermess M, Doppman JL, Sugarbaker P, Fisher RJ, Chatterji DC, Luetzeler J, Grimes G, Girton M, Adamson RH: Clinical trials with a newly developed intravenous liposoluble contrast material for computed tomography examination of the liver and spleen. Radiology 137: 217-222, 1980.
12. Havron A, Seltzer SE, Davis MA, Shulkin P: Radiopaque liposomes: A promising new contrast material for computed tomography of the spleen. Radiology 140: 507-511, 1981.
13. Lewis E, AufderHeide JF, Bernardino ME, Barnes PA, Thomas JL: CT detection of hepatic metastases with ethiodized oil emulsion 13. J Comput Assist Tomogr 6: 1108-1114, 1982.
14. Thomas JL, Bernardino ME, Vermess M, Barnes PA, Fuller LM, Hagemeister FB, Doppman J, Fisher RI, Longo DL: EOE-13 in the detection of hepatosplenic lymphoma. Radiology 145: 629-634, 1982.
15. Miller DL, Vermess M, Doppman JL, Simon RM, Sugarbaker PH, O'Leary TJ, Grimes G, Chatterji DG, Willis M: CT of the liver and spleen with EOE-13: Review of 225 examinations. Am J Radiol 143: 235-243, 1984.
16. Prando A, Wallace S, Bernardino ME, Lindel MM: Computed tomographic arteriography of the liver. Radiology 130: 679-701, 1979.
17. Freeny PC, Marks WM: Computed tomographic arteriography of the liver. Radiology 148: 193-197, 1983.
18. Matsui O, Kadoya M, Suzuki M, Inoue K, Itoh H, Ida M, Takashima T: Work in progress: Dynamic sequential computed tomography during arterial portography in the detection of hepatic neoplasms. Radiology 146: 721-727, 1983.
19. Alspaugh JP, Bernardino ME, Sewell CW, Sones PJ, Berkman WA, Price RB: CT directed hepatic biopsies: Increased diagnostic accuracy with low patient risk. J Comput Assist Tomogr 7: 1012-1017, 1983.
20. Stark DD, Bass NM, Moss AA, Bacon BR, McKerrow JH, Cann CE, Brito A, Goldberg HI: Nuclear magnetic resonance imaging of experimentally induced liver disease. Radiology 148: 743-751, 1983.
21. Doyle FH, Pennock JM, Banks LM, McDonnell MJ, Bydder GM, Steiner RE, Young IR, Clarke GJ, Pasmore T, Gilderdale DJ: Nuclear magnetic resonance imaging of the liver: Initial experience. Am J Radiol 138: 193-200, 1982.
22. Margulis AR, Moss AA, Crooks LE, Kaufman L: Nuclear magnetic resonance in the diagnosis of tumors of the liver. In: Felson B, Wiot FJ (eds). Seminars in Roentgenology. Grune & Stratton, Inc, New York, 1983, pp 123-125.

16

PREDICTIVE ASSAYS OF CLINICAL RESPONSE FOR PRIMARY AND METASTATIC COLORECTAL CANCER

Daniel D. Von Hoff

SUMMARY

An in vitro soft agar cloning technique was utilized to attempt to culture 762 patients' colorectal carcinoma tissue samples. Overall, only 244 of the specimens (33%) formed enough colonies in soft agar on which to perform reliable drug sensitivity tests. There were no differences in evaluable growth for primary versus metastatic lesions. One method to improve this evaluable growth appears to be culture of the tumor cells in capillary tubes rather than in Petri dishes. Culture in capillary tubes allows increase in evaluable growth, improved plating efficiencies, and requires fewer cells for drug sensitivity testing. In vitro drug sensitivity testing has revealed that colorectal carcinoma is resistant to most standard and investigational anticancer agents. These in vitro findings clearly mimic the clinical findings. Drugs with slightly higher in vitro response rates worthy of trials in the clinic include the standard agent vinblastine and the new agents, vinzolidine and trimetrexate. Exploration of dose response curves indicate that vinblastine, vincristine, or mitoxantrone might be worth studying in high-dose or regional therapy regimens. Even though, in this study, the in vitro-in vivo correlations look reasonable, the use of the cloning assay to predict for response or lack of response of colorectal carcinoma, is not yet practical. This is attributed to the lack of consistent growth in the cloning assay and the high resistance noted for the tumors. Despite these limitations, the human tumor cloning system can still be a useful tool as the basis for the clinical study of colorectal carcinoma.

INTRODUCTION

There are currently a number of in vitro and in vivo assay systems designed to predict for response or lack of response of an individual patient's tumor to a particular antineoplastic agent (1). The most studied in vitro assays include thymidine incorporation, dye exclusion, and cloning assays, while the most studied in vivo assays include human tumors growing in nude mice or in the subrenal capsule system (2).

In this chapter, we describe our experience utilizing a human tumor cloning system to perform drug sensitivity testing on primary and metastatic colorectal cancer. This system was most recently described by Hamburger and Salmon (3,4). Other groups have also reported growth of human colorectal carcinoma utilizing similar systems (5-11).

OVERALL GROWTH OF COLORECTAL CANCER IN SOFT AGAR

By the fall of 1984, our laboratory had received a total of 11,021 patients' tumor specimens for culture in soft agar. A total of 762 of these 11,021 specimens (7%) were from patients with colorectal carcinoma. Of these 762 specimens, 349 were from primary lesions, 332 from metastases, 63 were liver metastases, and 18 were colorectal carcinomas from unknown biopsy sites. All colorectal tumors were collected as previously described (12) and cultured in the routine soft agar cloning system (3,4,12).

As noted in Table 1, evaluable growth ($\geq$ 30 colonies per plate or per 500,000 cells plated) was achieved in 33% of primary lesions, 32% of nonliver metastases, and 35% of liver metastases. Table 2 details the median number of colonies noted for specimens from the different sources. There are no significant differences in the median number of colonies that form from primary tumor specimens versus metastases or versus liver metastases.

Table 1. Evaluable Growth ($\geq$ 30 colonies) by Source of Tumor

Source	No. with growth/ No. attempted	% evaluable growth
Primary	116/349	33
Metastases (non liver)	106/332	32
Lymph node	71/198	36
Fluid (ascites, pleural, pericardial)	15/47	32
Solid peritoneal/omental/subcutaneous	20/87	23
Liver metastases	22/63	35

Table 2. Median Number of Colonies by Source of Tumor

Source	n	Median number of colonies
Primary	116	89
Metastases (nonliver)	106	81
Liver metastases	22	75

In previous work, a number of factors were examined to determine if they affected the number of colorectal tumors that gave evaluable growth (10). Two factors that definitely influenced evaluable growth were sex (tumors from females had a higher percentage of evaluable growth rate than tumors from males, $P < .006$) and Dukes' stage at diagnosis (Dukes' stage C disease tumors had a higher percentage of evaluable growth than stage A and B tumors, $p < .02$) Factors that did not influence evaluable growth included age, degree of tumor differentiation, carcinoembryonic antigen (CEA) (< 2.5 vs > 2.5) level, and prior radiation therapy to the tumor.

Based on the above results, it was clear that not all patient tumors form colonies in soft agar. In addition, the number of colonies formed per number of cells plated (plating efficiency) was quite low. These problems have hampered utilizing the cloning system for clinical trials. In addition, these problems have caused many investigators to believe that the cloning system was too selective and did not represent the entire cell population of the patients' tumors. Finally, the cloning technique requires a large number of tumor cells for drug sensitivity testing. A 1 cm^3 piece of tissue only allows testing of two to four drugs.

METHODS FOR IMPROVING GROWTH IN SOFT AGAR

There have been many methods explored to improve growth of tumor cells in soft agar (13-15). Most have utilized changes in culture media or growth under hypoxic conditions. To date, none of these methods have dramatically improved evaluable growth and plating efficiences.

Recently, our group described a microcapillary method for improving growth of primary human tumors (16). In this method tumor cells are suspended in soft agar in square 100 µl capillary tubes. The tubes are sealed with clay on each end. Colonies that formed in the tubes could easily be recognized under the inverted microscope or identified with an automated scanner (Cellscan-Triton Bioscience, Alameda, California) Texas).

To determine if the capillary cloning system is superior to the conventional Petri dish technique for growing patients' malignancies, a total of 18 patients' colorectal carcinoma specimens were divided in half and plated in each system (capillary system versus Petri dish). A total of 50,000 cells were plated in each 100 µl tube, and 500,000 cells were plated in the Petri dish. Seven of the 18 tumors had evaluable growth (defined as ≥ 30 colonies/plate) utilizing the Petri dish technique, while 16 of the same 18 tumors had evaluable growth in the capillary system. In addition to improved evaluable growth, the average increase in plating efficiencies for the capillary system was tenfold (median threefold improvement).

189

In summary, the newly developed capillary cloning system appeared to allow improved growth of primary human colorectal carcinoma in soft agar. In addition, plating efficiences are improved with the capillary system, and the number of tumor cells needed per drug test is 1/10 that used with the conventional Petri dish technique.

DRUG SENSITIVITY TESTING

Despite the difficulties in consistently growing human colorectal carcinoma in soft agar, we have been performing drug sensitivity testing on the tumors that did form ≥ 30 colonies per 500,000 cells plated. In the total of 244 specimens with adequate growth (out of 762 specimens received) a total of 1,583 drug tests were performed (an average of six drugs per specimen). Table 3 details the in vitro activity of standard agents against the colorectal specimens. All drug exposure times were for a period of one hour at 1/10 the clinically achievable concentration. As noted in that table, most of the in vitro response rates were in the 10-18% range. This in vitro activity closely parallels the known clinical activity of these agents. It is of interest that the in vitro activity of vinblastine was higher, 29%. A review of the literature on the activity of vinblastine against colorectal carcinoma reveals that most of the clinical trials were performed between 1960 and 1965 (17). In addition, most of the studies were performed utilizing suboptimal schedules (not continuous infusions). Despite the problems with these initial trials, some responses were noted. Based on our in vitro findings, vinblastine would appear to be worthy of another clinical trial in patients with colorectal carcinoma.

Table 3. In Vitro Activity of Standard Agents Against Colorectal Carcinoma

Drug	Concentration (μg/ml)	No. Responders/ No. Evaluable	% Response
5-Fluorouracil	6.0	20/154	12
BCNU*	0.1	11/101	10
Mitomycin C	0.1	21/137	15
Doxorubicin	0.04	5.41	12
Methotrexate	0.3	6/33	18
Cisplatin	0.20	4/28	14
Melphalan	0.01	3/19	16
Vincristine	0.01	1/10	10
Vinblastine	0.05	5/17	29

*   BCNU - bis-cloroethyl nitrosourea

A large number of investigational agents have also been tested in vitro (1 hour exposure times at 1/10 the clinically achievable concentration). Table 4 details these results. As noted in that table, vinzolidine (a new Vinca alkaloid closely related to Vinblastine), trimetrexate (a new antifolate), and tiazofurin (a nicotinic acid analog) have higher in vitro responses than the other agents. These are the only compounds that look promising enough to justify phase II studies in the clinic. The other agents have the same marginal in vitro activity noted for the standard agents listed in Table 3.

Table 4. In Vitro Activity of Investigational Agents Against Colorectal Carcinoma

Drug	Concentration (µg/ml)	No. Responders/ No. Evaluable	% Response
Vinzolidine	1.0	5/10	50
Trimetrexate	1.0	4/10	40
Tiazofurin	10.0	8/27	30
Echinomycin	0.01	4/17	23
Menogarol	0.02	3/15	20
Elliptinium	0.04	2/10	20
Mitoguazone	10.0	13/69	18
Bisantrene	0.50	2/13	15
Fludarabine	1.0	3/20	15
Mitoxantrone	0.05	3/30	10

DRUG SENSITIVITY OF THE PRIMARY TUMOR VERSUS METASTASIS

To determine the in vitro drug sensitivities of a primary tumor and its metastasis, a study was performed utilizing simultaneous sampling of tumors in the same patient. As a baseline measurement to assess the variability in the cloning system, the same specimen was divided in half, and each half was processed separately. Drug tests were performed with the same drugs on each half of the specimen. As noted in Table 5, when the same specimen was processed twice, the correlation coefficient for the percentage of survivals for the paired biopsies was 0.80 ($P < .01$). Therefore, there was good agreement in drug sensitivities for the same specimen. When two different areas of the same tumor were tested (central and peripheral parts of the tumor), the correlation coefficient showed less agreement (r=0.51). However, when a metastasis was introduced into the pair, there was

191

essentially no correlation between drug sensitivities in the primary and the metastasis or metastasis and metastasis (r=0.03 and -0.10 respectively). Thus, if one takes a biopsy from a primary tumor, the drug sensitivity spectrum of that tumor will not reflect the drug sensitivity spectrum of the metastasis.

Table 5. Correlation Coefficients for Drug Sensitivity Studies in Colorectal Cancer

Category	n	Number of paired drug tests	r*	P
Same specimen processed twice	12	21	0.80	.01
Two different areas, same primary	5	15	0.51	.04
Primary vs metastasis	4	12	0.03	.1
Primary vs liver metastasis	2	6	0.02	.1
Metastasis vs. metastasis	5	18	-0.10	.7

* Spearman rank order

IN VITRO - IN VIVO CORRELATIONS

To determine if the cloning system could be utilized to predict for response (or lack of response) of an individual patient's colon cancer to a particular antineoplastic agent, tumors from 27 patients (out of a total of 762) were sent for culture in the cloning system and were treated with the most active single agent in the cloning assay (even if it produced very little decrease in survival of tumor colony forming units). Four times there were tumors that were sensitive in vitro ($\leq$ 50% survival of tumor colony forming units), and the patient responded. In four other cases, the tumors were sensitive in the culture plate, but the patient did not respond. There was one instance in which the tumor was resistant in culture, but the patient responded to the drug 5-fluorouracil (5-FU) and 18 instances in which the tumors were resistant in culture and the patient did not respond. Overall, the percentage of true positives for the assay was 4 of 8 (50%), while the percentage of true negatives was 18 of 19 (95%). To put these results into perspective, it must be remembered that tumors from a total of 762 patients were sent in for cloning in soft agar, but only 248 formed colonies in agar, 8 were sensitive in vitro to the same agent, and only 4 responded to that agent (all 4 responses were partial responses of < 4 months duration). Overall, only 4 of the 762 specimens attempted (0.5%) had any possible benefit. Based on these results, it does not seem practical to introduce the current Petri dish cloning system into routine use for care of the patient with colorectal carcinoma.

192

STUDIES OF MECHANISMS TO BYPASS RESISTANCE

From the above studies, it is obvious that colorectal carcinoma has extreme in vitro resistance to a variety of antineoplastic agents. To determine if there might be a way to bypass this resistance, collateral sensitivity and dose response effects were explored.

Collateral Sensitivity

Collateral sensitivity is defined as development of resistance to one drug with development of concomitant sensitivity to another drug. To determine if primary colorectal carcinomas exhibited collateral sensitivity, a total of 349 primary colon cancers were examined. One hundred sixteen of the tumors formed at least 30 colonies per plate and were deemed evaluable. A total of 10 drugs including 5-FU, BCNU, mitomycin C, doxorubicin, methotrexate, cisplatin, melphalan, vincristine, vinblastine and bisantrene were simultaneously tested against these specimens. If the tumor sample was small, as many drugs as possible were tested against the tumor. Typical results are noted in Table 6 for tumors resistant to 5-FU. As an example, none of 84 tumors resistant to 5-FU were sensitive to BCNU. As one scans Table 6, it is impressive that for the most part none of the tumors resistant to 5-FU were sensitive to any of the other drugs. When all permutations are examined, it is clear that colorectal carcinomas do not exhibit collateral resistance. This finding may be the reason that clinical response rates of colorectal carcinoma are not improved by utilizing combination chemotherapeutic regimens.

Table 6. Collateral Sensitivities of Tumors Resistant to 5-Fluorouracil (5-FU)

Resistant to	Sensitive to	No. Sensitive/ No. Tested	% Collateral sensitivity
5-FU	BCNU[*]	0/84	0
5-FU	Mitomycin C	0/92	0
5-FU	Doxorubicin	0/27	0
5-FU	Methotrexate	0/25	0
5-FU	Cisplatin	0/21	0
5-FU	Melphalan	0/18	0
5-FU	Vincristine	1/15	7
5-FU	Vinblastine	0/12	0
5-FU	Bisantrene	0/12	0

[*] BCNU - bis-cloroethyl nitrosourea

Dose Response Effects

To determine which anticancer agents have the steepest dose response curves against colorectal carcinoma, a total of 14 drugs were tested at various concentrations against colorectal carcinoma. Dose response curves were constructed using the concentration of drug plotted on the x axis and the percentage of response in vitro (number of responses/number of tumors cultured) plotted on the y axis. To quantitate the steepness of the curves, a slope was calculated

$$\left[\frac{\% \text{ response}}{\text{concentration}} \right]$$

Table 7 details the slopes for the 14 antineoplastic agents tested. The slopes for BCNU and melphalan are quite flat, indicating that these agents would not be as useful in higher doses as would higher doses of the Vinca alkaloids, vinblastine, or vincristine. Of particular note is the steep dose response curve for the new agent mitoxantrone. These findings indicate that there are other drugs that should be tried either for regional therapy (where one can exploit delivery of higher concentrations of drug to a confined area) or for high-dose regimens with bone marrow rescue. Certainly, mitoxantrone or the Vinca alkaloids should be considered for dose escalation regimens (provided toxicities other than myelosuppression do not interfere with their administration).

Table 7. Dose Response Effects in Colorectal Carcinoma

Drug	Slope
BCNU	0.34
Melphalan	0.24
Bisantrene	1.11
Tiazofurin	1.44
Fludarabine	2.75
Methotrexate	3.40
5-Fluorouracil	8.25
Vinzolidine	14.44
Cisplatin	15.00
Busulfan	39.47
Doxorubicin	41.66
Vinblastine	219.99
Vincristine	266.67
Mitoxantrone	1799.99
Mitomycin C	Not done

CONCLUSIONS

From the above results, it is clear that colorectal carcinoma specimens taken directly from patients will form colonies in soft agar approximately 33% of the time. The capillary cloning system appears to be a method for considerably improving this evaluable growth rate.

Colorectal carcinoma is highly resistant to antineoplastic agents in vitro, which closely mimics the clinical situation. Based on results of testing standard and investigational antitumor agents, only vinblastine, vinzolidine, and trimetrexate appear worthy of phase II clinical trials in patients with advanced colorectal carcinoma. In addition, based on in vitro dose response data, the Vinca alkaloids and the anthracene derivative, mitoxantrone should be studied for regional or high-dose regimens.

At the present time, based on the significant problems associated with the cloning assay plus the substantial in vitro resistance manifested by colon tumors, the human tumor cloning assay has no place in the clinical management of patients with colorectal carcinoma. However, the cloning assay can be utilized to study the biology of colorectal carcinoma as well as to screen new antineoplastic agents for activity against colorectal carcinoma.

ACKNOWLEDGMENT

This study was supported in part by grant CA 27733 from the Department of Health and Human Services and Grant CH 162C from the American Cancer Society.

References

1. Von Hoff DD, Weisenthal LM: In vitro methods to predict for patient response to chemotherapy. Adv Pharmacol Chemother 17: 133-156, 1980.
2. Bogden AE, Von Hoff DD: Comparison of the human tumor cloning and subrenal capsule assays. Cancer Res 44: 1087-1090, 1984.
3. Hamburger AW, Salmon SE: Primary bioassay of human tumor stem cells. Science 197: 461-463, 1977.
4. Hamburger AW, Salmon SE: Primary bioassay of human myeloma stem cells. J Clin Invest 60: 846-854, 1977.
5. Buick RN, Fry SE, Salmon SE: Application of in vitro soft agar techniques for growth of tumor cells to the study of colon cancer. Cancer 45: 1238-1242, 1980.
6. Perkins M, Von Hoff DD: Experience with a two-layer soft agar system for growing gastrointestinal tumors. In: JR Stroehlein (ed), Gastrointestinal Cancer. Raven Press, New York, 1981, pp 381-389.
7. Laboisse CL, Augeron C, Potet F: Growth and differentiation of human gastrointestinal adenocarcinoma stem cells in soft agarose. Cancer Res 41: 310-315, 1981.

8. Kern DH, Campbell MA, Cochran AJ, Burk MW, Morton DL: Cloning of human solid tumors in soft agar. Int J Cancer 30: 725-729, 1982.
9. Agrez MV, Kovach JS, Beart RW Jr, Rubin J, Moertel CG, Lieber MM: Human colorectal carcinoma: Patterns of sensitivity to chemotherapeutic agents in the human tumor stem cell assay. J Surg Oncol 20: 187-191, 1982.
10. Loesch DM, Von Hoff DD, Page CP, Rodrigues V: Direct cloning of human adenocarcinoma of the colon in soft agar: Relationship to negative clinical correlates and level of CEA titer (Abstract). Proc Am Assoc Cancer Res 23: 187, 1982.
11. Bertelsen CA, Sondak VK, Mann BD, Kurn EL, Kern DH: Chemosensitivity testing of human solid tumors. Cancer 53: 1240-1245, 1984.
12. Von Hoff DD, Clark GM, Stogdill BJ, Sarodsky MF, O'Brien MT, Casper JT, Mattox DE, Page CP, Cruz AB, Sandback JF: Prospective clinical trial of a human tumor cloning system. Cancer Res 43: 1926-1931, 1983.
13. Pathak MA, Matrisian LM, MaGun BE, Salmon SE: Effect of epidermal growth factor on clonogenic growth of primary human tumor cells. Int J Cancer 30: 745-750, 1982.
14. Sloman JC, Murphy MJ Jr.: Dexamethasone-induced increase in in vitro clonogenicity of human neoplasms. J Clin Oncol 2: 944-947, 1984.
15. Kern DH, Chien F-W, Morton DL: Selective effects of insulin and hydrocortisone on colony formation and chemosensitivity of human tumors in soft agar. Int J Cancer 33: 807-812, 1984.
16. Von Hoff DD, Huoang M: Perfused capillary cloning system for improved growth of human tumors (Abstract). Proc Am Assoc Cancer Res 24: 86, 1983.
17. Livingston RB, Carter SK: Single agents in cancer chemotherapy. Plenum Publ Corp, New York, 1970, pp 405.

17

RADIOLABELED ANTIBODIES FOR GASTROINTESTINAL MALIGNANCIES

Stanley E. Order

SUMMARY

The specialized requirements for the therapeutic application of radiolabeled antibodies in contrast to diagnostic applications are reviewed. The major variables influencing therapeutic efficacy, i.e., tumor concentration of radiolabeled antibody, tumor effective half-life, species of derivation of antibody, and other pertinent features are reviewed in light of presently successful clinical programs. The scientific basis and evaluation of new protocols, with radiolabeled antibodies in the treatment of liver metastasis from colorectal carcinoma are discussed based on clinical research and new information concerning radiolabeled antibody.

INTRODUCTION

The therapeutic use of radiolabeled antibodies for the treatment of gastrointestinal malignancies has been of benefit in over 100 patients with hepatoma (50% remission) and in 20 patients with intrahepatic biliary cancer (50% remission rate) (1-3). In the development of appropriate radiolabeled antibodies for diagnostic purposes for other gastrointestinal malignancies, scientists familiar with immunology and nuclear scanning have not translated their data into the quantitative terms that will allow evaluation for potential therapy (4,5).

In this chapter, we will use the knowledge gained from present day experience in the use of radiolabeled antibodies for therapeutic purposes to analyze those factors that must be addressed in order to expand and continue progress with this new modality.

PRIMARY LIVER MALIGNANCIES: A MODEL FOR RADIOLABELED ANTIBODY THERAPY

There are two major considerations in the therapeutic use of radiolabeled antibodies. The first is the antibody as the isotope carrier (6), and the second is the physical characteristic of the isotope, e.g., the physical half-life, decay schema, radiation energy, dose rate, total tumor dose, and normal tissue dose.

ANTIBODY AS AN ISOTOPE CARRIER

A number of factors must be evaluated in assessing the therapeutic potential of antibodies as isotope carriers. These variables, considered in greater detail in the following sections, extend to antibody specificity, including characteristics of the tumor antigens, their cross-reactivity, and concentration at the tumor site, the species of antibody derivation, the molecular state of the antibody, its labeling index, and host immune recognition of the antibodies. In addition, characteristics of the isotope must be taken into consideration.

Characteristics of Tumor Antigens

In the early years of investigation of radiolabeled antibodies, the prerequisite was for immune specificity not represented in other tissues, and the absence of such determinants discouraged many investigators. It was often expressed that antigen-antibody reactions of tumor-associated antigens would lead to untoward responses in normal tissues because of antigenic cross-reactions and that such antigens were of no therapeutic interest (7). When using a radioimmunoassay for diagnosis, antigenic uniqueness would be of extreme importance and value; however, the quantitation of antigen in the tumor would determine its potential value as a target for radiolabeled antibodies.

In diagnosing tumors using radiolabeled antibodies, the scanning techniques require a differential count between the tumor-bearing region (foreground) and the normal tissues (background). Therefore, any technique that amplifies these differences by concentration, altered kinetics, or scanning technique would be valuable for diagnosis, even though absolute dose deposition for therapy might be reduced. An example of such altered kinetics is the use of the Fab fragment of the immunospecific IgG, where rapid background clearance enhances scanning potential, but would also reduce therapeutic potential from lessened tumor dose due to more rapid radiolabeled-antibody clearance (8,9).

In the therapeutic use of radiolabeled antibodies, it is quantitative deposition of radiolabeled antibodies and the tumor effective half-life (retention of the antibodies at the tumor site) that determines the tumor dose and the consequent cytotoxicity and response (7). Therefore, contrary to reports in the literature, a positive tumor scan is not necessarily a sufficient requirement for therapeutic application of the radiolabeled antibody (8).

Tumor-specific or unique antigens remain desirable, but in therapeutic application, this is true only if the radiolabeled antibody deposition leads to a significant tumor dose. Our clinical experience to date with tumor-associated antigens has indicated that:

1. Cross-reactivity in normal tissue does not affect the cytotoxic value of ^{131}I antiferritin, since a "biologic window" exists in the tumor that allows high tumor dose deposition, e.g., in clinical hepatoma 8.4 µCi/g versus 1.8 µCi/g in the normal liver (10).

2. Characteristics of the "biologic window" include the neovasculature of tumors, ferritin tumor synthesis and secretion, and slow blood flow (11-13).

3. An antigen relegated to a specific tumor product (alpha fetoprotein; AFP) was reportedly an excellent target for diagnostic scanning, but when tested for therapeutic value, it deposited 2.7 µCi/g in the hepatoma in comparison to 2.7 µCi/g in the normal liver (10,14). This does not imply that in other AFP-positive tumors, or perhaps other antibody preparations, that radiolabeled anti-AFP might not have value.

4. The same antigen in different tumors might behave as a different target. Thus, our experience with ^{131}I anticarcinoembryonic antigen (CEA) (10) in intrahepatic biliary cancer with a deposition of 4.7 µCi/g contrasts to colorectal metastasis to the liver with a deposition of 2 µCi/g which was not of therapeutic value (15).

It has become clear that intercomparisons of the varied antigenic specificities will be a necessary evaluation for therapy and potentially includes multiple antigenic targets for both polyclonal and monoclonal radiolabeled antibodies. The evaluation will be based on dose rate and total tumor dose, and normal tissue dose. When the physical methods of calculation become more widely utilized, then progress will be based on radiation therapy dosimetry, a standard in the field of radiation oncology.

Concentration of Antigen

The concentration of a tumor-associated antigen is a more complex relationship than it may seem at first evaluation because of the kinetics of antigen transport and circulation (7,10,11-13). AFP transits the intra- and extracellular compartments rapidly, which leads to a high blood titer (14). Antibody bound to the antigen elutes as a complex rather easily. The molecular weight of AFP, 71,000, may also play a role in the elution of antigen-antibody complexes.

In contrast, ferritin is also synthesized and secreted by the tumor cells and is retained in the stroma, as well as equilibrated to some extent with the blood stream (17,18). Ferritin's molecular weight is 440,000 and antigen-antibody complexes are, in fact, more completely bound at the tumor site. In hepatoma, the labeled antibodies ^{131}I anti-AFP concentrate to 2.7 μCi/g, whereas ^{131}I antiferritin leads to 8.4 μCi/g when the same specific activity and species for derivation of the antibody are used (10).

When tumors have significant antigenic content, and the isotope has a reasonable linear energy range, then the dosimetry of such radiation will irradiate nonantigenically tagged cells. The principles of dosimetry dominating such a biologic implant are best explained by traditional radioactive implant dosimetry, where radioactive scattering is additive, even where the isotope is not implanted (Figure 1).

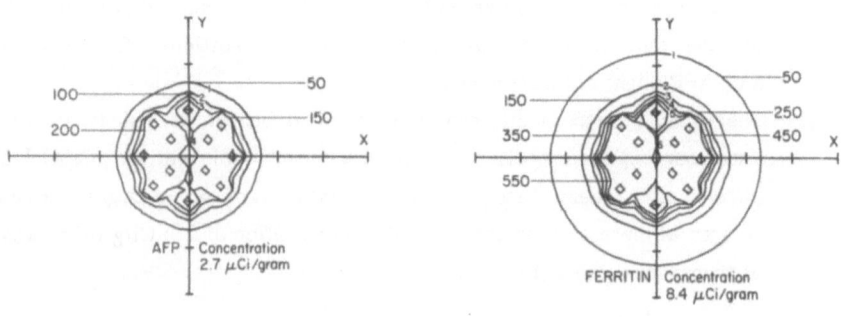

FIGURE 1. To demonstrate the comparison of dosimetry for a physical implantation, an ^{125}I seed implant was simulated on our computer in a 3 cm tumor with the specific activity of antiferritin and anti-AFP. Twelve seeds were distributed in both cases. This example does not deal with ^{131}I or with tumor-effective half-life and assumes complete disintegration of the isotope [125]I. Nonetheless, the principles of saturation, if all other variables are stable, demonstrate 50-200 rad for anti-AFP, and 50-550 rad for antiferritin.

Concentration of Radiolabeled Antibodies at the Tumor

The concentration of radiolabeled antibodies at the tumor target (μCi/g) or tumor saturation and tumor-effective half-life (physical and biologic half-lives) determine tumor dose. Therefore, a reduction in tumor-effective half-life means a reduced tumor dose, and species of derivation must be evaluated in therapeutic applications of radiolabeled antibodies.

200

SPECIES OF DERIVATION OF ANTIBODY

In the ^{131}I antiferritin treatment of hepatoma, cyclic therapy was carried out every two months by altering the species from which the antibody was derived (2,19). The effect of the species was soon to become apparent. All of the antibodies bound ferritin in vitro and were inhibited by comparing rabbit antiferritin as a standard to other species of ^{131}I antiferritin. In vitro Ouchterlony assay, radioimmunoassay, and electrophoresis of the antibodies demonstrated ferritin binding. However, in vivo tumor-effective half-life, which depended on biodegradability of the radiolabeled antibody, demonstrated the superiority of rabbit, pig, monkey, and bovine antibodies (3-4.5 days) to sheep and goat (2-2.5 days) and chicken and turkey (1-1.5 days) antibodies. Those interested in using murine monoclonal antibodies must appreciate the shortened effective half-life of murine antibodies (2 days or less).

MOLECULAR STATE

Tumor-effective half-life is altered not only by the species of derivation, but also by any one of several molecular manipulations. Enzymatic cleavage to Fab_1 or Fab_2 improves tumor imaging, heightens antibody clearance, and reduces immunogenic properties of foreign IgG (9). However Fab_1 and Fab_2 have shortened tumor-effective half-lives and are not ideal isotope carriers.

Affinity purification increases specificity of polyclonal antibodies and reduces tumor-effective half-life (20). In our experience, the curve is biphasic, and the first half-life is less than 24 hours (20). Affinity purification is superior for scanning and inferior for therapy (4,20).

Subclass of IgG

Monoclonal antibodies offer the advantage of unique subclass selection. To date, several laboratories have indicated a preference for the IgG_{2A} antibody carrier (personal communication, Carlo D, Hybritech Inc., La Jolla, California).

LABELING INDEX (SPECIFIC ACTIVITY mCi/mg IgG)

In the analysis of experimental or clinical tumors, the milligrams of IgG required to saturate the tumor site is basic information that allows consideration of an increase of specific activity for isotopic linkage in millicuries per gram of IgG for maximum tumor

201

dose. However, in our clinical experience, when specific activity exceeds 8-10 mCi/g, radiolysis of the antibody occurred, particularly with storage.

Experimental studies preferably should use single specific activities unless the questions address specific activity itself. Altering specific activity and administering radiolabeled antibodies in escalating doses creates two variables, concentration of antibody and the isotope carried, rather than a fixed antibody concentration with variable isotopic activity.

IMMUNE RECOGNITION

In some laboratories, investigators are attempting to select preferential monoclonal antibodies by intrinsic biologic behavior, such as T-cell dependent antibody toxicity and macrophage activation (personal communication, Carlo D, Hybritech Inc., La Jolla, California). Would these antibodies be better isotopic carriers by combining immunity and radiation? Although presently speculative, this remains a potentially important area of research.

Host immune recognition of the antibodies also affects the therapeutic application. Of seven patients given two cycles of similar antibodies, tumors were recognized by the radiolabeled antibody in four patients. This led to the absence of tumor targeting in the second treatment, reduced the effective half-life to less than one day, and even resulted in dehalogenation of the antibody. In three patients lacking immune recognition, the second treatment was the same as the first regarding tumor targeting and appropriate tumor-effective half-lives.

Human monoclonal antibodies remain very useful because of the lack of immune recognition and the potentially prolonged tumor-effective half-lives.

ISOTOPE CHARACTERISTICS

The physical half-life of an isotope is a convenient description of the rate of decay that ultimately leads to complete radiodecay. Radiolabeled antibody has a persistence at the tumor target based on its biologic half-life (degradation of the antibody) and the physical decay of the isotope. The selection of an isotope must be based in part on the efficiency of radiation deposition during the persistence of the antibody at the tumor target; the composite effects is described by the tumor-effective half-life.

202

$$\text{Tumor Effective Half-Life} = \frac{\text{Physical} \times \text{Biologic Half-Lives}}{\text{Physical} + \text{Biologic Half-Lives}}$$

Thus, ^{125}I with a 60-day physical half-life would require a biologic half-life exceeding any realistic expectation. ^{131}I with a physical half-life of eight days and a biologic half-life of eight days would yield a tumor-effective half-life of four days which has been consistent with therapeutically valuable ^{131}I radiolabeled antibody. Limitations that have occurred were due to individual tumor saturation (21).

Isotopic linear energy describes the range of radiation energy from the isotopic source in Mev (^{131}I = 0.36 Mev; ^{90}Y = 0.9 Mev). ^{131}I is both a gamma and a beta emitter with a physical half-life of eight days, whereas ^{90}Y is a pure beta emitter with a half-life of 64.6 hrs. Administration of ^{131}I requires patient hospitalization. High doses are given to facilitate gamma decay (scanning), while the beta decay provides the therapeutic source. The ^{90}Y will deposit its energy at a higher dose rate, will not require patient hospitalization, and will require a second isotope for scanning. The energy of ^{90}Y will allow it to penetrate several millimeters of the tissue where it is deposited, an advantage for radiation cytotoxicity of cells without antigen-antibody deposition on their surface. Dose to the total body from a gamma plus beta emitter (^{131}I) would be greater than with a pure beta emitting isotope, owing to the longer range of gamma radiation.

The radiobiology of dose rate effects seem to indicate that in equivalent doses, a lower dose rate allows for greater tumor cell replication, i.e., tumor regrowth (22). Determination of the total doses to both tumor and normal tissues is a consistent feature of modern-day radiation oncology dosimetry, and these known factors could be used to guide clinical protocols.

RESULTS OF PRESENT TRIALS WITH ^{131}I-LABELED ANTIBODIES

^{131}I antiferritin has been used extensively in over 100 hepatoma patients, and the physics, dosimetry, and toxicity has been described (1,2,23) (Figure 2). The use of doxorubicin (Adriamycin), 15 mg, and 5-fluorouracil, 500 mg, 24 hr prior to administration of radiolabeled antibodies has been a successful combination. There has been a 50% remission rate and a median survival for AFP-negative patients of 6 months and 11 months for AFP-positive patients. The longest survival time is now five years, and disease-free survival time is three years. Thrombocytopenia remains the major toxicity (23), and only one patient in remission over two years has had significant pancytopenia.

203

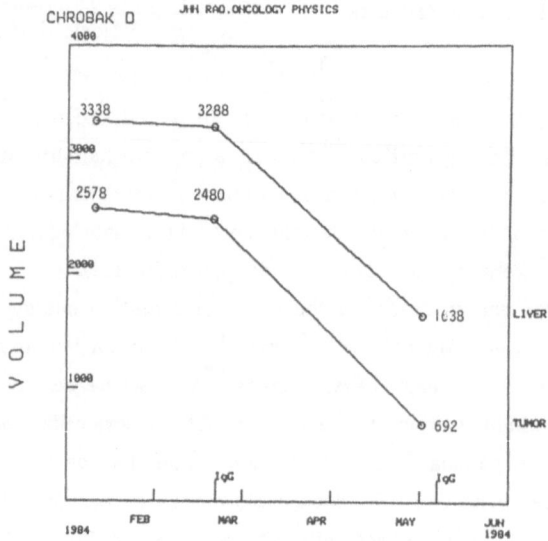

FIGURE 2. Total liver volume and tumor volume reconstruction from computed tomographic scans were carried out using a second computer. This patient's tumor decreased from 2480 cc to 692 cc, and the reduction correlated with all of the clinical, physical, and laboratory signs of remission.

Cyclic therapy was accomplished every two months by altering the species from which the antibodies were derived. Rabbit, pig, monkey, and bovine antibodies had the longest tumor-effective half-lives.

Those patients in remission who went through the program and continued to have adequate blood counts have been candidates for retreatment with the original effective antibodies. Preliminary experience with one dosage developed in our laboratory indicates that those patients without anti-antibodies are candidates for retreatment.

In intrahepatic biliary cancer, 20 patients to date have been treated with ^{131}I anti-CEA and the dosimetry, and principles of application coincide with the hepatoma experience. Remission in both hepatoma and intrahepatic biliary cancer has as its main criteria, tumor volume reconstruction and consistency with the clinical course.

In Hodgkin's disease the ^{131}I antiferritin was given to patients who have exhausted conventional treatment including chemotherapy. In 23 patients, a 43% partial response and 73% remission of B symptoms were reported (24). A more extensive study of ours is presently being analyzed at our institution.

204

Clinical trials have been carried out at three institutions, Johns Hopkins, University of California - San Francisco, and Albert Einstein Hospital in Philadelphia. This demonstrates the ability to export this technology and to achieve similar results.

The routine use of single photon emission tomography scanning has vividly demonstrated the contrast of normal (Tc^{99m}) and tumor (^{131}I) tissue selectivity of the antibodies (Figure 3). In addition, in Hodgkin's disease the smaller collections of tumor, nodal disease, has been demonstrated by this technique because of reduction of background counts, but not by the conventional scans.

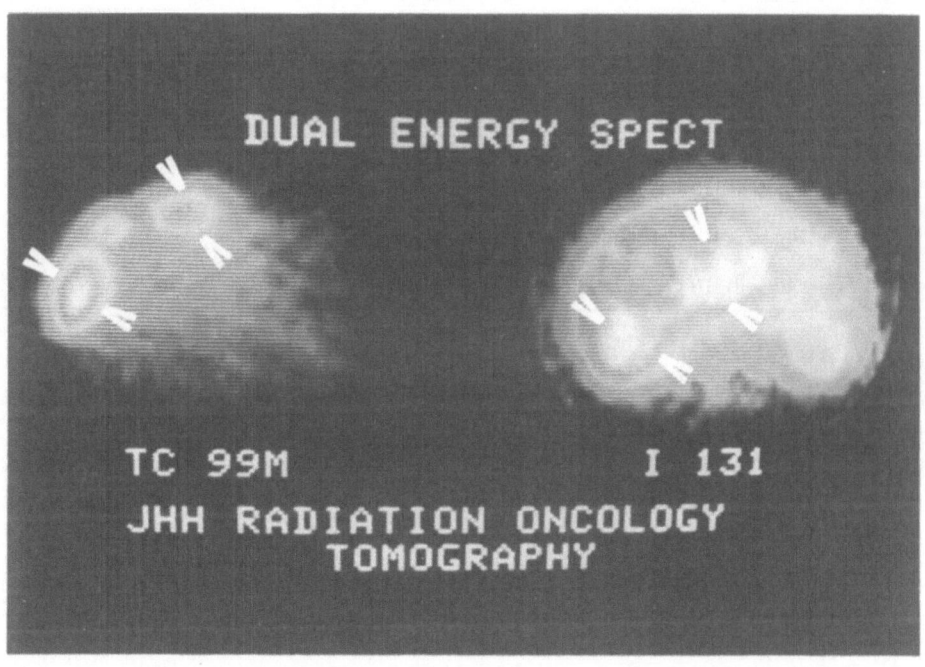

FIGURE 3. Single photon emission tomographic scanning demonstrates minimal normal liver Tc^{99m} and tumor uptake in the abnormal region with ^{131}I antiferritin.

PRINCIPLES FOR DEVELOPMENT OF FORMAL GASTROINTESTINAL TUMOR STUDIES

Table 1 enumerates the sequence of steps necessary to implement the clinical application of radiolabeled antibodies to gastrointestinal tumors. The laboratory and clinical experience gained indicates that high-concentration antigens should be looked for in gastrointestinal malignancies. Then, quantitative studies of the dosimetry of the radiolabeled antibodies should be carried out. Improved isotopic linkages with beta-emitting isotopes will then allow formal phase I, II, and III studies to be carried out in multi-institutional clinical cooperative groups. Under the auspices of the American Cancer Society and the Radiation Therapy Oncology Group, we are currently carrying out a phase III randomized prospective study in hepatoma patients, comparing the use of chemotherapy to radiolabeled antibodies.

Table 1. Radiolabeled antibodies in gastrointestinal malignancies

Determine high concentration antigen

Create appropriate radiolabeled antibodies

Determine tumor and normal tissue dosimetry and kinetics

Central laboratory for supply

Phase I, II pilot studies

Phase II, III group studies

The need for better therapy in metastatic colorectal cancer and the ability to quantitate liver tumors suggest this as an ideal site for study. We will be examining ^{111}Indium-labeled monoclonal antibodies for the quantitative distribution as a first step in this direction. Present day clinical application and results indicate the viability of this approach and gives us cause for anticipation of new and beneficial clinical results.

ACKNOWLEDGMENT

This work is supported by American Cancer Society grant PPD 227, National Cancer Institute grants CA 06973-22 and CA 29536-04, and Hybritech, Inc.

References

1.   Order SE, Klein JL, Ettinger DS, Alderson P, Siegelman S, Leichner P: Phase I-II study of radiolabeled antibody integrated in the treatment of primary hepatic malignancies. Int J Radiat Oncol Biol Phys 6: 703-710, 1980.

2. Order SE, Klein JL, Leichner PK, Wharam MD, Chambers J, Kopher K, Ettinger DS, Siegelman S: Radiolabeled antibodies in the treatment of primary liver malignancies. In: B Levin and R Riddell (eds), Gastrointestinal cancer. Elsevier North-Holland, New York, 1984, pp 222-232.

3. Order SE, Klein JL, Leichner PK, Self S, Leibel S, Ettinger DS: I-131 radiolabeled antibody (antiferritin) in the treatment of hepatoma - An update (Abstract). Proc Am Soc Clin Oncol 3: 138, 1984.

4. Goldenberg D, Kim E, Bennett S, Nelson M, DeLand F: CEA radioimmunodetection in the evaluation of colorectal cancer and the detection of occult neoplasms. Gastroenterology 84: 524-532, 1983.

5. Mach J, Chatal J, Lumbroso S, Bacheggi F, Forni M, Pritchard J, Beiche C, Douillard J, Carrel S, Herlyn M, Steplewski Z, Koprowski H: Tumor localization in patients by radiolabeled monoclonal antibodies against colon cancer. Cancer Res 43: 5593-5600, 1983.

6. Order SE: The history and progress of serologic immunotherapy and radiodiagnosis. Radiology 118: 219-223, 1976.

7. Leichner P, Klein J, Garrison J, Jenkins R, Nickoloff E, Ettinger D, Order SE: Dosimetry of I-131 labeled antiferritin in hepatoma: A model for radioimmunoglobulin dosimetry. Int J Radiat Oncol Biol Phys 7: 323-333, 1981.

8. Larson S, Carrasquillo J, Krohn K, Brown J, McGaffin R, Ferens J, Graham M, Hill L, Beaumier P, Hellstrom K, Hellstrom I: Localization of ^{131}I labeled p97-specific Fab fragments in human melanoma as a basis for radiotherapy. J Clin Invest 72: 2101-2114, 1983.

9. Smith TW, Haber E, Yeatman L, Butle V: Reversal of advanced digoxin intoxification with Fab fragments of Digoxin-specific antibodies. N Engl J Med 294: 797-800, 1976.

10. Leichner P, Klein J, Fishman E, Siegelman S, Ettinger D, Order SE: Comparative tumor dose from I-131 labeled polyclonal antiferritin, anti-AFP, and anti-CEA in primary liver cancer. Cancer Drug Delivery, 1: 321-328, 1984.

11. Rostock R, Klein J, Leichner P, Kopher K, Order SE: Selective tumor localization in experimental hepatoma by radiolabeled antiferritin antibody. Int J Radiat Oncol Biol Phys 9: 1345-1350, 1983.

12. Rostock R, Klein J, Kopher K, Order SE: Variables affecting the tumor localization of I-131 antiferritin in experimental hepatoma Am J Clin Oncol 6: 9-18, 1984.

13. Rostock R, Klein J, Leichner P, Order SE: Distribution of and physiologic factors that affect I-131 antiferritin tumor localization in experimental hepatoma. Int J Radiat Oncol Biol Phys 10: 1135-1141, 1984.

14. Abelev G: Alpha-fetoprotein in oncogenesis and its association with malignant tumors. Adv Cancer Res 14: 295-358, 1971.

15. Goldenberg D, DeLand F, Kim E, Bennett S, Primus F, van Nagell J, Estes N, DeSimone P, Rayburn P: Use of radiolabeled antibodies to carcinoembryonic antigen for the detection and localization of diverse cancers by external photoscanning. N Engl J Med 298: 1384-1388, 1978.

16. Order SE, Kopicky J, Leibel S: Principles of successful radiation therapy. GK Hall Publishers, Boston, 1979, pp 1-191.

17. Katz D, Order SE, Graves G, Benacerraf B: Purification of Hodgkin's disease tumor associated antigens. Proc Natl Acad Sci USA 70: 369-400, 1973.

18. Eshhar T, Order SE, Katz D: Ferritin: A Hodgkin's disease associated antigen. Proc Natl Acad Sci USA 81: 3956-3960, 1974.

19. Order SE, Ettinger D, Leibel S, Klein J, Leichner P: Cyclic radiolabeled I-131 antiferritin in multimodality therapy of hepatocellular carcinoma (Abstract). Proc Amer Soc Clin Oncol 2: 119, 1983.

20. Order SE: Monoclonal antibodies potential in radiation therapy and oncology. Int J Radiat Oncol Biol Phys 8: 1193-1201, 1982.

207

21. Leichner P, Klein J, Siegelman S, Ettinger D, Order SE: Dosimetry of I-131 labeled antiferritin in hepatoma: Specific activities in the tumor and liver. Cancer Treat Rep 6: 647-657, 1983.
22. Shipley W, Peacock J, Steele G, Stephens T: Continuous irradiation of the Lewis lung carcinoma in vivo at clinically 'ultra' low dose rates. Int J Radiat Oncol Biol Phys 9: 1647-1653, 1983.
23. Ettinger E, Order SE, Wharam MD, Parker M, Klein K, Leichner P: Phase I-II study of isotopic immunoglobulin therapy for primary liver cancer. Cancer Treat Rep 65: 639-646, 1981.
24. Lenhard R, Order SE, Spunberg J, Ettinger D, Asbell S, Leibel S: Radioimmunoglobulins: A new therapeutic modality in Hodgkin's disease (Abstract). Proc Am Soc Clin Oncol 2: 211, 1983.

SECTION IV.

CRITERIA OF RESPONSE

18

PROBLEMS WITH RESPONSE CRITERIA

Philip T. Lavin

SUMMARY

During the past 20 years of oncologic research, objective tumor response has become an important study endpoint for phase II and phase III studies involving advanced solid tumors. A variety of factors are changing the basic assumptions behind the response criteria. With the development of new methods for disease visualization, patients formally classified as having unevaluable or nonmeasurable disease are now considered to have measurable disease. Disease can also be visualized more accurately than ever before. Similarly, new methods for the delivery of disease-directed therapy have given new importance to the concept of stable disease. These changing perspectives require sensitivity to the biologic principles of tumor growth and the therapeutic mechanism of action and, in turn, the application of new analytic methodologies to exploit more precise measurements of disease and to model serial measurements. These needs will provide significant opportunities to the oncologist and biostatistician in the formulation of more sophisticated models and analyses.

A variety of issues must be addressed as both disease evaluation methods and therapeutic modalities evolve and they pose the following questions: 1) What are the flaws with the current objective response criteria? 2) What biologic principles should be included in models of tumor growth? 3) What data analysis alternatives are there to the presentation of response rates? 4) How can the actual tumor measurements be utilized to reduce sample size needs? Suggested answers are presented for each of these questions. These proposed remedies will promote more meaningful evaluations of new drugs and modalities, while taking advantage of the increased precision with which the disease can be visualized.

INTRODUCTION

In 1965, A. Bradford Hill stated " . . . all scientific work is incomplete whether it be observations or experimental. All scientific work is liable to be upset or modified by advancing knowledge." His comments apply aptly to the evaluation of disease-directed therapy in clinical studies of advanced cancer, where objective tumor response is a primary study endpoint. The purpose of this chapter is to point out many of the difficulties associated with the definitions of tumor response and some of the newly developed analytical approaches for the analysis of tumor response.

The concept of objective tumor response has been an accepted part of phase II and phase III cancer clinical trials involving patients with advanced measurable disease. In this evaluation process, the disease being measured could be the primary tumor mass, metastatic disease such as hepatomegaly or ascites, or perhaps some tumor marker such as carcinoembryonic antigen (CEA) or CA19-9. For the indicator selected for periodic monitoring, a set of standardized response criteria have been adopted to promote interpretation of the numerous studies conducted and reported in the literature. The criteria used by the Eastern Cooperative Oncology Group (1) are representative of response criteria currently in use by the clinical oncology research community.

These response criteria consist of four major categories, complete response, partial response, no change, and progression. The definitions are presented in Table 1. The categories have a well-established hierarchy in that if progression occurs first, then the patient is so classified; if a complete response occurs after a partial response, then the patient is classified as a complete responder; and if no partial response and no progression are seen, the patient is classified in the "no change" category. The criteria have been broadly applied to many different cancers such as sarcomas, myelomas, and lymphoma, in addition to the more traditional applications to breast, colon, and lung cancers.

Table 1. Response Criteria of the Eastern Cooperative Oncology Group

Category	Criteria
Complete response	Complete disappearance of all malignant disease
Partial response	$\geq 50\%$ reduction in the product of the longest perpendicular diameters of the most clearly measureable tumor mass
No change	$< 50\%$ reduction or $< 25\%$ increase in the product calculated above
Progression	$\geq 25\%$ increase in the product calculated above or new malignant disease

In the literature, the most traditional and widely used method of reporting tumor response is response rates. This is highly limiting in that a variety of other measures can be reported without any change to the current response criteria definition.

This chapter identifies: 1) the problems with the current response criteria, 2) the biologic principles that should be included in models of tumor growth, 3) data analysis alternatives to the presentation of response rates, 4) actual tumor measurements to reduce sample size.

PROBLEMS WITH THE CURRENT RESPONSE CRITERIA

The use of these criteria do not appear problematic until a closer inspection of them takes place. Lavin and Flowerdew (2), in a tumor simulation experiment, were able to provide an idealized setting in which to test these response criteria. They concluded that the criteria for response and progression should be revised so that a 50% reduction for response should correspond to a 100% increase for progression in the measurement of solid tumors. They also found that the chances of declaring a response or progression depend on the number and frequency of measurements, i.e., the chance of falsely declaring progression using the existing 25% increase criteria leads to a situation where there is an 86% chance of falsely declaring progression if eight follow-up measurements are taken of disease that is truly unchanged. Finally, they saw that stable disease (no change) can be a meaningful study endpoint that could be overlooked when stable disease cannot be an absorbing state. Lavin and Flowerdew concluded that the chances would be very high of dismissing a drug that totally stabilized disease. Table 2 displays the effect of the number of measurements and the choice of progression threshold criteria on the probability of declaring progression when disease being measured was actually stable.

Table 2. Probability of Declaring Progression When Disease is Stable

Number of Follow-up Observations	Progression > 25% Increase	Threshold Criteria > 100% Increase
1	26%	2.5%
2	45%	4.9%
4	68%	9.3%
8	86%	16.8%

The problem also extends into the changing technology associated with disease measurement. Ten years ago, palpation and x-ray were the principal means used to measure disease. Today, computed tomographic (CT) scans, contrast procedures, and monoclonal antibody products offer additional methods for measuring disease. As a result, more disease sites can be visualized much more accurately than before. Thus, more populations with earlier stage disease can qualify for response evaluation. Table 3 illustrates such a situation for two hypothetical studies opened to patients with different

213

forms of evaluable disease. Patients in the 1984 study are likely to have higher response rates simply because of a more favorable population selection. Thus, response rates will need to be adjusted when new technologies are applied and new populations are studied. Table 3 illustrates how higher response rates might result without adjusting.

These flaws are not difficult to overcome. Through recognition of the biologic principles associated with tumor response, statistical models and analyses can proceed in spite of the above problems.

Table 3. Response Rates Comparison for Two Hypothetical Studies of Colorectal Cancer

Response Indicator	1974 Study	1984 Study
Palpable mass	30% (6/20)	30% (3/10)
Nonpalpable mass visualized by CT scan	–	60% (3/5)
Microscopic disease measurable by the monoclonal antibody CA 19-9	–	90% (4/5)
Overall response rate	30% (6/20)	50% (10/20)

BIOLOGIC PRINCIPLES FOR TUMOR RESPONSE MODELS AND ANALYSES

A variety of practical constraints govern tumor response analyses and models. A recognition of these limitations can point the biostatistician in the direction most appropriate for each clinical study. Consider the specific problems associated with the phase II testing of drugs on patients with liver metastases from colon cancer. These patients might be suitable candidates for hepatic infusion therapy or for more traditional forms of chemotherapy. Patient selection processes can clearly bias study results if the hepatic infusion group must meet special eligibility requirements that are not imposed on patients undergoing more traditional chemotherapy. An understanding of these selection requirements is clearly necessary in order to begin the task of comparing the results of a hepatic infusion trial to other therapies under phase II testing.

Table 4 demonstrates the results from hypothetical studies in which patients receive hepatic infusion therapy in one study and traditional chemotherapy in the second study. While response rates are the same for patients with metastatic disease sites, the overall response rates are higher for the hepatic infusion study because of the inherent selection bias. The message of this example is that a rate adjustment is required before a claim of superiority can be made.

214

Table 4. Response Rates Comparison for Two Hypothetical Studies Involving Hepatic Infusion Therapy and Traditional Chemotherapy

Degree of Metastatic Disease Involvement	Hepatic Infusion	Traditional Chemotherapy
Hepatomegaly only	40% (8/20)	40% (2/5)
Hepatomegaly and local metastatic spread	-	10% (1/10)
Hepatomegaly and distant metastatic spread	-	0% (0/5)
Overall Response Rate	40% (8/20)	15% (3/20)

The biologic principles under study can be more complex in the above example if site-specific responses are considered. Patients with hepatic infusion therapy might be expected to have more pronounced reductions in hepatomegaly, given the route of drug administration. Here, the reporting of overall response rates might be of lesser interest than the response rates for liver metastases and the life table for the time to progression.

An examination of the sources of error generated through the process of tumor measurement leads naturally to the methods of evaluation. A deep pelvic mass in a patient may be difficult to measure by palpation, but it can be precisely measured using a CT scan. A 10% increase in size of the tumor as seen on CT scan would be certain progression, but it would be within chance variation when measured by palpation. The increased precision allows for the modeling of serial tumor data according to a growth model for the patient-specific tumor. The growth model could exploit the obvious correlations between successive measurements. A fully developed growth model would allow for the identification of optimal time points for measuring disease once classes of growth models were identified. The models of Laird and Ware (3), which were designed for the analysis of serial measurements, adapt nicely to the missing data problems frequently encountered in these analyses. Growth models, such as those proposed by Schnacky (4) for tumor doubling times, can be reanalyzed with more efficiency. These models can also accept concomitant baseline factors to control for imbalances in these factors or to adjust to a standard population.

These biologic factors can influence the selection of an appropriate statistical technique or model in order to utilize the data fully for study planning and analysis.

To provide some general rules for the consideration of analyses and modeling, a variety of factors could influence the process. These factors include:

(1)   site-specific therapy, depending on the mode of administration;

(2)   different error sources in tumor measurements, i.e., method of measurement, location of disease, investigator interpretation, or missing data;

(3)   trends in serial tumor measurements, i.e., a steadily increasing sequence of measurements for progression, a steadily decreasing sequence of measurements for partial response;

(4)   observations of tumor responses following therapy initiation, i.e., after 2-3 cycles of therapy;

(5)   reporting of concomitant factors such as the initial performance status, degree of weight loss in the previous six months, sites of metastatic disease, liver function, and disease volume and comparison with other findings; and

(6)   endpoints that can include duration of disease stabilization, proportion in response at a given point in time, site-specific response rates, or mean tumor reduction after each cycle of therapy.

These six factors each represent challenges to the clinical oncologist and biostatistician in finding optimal ways to look at the data.

DATA ANALYSIS ALTERNATIVES TO RESPONSE RATES

Simply reporting the response rates can fail to provide insights into the antitumor activity of therapeutic regimens. For example, in two recent Eastern Cooperative Oncology Group clinical trials in advanced gastric cancer, the response rates for the 5-fluorouracil (5-FU) plus methyl chloroethyl cyclohexyl nitrosourea (CCNU) regimens were 40% in the first study (5) and 24% in the second study (6). The sample sizes in each study were large enough to cast doubt on whether the results were consistent across the two studies. To gain further insight into the different results, the distributions of the ratio of the indicator tumor area after one month to that at baseline was plotted for each 5-FU plus methyl CCNU regimen. The analysis (7) demonstrated that a simple measurement error could have explained the difference, as the two regimens had very similar distributions except for the 30-70% reduction region. Figure 1 illustrates these

216

distributions. By recognizing that the one-month tumor-area ratio obeyed a log-normal distribution, as depicted in Figure 2, statistical modeling could be employed as a way to pool and compare the two studies. Alternative methods analysis helped to clarify the reasons for the apparent differences between the two 5-FU plus methly CCNU regimens.

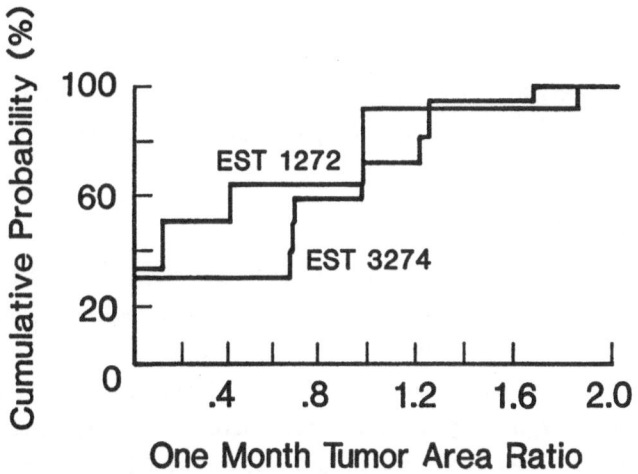

FIGURE 1. Cumulative distribution for the one-month solid tumor-area ratio, one-month baseline for two plus 5-FU plus methyl CCNU programs.

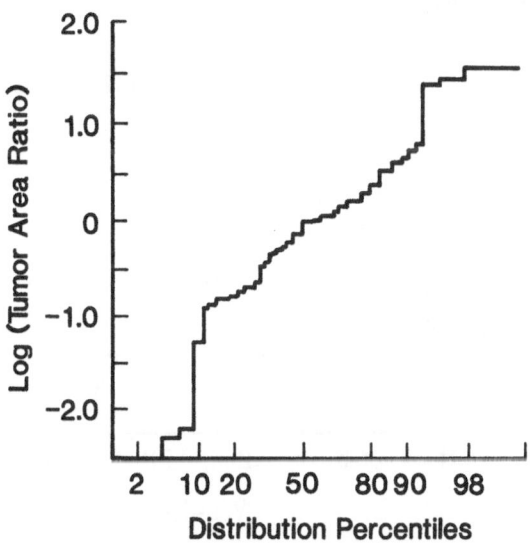

FIGURE 2. Demonstration of log-normal distribution for the one-month tumor-area ratio (46 patients).

Linear Logistic Model

The linear logistic model (8) is useful for representing the probability of response P as a logistic function of baseline covariates. The equation can be written as:

$$\ln \left[\frac{P}{1-P} \right] = \alpha_1 X_1 + \alpha_2 X_2 + \ldots + \alpha_n X_n$$

where X_1, X_2, ···, and X_n are the baseline covariate levels. This model can be used to pool data from several studies, to adjust response rates from one study to another, and to identify prognostic factors.

Probability of Being in Response Model

This model is a two-stage exponential model for representing the probability of being in response as a function of time. The time to response is modeled as an exponential distribution with parameter λ_1, while the duration of response is modeled as another exponential distribution with parameter λ_2. The parameters λ_1 and λ_2 can be estimated numerically from data. This model, developed by Begg and Larson (9), is illustrated in Figure 3 for patients with advanced measurable colorectal cancer. The principle behind the model can be readily applied to data to plot the empiric probability of being in response if there is no need for data pooling, probability model adjustment, or prognostic factor identification.

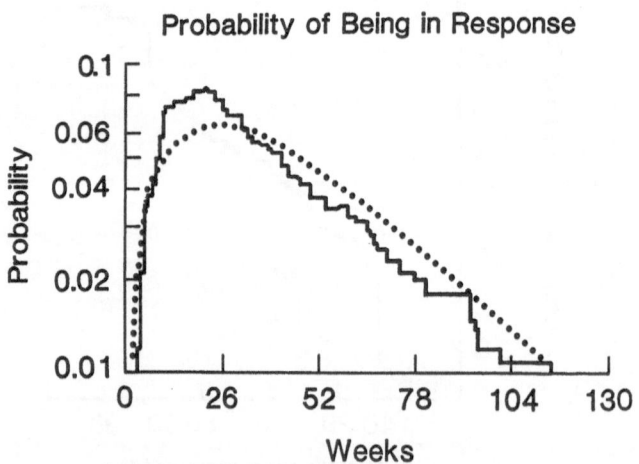

FIGURE 3. Estimates of probability of being in response function from an exponential model, together with nonparametric estimates, for advanced measurable colorectal cancer.

218

Tumor Area Ratio Distributions

The measurement of different solid tumors in different patients at different points in time can be overcome in part by normalizing tumor areas. This can be achieved by dividing subsequent tumor-area measurements by the baseline measurement. This technique allows for the construction of tumor-area ratios at fixed points in time. Figure 1 displays the advanced gastric tumor-area ratio data at one month. Other tumor-area ratio distributions can be calculated at the end of therapy cycles. If log normality applies, as was seen in Figure 2, models of the tumor-area ratio can be readily constructed.

Another alternative is to compute the tumor-area ratios at the end of each therapy cycle, and to then construct the area under the tumor-area ratio curve for each patient. This has the advantage of compensating for the high correlation between successive tumor-area ratios for the same patient. In this setting, log-normal distributions can also be considered for modeling these summary measures.

Landmark Analyses

The survival of responding patients versus non-responding patients can also be evaluated using a Landmark analysis technique devised by Anderson, et al. (10). This technique adjusts for the biases associated with responding patients with a guaranteed survival and patients living long enough to respond. This technique allows for bias elimination. The National Prostatic Cancer Project (11) presented a survival curve for response categories to show the survival advantages experienced by advanced prostatic cancer patients in the stable disease category (Figure 4).

Tumor Growth Models

A very promising class of tumor growth models can be developed from the random effects models proposed by Laird and Ware (3). In these models, the individual tumor measurement (or normalized outcome) becomes the dependent variable, which allows for different numbers of observations for different patients. These models are also specially designed for the case of correlated serial measurements. The models can, therefore, handle missing data, measurements collected at different time points, and covariates such as the patient, investigator, measurement, and technique, as well as known prognostic factors. These models are already being used successfully in environmental monitoring data.

219

These models are particularly promising in that they permit more precise calibration and evaluation of serial tumor markers for disease monitoring, second look at old drug data for disease stabilization potential, and reduced sample size needs for phase II and phase III study design.

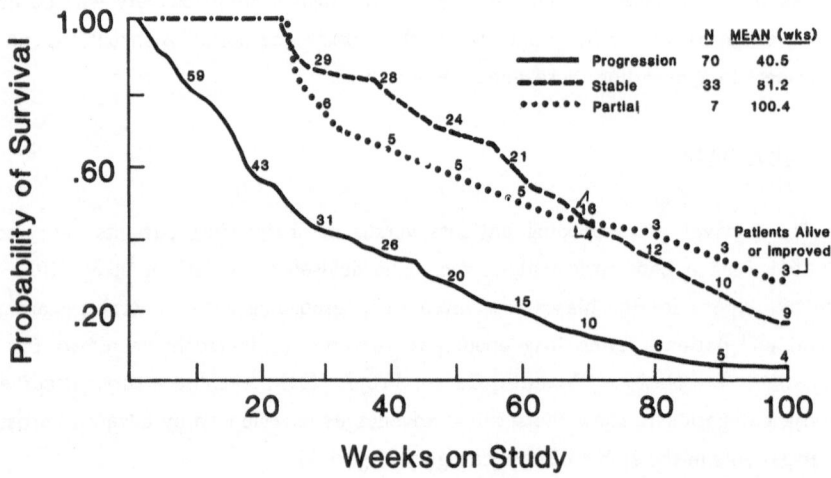

FIGURE 4. Survival life table for response categories in advanced prostatic cancer. (National Prostatic Cancer Project Trial 100)

220

The identification of statistical models permits the application of these models for planning phase II and phase III studies. It is possible to test for disease stabilization in advanced gastric cancer in a single phase II agent study and to compare levels of reduction in a phase III study in which two treatment regimens are being compared. It will be assumed that the endpoint of interest will be the tumor-area ratio after one month on therapy. A further assumption is that the tumor-area ratio obeys a log-normal distribution with a given standard deviation $\sigma = .64$ from Figure 2.

Phase II Testing
Let M = Mean tumor-area ratio at one month.

To Test H_o: $M = 1$ versus $H_A = M > 1$

with .05 level of significance, a Z test can be used to obtain the rejection region $\overline{X} > 1.25/\sqrt{N}$, where $\overline{X}$ is the geometric mean of the one-month tumor-area ratios and N is the sample size. Table 5 gives rejection rules for different sample sizes to test the hypothesis of disease stabilization. With as few as eight subjects, the hypothesis of disease stabilization could be rejected if the geometric mean of the tumor area ratios exceeded 1.5.

Table 5. Phase III Treatment Evaluation for Disease Stabilization Potential

Sample Size Requirements One-Sided Test of Hypothesis (5% Type I Error, $\sigma = 0.64$)	
Sample Size	Log-Normal Rejection Rule
10	40% Increase
25	23% Increase
50	16% Increase

Phase III Comparisons
Let M_1 = Mean tumor-area ratio for program 1 at one month
Let M_2 = Mean tumor-area ratio for program 2 at one month

To test H_0: $M_1 = M_2$ versus H_A: $M_1 < M_2$

with .05 level of significance, a Z test can be used to obtain the rejection $\overline{X}_1 - \overline{X}_2 > 1.76/\sqrt{N}$, where $\overline{X}_1$ and $\overline{X}_2$ are the geometric means of programs 1 and 2 for the one-month tumor-area ratios, and N is the sample size per group. Sample size requirements for the test can be based on a 20% Type II error. Results of the calculations, presented in Table 6, demonstrate considerable savings in reduced sample size over the comparable test formulated according to a binomial model.

Table 6. Phase III Comparison of Two Therapy Programs

Sample Size Requirements
One-Sided Test of Hypothesis
(5% Type I Error, 20% Type II Error, $\sigma = 0.64$)

Response Rate Comparisons	Binomial Model	Log-Normal Model
	REQUIREMENT PER GROUP	
20% vs 30%	290	125
20% vs 40%	75	36
20% vs 50%	36	18

DISCUSSION

A variety of factors are changing the way that disease is measured, therapy is delivered, and who is being treated. Sophistication in the visualization of disease, marked by technologic breakthroughs in scanning techniques and monoclonal antibodies, have made it easier to decide if therapies are working and have provided prompter feedback when these therapies work. New methods for therapy delivery, such as hepatic infusion and monoclonal antibodies, represent parallel advances. Finally, national cancer activities have brought these new technologies to more oncologists in more hospitals than ever before. In spite of these major advances, the criteria for evaluating the success of the therapy have remained unchanged.

The need for revised criteria goes hand and hand with the need for new ways to look at tumor measurement data. The criteria need revisions in the definition of progression (a 100% increase is recommended instead of a 25% increase for solid tumors); the ability to drop the partial and complete response categories for diseases like prostatic cancer and breast cancer where survival with metastatic disease is more important than response; and the handling of multiple sites of measurable disease through a cumulative index of involved disease sites.

The need for new ways to analyze the data is a challenging problem to the biostatistician and the oncologist, who must ensure that the analyses and models are valid. The new ways must address the biology of the treatment delivery and the disease, the technology used to measure disease, and the meaningful endpoints to consider in light of the disease, its treatment, and its measurement. In addition, the selection of appropriate and efficient statistical techniques and models to suit the data being analyzed, the recognition of population selection biases that can require adjustment of results to compare to other findings, and the application of models to achieve more efficient designs in the planning of studies must also be addressed. Thus, the problem at hand requires a multidirectional approach.

The implications associated with the use of the response criteria could be quite far reaching. Depending upon the number of measurements per patient per study, for every one promising cancer agent undergoing phase II testing that has come along so far, there could be three to five other phase II study agents that had stabilization potential, but were dismissed from further study because no responses were seen. Investigators may wish to review completed studies to see if this stabilization potential was missed. Plots of tumor-area ratios after each drug cycle could be constructed for treatments of interest for comparison to other active agents in phase II study. This process would not require any additional data from that which was already recorded in the patient's medical history.

Another area of research that can benefit from improved visualization techniques is the use of tumor markers. Since extent of disease is itself a tumor marker, any promising tumor marker should correlate closely with the extent of disease. In turn, accurate tumor markers can then lead the way in determining if therapies were inactive before progression was reached. Again, by incorporating prognostic factors and baseline characteristics into the analytic models, tumor markers can be better calibrated with tumor size and can be designed to provide lead time. Monoclonal antibodies may also be tailored to deliver therapy from an improved understanding of disease measurement.

In closing, the biology of the metastases and the treatment of disease is vitally linked to the choice and direction of the response criteria. Improvements in medical technology now necessitate improvement in defining response criteria.

223

References

1. Oken MM, Creech RH, Tormey DC, Horton J, Davis TE, McFadden ET, Carbone PP: Toxicity and response criteria of the Eastern Cooperative Oncology Group. Am J Clin Oncol 5: 649-655, 1982.
2. Lavin PT, Flowerdew G: Studies in variation associated with the measurement of solid tumors. Cancer 46: 1286-1290, 1980.
3. Laird NA, Ware JH: Random effects models for longitudinal data. Biometrics 38: 963-974, 1982.
4. Schnacky SE, McCormack GW, Cuchural GJ: Growth rate patterns of solid tumors and their relation to responsiveness to therapy. Ann Intern Med 89: 107-121, 1978.
5. Moertel, CG, Mittelman JA, Bakemeier RF, Engstrom PF, Harley JA: Sequential and combination chemotherapy of advanced gastric cancer. Cancer 38: 678-682, 1976.
6. Moertel CG, Lavin PT: Phase II-III chemotherapy studies in advanced gastric cancer. Cancer Treat Rep 63: 1863-1869, 1979.
7. Lavin PT: An alternative model for the evaluation of antitumor activity. Cancer Clinical Trials 4: 451-457, 1981.
8. Cox DR: Analysis of binary data. Halsted Press, New York,1970, pp 16-27.
9. Begg CB, Larson, M: A study of the use of probability of being-in-response function as a summary of tumor response data. Biometrics 38: 59-66, 1982.
10. Anderson JR, Cain KC, Gelber RD: Analysis of survival by tumor response. J Clin Oncol 1: 710-719, 1983.
11. Slack NH, Mittelman A, Brady MF, Murphy GP (for the National Prostatic Cancer Project): The importance of the stable category for chemotherapy treated patients with advanced and relapsing prostate cancer. Cancer 46: 2393-2402, 1980.

19

ACCURACY OF DIAGNOSTIC TECHNIQUES WITH FOLLOW-UP AND EVALUATION OF DISEASE RECURRENCE

Michael E. Bernardino

SUMMARY

The impact of disease extent on survival is clear. Thus, the accurate assessment and reporting of the extent of metastatic disease in the liver and its response to therapy are critical in interpreting and comparing data from individual studies. The criteria for evaluating therapeutic response are dependent on the sensitivity and accuracy of the diagnostic techniques used for follow-up and evaluation of recurrent disease. Recent innovations in technology have made newer approaches possible. This chapter will review those diagnostic techniques available for patient follow-up and for evaluating tumor recurrence. An overview is provided on the diagnostic accuracy of radionuclide imaging, sonography, computed tomography, and magnetic resonance imaging.

COMPUTED TOMOGRAPHY

Imaging Recurrent Disease

Since the majority of recurrent colorectal carcinomas occur at the suture line, evaluation for recurrence should start in this area (1-3) (Figures 1,2). Barium studies of the rectum and intravenous pyelography may be useful, but only when gross changes occur. They are also limited in their field of evaluation, although they are easy to obtain.

Cross-sectional imaging offers the advantage of visualization of the entire pelvis. Moss et al. described a new staging technique for local recurrence (4). Stage I is an intraluminal polypoid mass without thickening of the colon wall (less than 1 cm) and no invasion of surrounding organs or pelvic sidewall. Stage II is a thickened colon wall (greater than 1 cm) or pelvic mass without extension to adjacent organs or extension to pelvic sidewalls. Stage III is a thickened colon wall or pelvic mass with invasion of adjacent organs, also, thickened colon wall or pelvic mass that extends to the pelvic

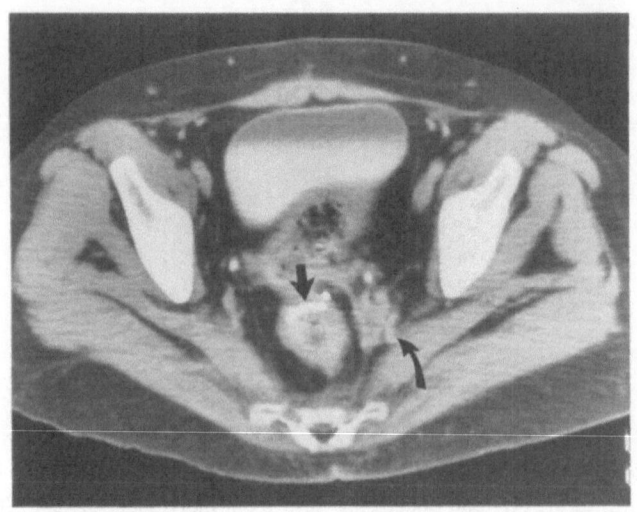

FIGURE 1: A computed tomographic scan demonstrates a local recurrence (curved arrow) adjacent to the suture line (arrow) from the patient's previous colonic surgery.

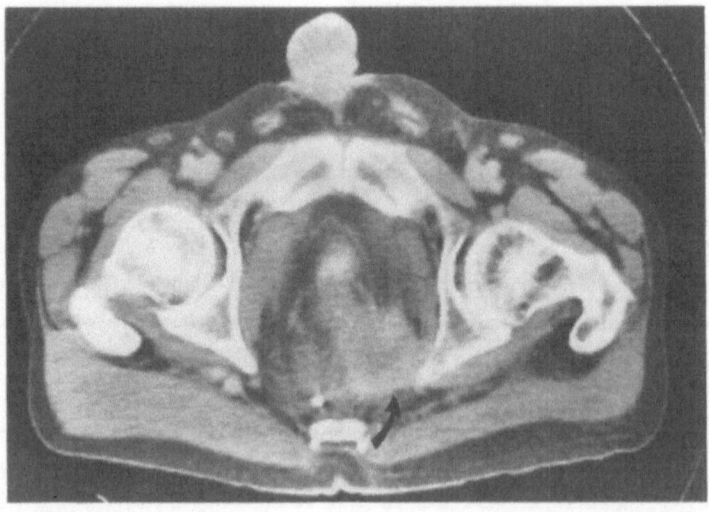

FIGURE 2. Large local pelvic recurrence (arrow) is noted. This recurrence is destroying the left acetabular cortex.

sidewalls. Stage IV is metastatic disease with or without local abnormality (Figure 3). Using the above criteria, the overall accuracy of staging recurrent rectal carcinomas with computed tomography (CT) was 95%. There was a 5% false-positive rate and a 0% false-negative rate. The majority of the recurrences found in this series were between 4.5 and 8.5 cm. However, there was a significant number of recurrences to areas outside the pelvis, such as the liver, bones, and retroperitoneal lymph nodes. In another study, by Mayes and Zornosa, the majority of the recurrences were within the pelvis; however, para-aortic nodes, the liver, and adrenal glands were also involved in many of the recurrent cases (5). Thus, cross-sectional imaging becomes an ideal technique not only for evaluating the most common site of recurrence (surgical site, pelvis), but also the other areas within the abdomen.

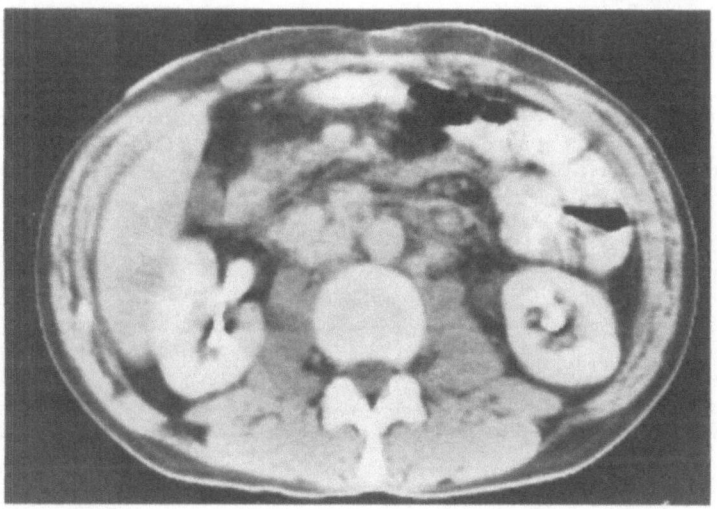

FIGURE 3. CT scan demonstrates multiple retroperitoneal nodes from recurrent metastatic colon carcinoma.

Evaluating Diagnostic Techniques for Therapeutic Response

CT has been used to determine whether lesions improve or worsen by determining the peripheral vascularity of the lesion or volumetric changes of the hepatic masses (6,7) (Figure 4A & B). Volumetric analysis of hepatic lesions via computer program is far more accurate than the radiologist's visual evaluation. In one series, the radiologist's evaluation of whether a lesion improved or worsened correlated with the computer volumetric changes within the lesion in only 41% of the cases (8). Thus, human error can be quite significant in the evaluation of therapy.

227

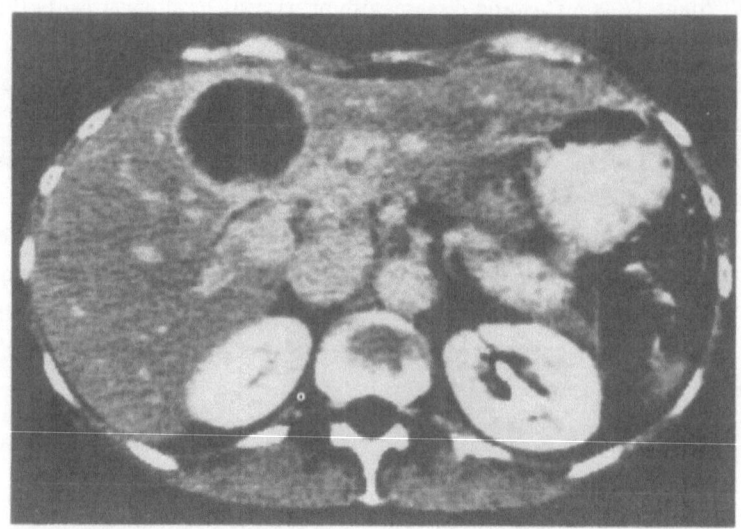

FIGURE 4A. CT scan demonstrates a low-density lesion in the liver from colon carcinoma. This lesion has been infarcted. However, it has a dense peripheral rim which is due to the vascularity of the tumor.

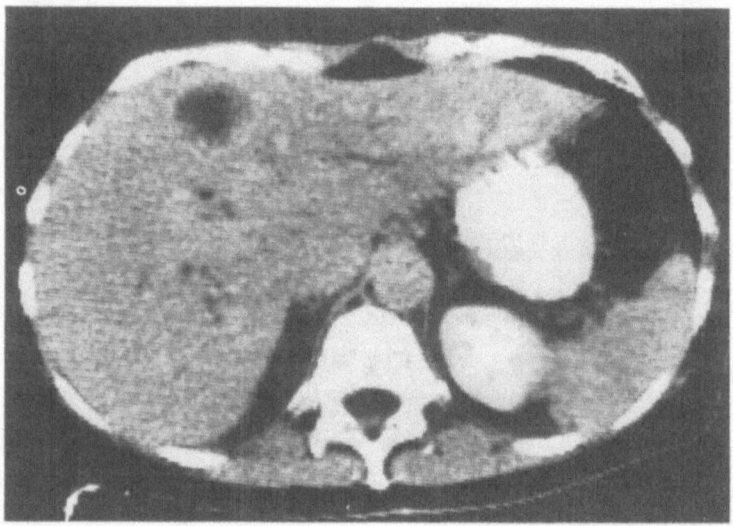

FIGURE 4B. Repeat examination three months later demonstrates that the lesion has decreased and has little vascular rim. Thus, the therapy has been partially beneficial.

Most tumors, after adequate therapy or embolization, decrease in density, become necrotic, and have no peripheral enhancement. When these findings are noted, the volume of the tumor may not change, even though significant tumor necrosis may be present. These findings are difficult to obtain by any other diagnostic tests short of angiography (8). If embolization is used as hepatic therapy, small air pockets may be noted immediately after the embolization process (9). These air or gas pockets may be due to the embolization process itself or the release of oxygen and nitrogen from dead tissue (Figure 5). These pockets do not represent an abscess, even in a patient who has a spiking temperature. The usual postembolization fever is due to the release of necrotic tissue. Postembolization syndrome may last up to 72 hours. Only in cases where the syndrome lasts longer or the patient has a grossly elevated white cell count with a shift should the possibility of an abscess be entertained.

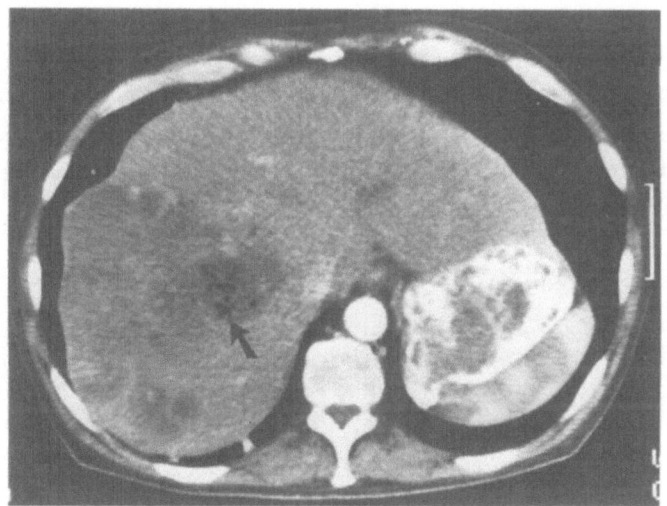

FIGURE 5. CT scan demonstrates a large hypoechoic lesion in the right hepatic lobe. This lesion has been infarcted. There are multiple punctate densities (arrow) within the liver. This is due to air introduced during the embolization procedure. It is not due to an abscess. This patient did have the clinical constellation of postinfarction syndrome.

Whichever technique is used to evaluate therapeutic response, at some point, the lesion may become stable. When a mass does stabilize is the tissue viable or nonviable (10,11)? Cross-sectional imaging modalities allow one to take a biopsy of the lesion in question at the time of the diagnostic evaluation. This significantly decreases the

229

patient's cost and provides the clinician with important information. In many cases, this can be done on an out-patient basis with a great deal of accuracy (12).

RADIONUCLIDE IMAGING AND ULTRASOUND

Radionuclide imaging is an accurate method of detecting lesions. However, without the use of tomographic imaging or special computer techniques to determine volumetric analysis, it is difficult to quantify the amount of tumor progression or regression within the liver in the patient on therapy. Again, evaluation of areas besides the liver for either progression or regression of disease is not possible.

Bernardino and Green showed that sonography was quite accurate at evaluating the chemotherapeutic response of hepatic metastases (13). Patients who improved, regressed, or remained unchanged showed a 98.6% correlation with other diagnostic modalities, such as angiography, CT, and radionuclide imaging (Figure 6A & B). However, another category of response was noted. These were lesions within the liver that changed their echogenic characteristics, but not the size of the lesion or the liver itself (Figure 7A & B). In these cases, there was absolutely no correlation with the other diagnostic modalities or the patient's clinical course. Some improved and some remained the same or worsened. Thus, if ultrasound is to be used to follow the response of hepatic metastasis to treatment in such patients, the clinical course should be relied upon to determine further therapy.

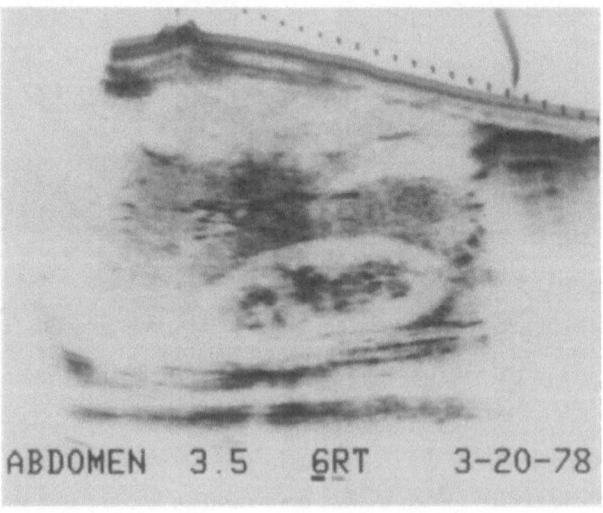

FIGURE 6A. Sonogram demonstrates a large hypoechoic mass in the anterior portion of the liver.

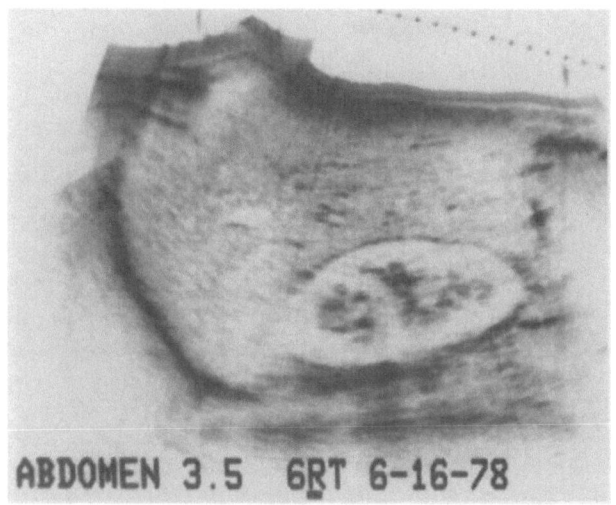

FIGURE 6B. Repeat examination three months later demonstrates resolution of the metastatic disease with therapy.

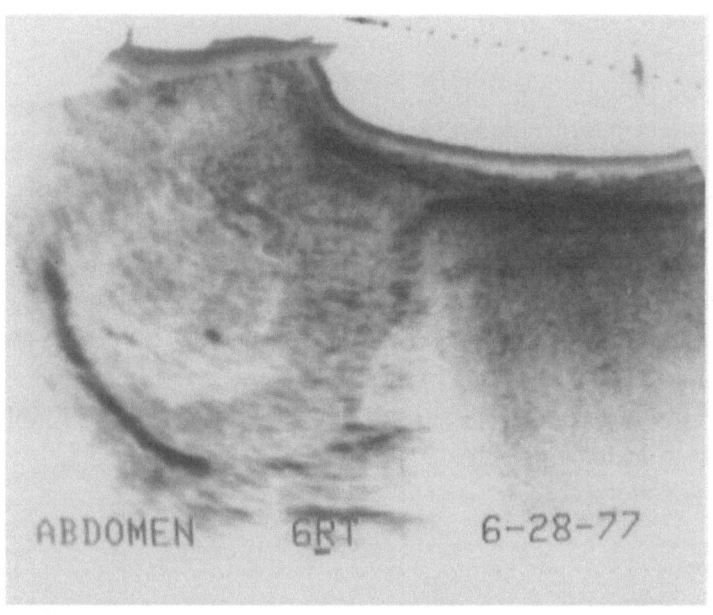

FIGURE 7A. Sonography demonstrates a hypoechoic mass in the right hepatic lobe.

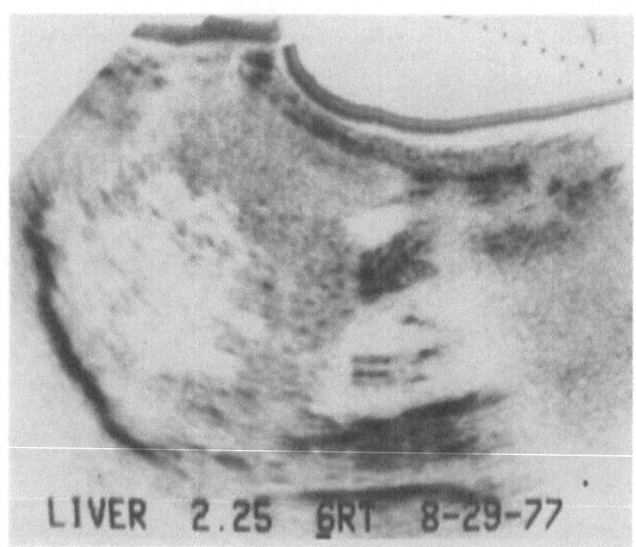

LIVER 2.25 6RT 8-29-77

FIGURE 7B. After two months of therapy the mass and liver remain the same size; however, the echogenic characteristics are different. This type of follow-up shows no correlation with the patient's other diagnostic studies. The clinician must rely on the patient's clinical condition.

MAGNETIC RESONANCE IMAGING

At the present time, little is known about whether magnetic resonance imaging (MRI) will help in the evaluation of tumor response to therapy. However, one should note that it is quite possible to obtain normal tissue samples from a grossly metastatic liver that will have abnormal T1 and T2 values (14). Therefore, after a certain threshold of tumor has been noted within the liver, this abnormality is seen. Such findings may have significant implications in the future. It may be quite possible to obtain abnormal MRI numbers from hepatic tumor involvement before they are detectable by conventional means. Such a finding would be extremely useful in assessing the benefits of therapy on metastases to the liver or to other sites.

References

1. Husband JE, Hodson NJ, Parsons CA: The use of computed tomography in recurrent rectal tumors. Radiology 134: 677-682, 1980.

2.   Hoth DF, Petrucci PE: Natural history and staging of colon cancer. Semin Oncol 3: 331-335, 1976.

3   Cass AW, Million RR, Pfaff WW: Patterns of recurrence following surgery alone for adenocarcinoma of the colon and rectum. Cancer 37: 2861-2865, 1976.

4.   Moss AA, Theoni RF, Schnyder P, Margulis AR: Value of computed tomography in the detection and staging of recurrent rectal carcinomas. J Comput Assist Tomogr 5: 870-874, 1981.

5.   Mayes GB, Zornoza J: Computed tomography of colon carcinoma. Am J Radiol 135: 43-46, 1980.

6.   Friedman MA, Resser KJ, Marcus TS, Moss AA, Cann CE: How accurate are computed tomographic scans in assessment of changes in tumor size? Am J Med 75: 193-198, 1983.

7.   Moss AA, Cann CE, Friedman MA, Marcus FS, Resser KJ, Berninger W: Volumetric CT analysis of hepatic tumors. J Comput Assist Tomogr 5: 714-718, 1981.

8.   Nakamura H, Tanaka T, Hori S, Yoshioka H, Kuroda C, Okamura J, Sakurai M: Transcatheter embolization of hepatocellular carcinoma: Assessment of efficacy in cases of resection following embolization. Radiology 147: 401-405, 1983.

9.   Bernardino ME, Chuang V, Wallace S, Thomas JL, Soo C-S: Therapeutically infarcted tumors: CT findings. Am J Radiol 136: 527, 1981.

10.   Lewis E, Bernardino ME, Salvador PG, Cabanillas FF, Barnes PA, Thomas JL: Post-therapy CT-detected mass in lymphoma patients: Is it viable tissue? J Comput Assist Tomogr 6: 792-795, 1982.

11.   Soo C-S, Bernardino ME, Chuang VP, Ordonez N: Pitfalls of CT findings in post-therapy testicular carcinoma. J Comput Assist Tomogr 5: 39-41, 1981.

12.   Bernardino ME: Percutaneous biopsy. Am J Radiol 142: 41-45, 1984.

13.   Bernardino ME, Green B: Ultrasonographic evaluation of chemotherapeutic response in hepatic metastases. Radiology 133: 437-441, 1979.

14.   Bernardino ME, Small W, Goldstein J, Sewell CW, Sones PJ, Gedgaudas-McClees K, Galambos JT, Wenger J, Casarella WJ: Multiple NMR T2 relaxation values in human liver tissue. Am J Radiol 141: 1203-1208, 1983.

20

THE EVALUATION OF SERIAL MARKER MEASUREMENTS FOR MONITORING PATIENTS AT RISK OF RECURRENT CANCER: APPLICATION TO COLORECTAL CANCER

Mitchell H. Gail

SUMMARY

In this chapter, three aspects of serial monitoring of cancer patients after resection are reviewed: (1) demonstrating that the marker profile is associated with increased risk of recurrence, (2) assessing the possible benefit of surgery in the marker-positive patient without other evidence of disease, and (3) evaluating the potential benefit of the marker for the entire population of patients with resected tumors. Points (2) and (3) are discussed with reference to colorectal cancer.

For demonstrating an association of marker profile with risk of recurrence, new statistical methods that take the time of recurrence into account are recommended, and design features for ideal clinical studies are discussed.

Available data suggest that second-look surgery following resection of colorectal cancer will improve five-year survival rates for the carcinoembryonic antigen (CEA) marker-positive, clinically negative patient from about 12% to about 21%, but the clinical evidence is scanty, especially regarding survival rates in patients with repeat resections. Sample size calculations for a clinical trial comparing immediate second-look surgery with watchful waiting suggest that such a trial is not feasible and indicate a need for more of the preliminary type of data used in this paper. The desirability of surgery for the marker-positive, clinically negative patient requires periodic reassessment because improvements in diagnostic technique are rapidly changing the definition of "clinically negative." The surgeon may encounter a decreasing proportion of untreatable recurrences and an increasing proportion of recurrence-free patients in future operations on marker-positive, "clinically negative" patients.

An extension of these analyses to all patients with resected disease shows that very little survival benefit is lost by eliminating or reducing conventional clinical follow-up. Instead, one can rely on a combined program of education to alert patients to important symptoms and of periodic CEA monitoring. This program captures practically all the survival benefit that could be obtained from a much more costly and inconvenient program, including both CEA monitoring and clinical follow-up.

INTRODUCTION

Biochemical markers for cancer have been used to monitor patients following resection who are at risk of recurrence, in the hope that early detection during follow-up will lead to more effective treatment and prolonged survival. In this chapter we discuss three questions central to the evaluation of serial marker measurements:

1. Are particular marker profiles indicative of increased risk of recurrence?

2. Can the use of markers in conjunction with second-look surgery improve survival for marker-positive patients without other evidence of recurrence?

3. Can the use of serial marker data in conjunction with second-look surgery improve overall five-year survival rates or otherwise improve management of the entire population of patients with initially resected disease?

In thinking about these questions, we shall use as an example the follow-up of patients with resected colorectal cancer, although the same issues arise more generally. These questions follow a natural sequence. One would not subject a group of marker-positive patients to second-look surgery in order to answer the second question unless previous evidence demonstrated an association between marker profiles and risk of recurrence. Likewise, one needs the answers to the second question in order to answer the third question.

One problem in evaluating serial marker data is deciding what feature of the marker profile (MP) should be used to predict risk of recurrence. We suppose that the entire MP from initial treatment at $t=0$ to follow-up time t is represented by $MP = \{Y(\tau); 0 \leq \tau \leq t\}$, where $Y(\tau)$ is the value of the marker at each instant τ. In order to make progress, we must examine some particular feature of the marker profile. For example, we might focus on the current value of the marker by studying $Z_1(t)=Y(t)$, or we might focus on the value of the marker ω months before t by choosing $Z_2(t)=Y(t-\omega)$. We could study whether the marker had ever exceeded a fixed value, η, by defining $Z_3(t)=1$, if $Y(\tau) \geq \eta$ for any $0 \leq \tau \leq t$ and $Z_3(t)=0$ otherwise. We could see whether the rate of change of the marker over the prior Δ months is important by studying $Z_4(t)= \{Y(t)-Y(t-\Delta)\}/\Delta$. The list of possible features of the marker profile is endless, and the art of these analyses is in choosing an appropriate feature, $Z(t)$, that captures the important information for monitoring and that is easy to define and use clinically. It is crucial that the investigator include in his publications a precise definition of the feature

236

of the marker profile used, Z(t), together with conventions used to accommodate missing data. Otherwise, the findings cannot be validated or used by other researchers or practitioners. I have previously discussed these issues (1).

ARE PARTICULAR MARKER PROFILES INDICATIVE OF INCREASED RISK OF RECURRENCE?

The question of whether particular marker profiles are indicative of increased risk of recurrence can be answered easily. If monitoring takes place only during a short period, three months, following resection, then, at three months, the survivors are grouped as having "favorable" or "unfavorable" marker profiles, and the subsequent disease-free intervals for these two groups are compared using standard methods of survival analysis.

However, monitoring is usually required for much longer periods, and marker measurements are obtained at irregular intervals so that at the time, t, of a recurrence a recent marker value may not be available. Moreover, in long-term clinical experiments, some patients are lost to follow-up or die of other causes before their recurrences are observed, and some patients remain disease-free until the study ends. In addition, the patients may have other risk factors for recurrence that must be taken into account when assessing the marker. Gail (1) proposed a method for dealing with these difficulties by regarding the marker feature Z(t) as a time-dependent covariate in the Cox (2) model. Rather than dwell on these mathematical details, we shall emphasize features of the ideal clinical study and illustrate the method by example.

Study Features

An ideal study design should consider and include each of the features described in this section.

- The procedures for diagnosing recurrence should not be allowed to depend on the patient's marker values, and, indeed, the clinician diagnosing recurrence should not have access to marker data. Otherwise, a detection bias may be introduced because, for example, whenever the marker increases, a special effort might be made to diagnose recurrence.
- The timing of marker measurements should, to the extent possible, follow a predetermined schedule and should not depend on the patient's clinical status. In particular, the investigator should avoid taking extra marker measurements when he believes the patient is about to have a recurrence. Likewise, laboratory personnel who carry out the marker assay should not be informed as to the patient's clinical status.

• One should study enough patients so that over the course of the experiment recurrence will be observed in at least 50 patients. This rough sample size calculation is based on the following model and method of analysis. We suppose that $Z(t)=1$ if the current marker value is "elevated" and $Z(t)=0$ otherwise. We suppose that the hazard of recurrence at time t for a patient with $Z(t)=1$ is θ times the hazard of recurrence for otherwise similar patients at time t for whom $Z(t)=0$. Here θ is the relative hazard exp $\{\alpha Z(t)\}$ in equation 1 of Gail (1). If there are roughly equal numbers of those in marker states $Z(t)=1$ and $Z(t)=0$ at the times, t, of recurrence, then the sample size calculations of Schoenfeld (3) for the Cox survival model (2) show that about 35 recurrences are needed to have power 90% to detect a threefold relative hazard ($\theta=3$) for a two-sided size $\alpha=0.05$ test of the null hypothesis $\theta=1$. As discussed by Gail (1) and Mantel and Byer (4), this test is the usual Mantel-Haenszel (5) or logrank test, except that patients can change "groups" in time, depending on the value of $Z(t)$. A few more recurrences are needed to compensate for incomplete marker data and for imbalances in the numbers at risk at time t with $Z(t)=1$ and $Z(t)=0$. To detect smaller values of θ, more recurrences would be required, but any good marker should show a relative hazard of three or more.

• The marker measurements should be made frequently enough so that when a recurrence develops at time t one will be able to determine the marker features $Z(t)$ of the patient who suffers recurrence and of a substantial number of other patients at risk. Unless the value of $Z(t)$ can be determined for the patient who recurs at t, the information from this recurrence is lost. The information is also lost unless there is at least one comparison patient at risk at t whose $Z(t)$ differs from that of the patient with recurring disease. Because we do not have marker measurements at every instant t, we must adopt conventions to decide when $Z(t)$ is known or not and to interpolate or extrapolate from known marker values to determine $Z(t)$. For example, if $Z(t)=\gamma(t)$, we might set $Z(t)$ as equal to the last available marker measurement prior to t, provided that measurement occurred no more than 100 days prior to t. In this case, our convention is to regard $Z(t)$ as unknown unless a prior measurement falls within the "window" of 100 days prior to t. The conventions used to define $Z(t)$ in terms of necessarily incomplete data and to reject $Z(t)$ as unknown should be clearly stated in any anaylsis. These points are essential to the complete definition of $Z(t)$.

• Other known risk factors, such as initial stage of disease, should be measured. The analysis will be adjusted to take these risk factors into account.

Serial markers, therefore, may be studied conveniently and economically in the context of a therapeutic clinical trial. Such protocols define a schedule of follow-up procedures to diagnose recurrence, and important risk factors are measured. A trial of respectable size will plan for 90 or more recurrences. Methods for assuring the quality of the clinical data and for data analysis are typically in place. One can often obtain the necessary information on serial monitoring by simply drawing serum for marker studies only at prescheduled follow-up visits and freezing it for later laboratory processing. The expensive part of the experiment, clinical follow-up and data acquisition, is already paid for.

For example, the Lung Cancer Study Group (6) studied whether serial white blood cell (WBC) counts were predictive of increased risk of recurrence in resected non-small cell lung cancer. The numbers of events in Table 1 represent patients with recurrences and with valid marker measurements, namely WBC counts taken within 100 days prior to the date of recurrence. The analyses were stratified on two important risk factors, tumor stage (T1 versus T2) and cell type (squamous versus nonsquamous). The data on "no lag" show that a patient with WBC > 9100 cells/mm^3 is 2.38 times as likely to have a recurrence at a time t as is another similar patient with WBC ≤ 9100. In this case, $Z(t)=1$ if $Y(t) > 9100$ and $Z(t)=0$ otherwise. The "six months' lag" analysis considers $Z(t)=1$ if $Y(t-6) > 9100$ and $Z(t)=0$ if $Y(t-6) \leq 9100$. These results show that the hazard for a patient at time t whose WBC count was elevated six months before is 2.04 times the hazard at time t of another patient whose WBC count was not elevated six months previously.

Table 1. Analysis of Serial White Counts (cells/mm^3) in Patients at Risk of Recurrent Non-small Cell Lung Cancer

	Number of Events	Relative Hazard	95% Confidence Interval	p-value
No lag time > 9100: 0-9100	115	2.38	1.62-3.50	p < 0.001
Six months lag time > 9100: 0-9100	85	2.04	1.27-3.27	p=0.002

These analyses indicate that elevations in WBC during follow-up are indeed associated with increased risk of recurrence. Similar analyses show that currently elevated CEA values are strongly associated with increased risk of recurrence of

239

colorectal cancer (1), and this conclusion was also reached with slightly different statistical methods by the investigators (7) who gathered the CEA data used by Gail (1). Steele, et al. (8) recently published data on monitoring CEA in 456 patients with colon cancer and 141 patients with rectal cancer. These patients were followed up in the course of therapeutic randomized clinical trials. An elegant ordering of increasing risk of overall recurrence was found for four categories: 1) maximum CEA ≤ 5 ng/mℓ and monthly CEA increase $\leq 3\%$, 2) maximum > 5 ng/mℓ, monthly increase $\leq 3\%$, 3) maximum ≤ 5 ng/mℓ, monthly increase $> 3\%$, and 4) maximum > 5 ng/mℓ, monthly increase $> 3\%$. It would be interesting to reanalyze these data to take prognostic factors and time of recurrence into account and to see whether similar changes that occur six months before the recurrence are also associated with increased risk.

In order to have potential clinical utility, the marker must show an association with increased risk of recurrence. However, much more is required in order for the marker to be useful for prolonging survival.

CAN THE USE OF MARKERS IN CONJUNCTION WITH SECOND-LOOK SURGERY IMPROVE SURVIVAL FOR MARKER-POSITIVE PATIENTS WITHOUT OTHER EVIDENCE OF RECURRENCE?

Figure 1 depicts various contingencies for the marker-positive, clinically negative patient. The symbols M, C, R, and T correspond to a positive marker profile (M), clinical evidence of recurrence (including sigmoidoscopy and other diagnostic procedures) prior to second-look surgery (C), disease recurrence detectable on the basis of all clinical, laboratory, and surgical evidence at the time of second-look surgery (R), and the fact that the recurrence is treatable (resectable) at second-look surgery (T). The symbols $\overline{M}, \overline{C}, \overline{R}$, and $\overline{T}$ represent complementary events. Thus $M\overline{C}R\overline{T}$ describes a marker-positive, clinically negative patient who has a nonresectable recurrence at the time of second-look surgery. The quantities a_1, a_2, and a_3 are the conditional probabilities $P(RT \mid M\overline{C})$, $P(R\overline{T} \mid M\overline{C})$, and $P(\overline{R} \mid M\overline{C})$ respectively. The three probabilities $p_r=0.02$, $p=0.921$, and $p_s=.30$ are respectively the probabilities of five-year survival measured from the time of potential second-look surgery for a patient with untreated R, for a patient with untreated $\overline{R}$, and for a RT patient who survives a repeat resection. The factor $\rho = .95$ is the probability of surviving the perioperative period.

If these various probabilities in Figure 1 are correct, one can calculate the probability of five-year survival of $M\overline{C}$ patients for the two strategies, no operation or operation. For no operation, the $M\overline{C}RT$ patient contributes .333 x .02=.007, whereas, if he undergoes second-look surgery, he contributes 0.333 x .95 x .30=.095. Note that the overall five-year survival rates are 20.6% for the operation strategy and 12.4% for the no operation strategy.

240

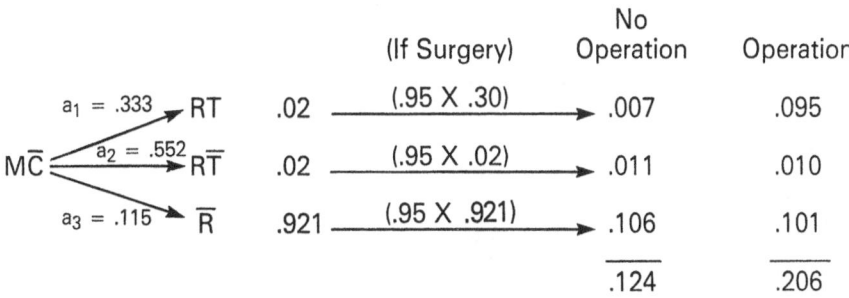

	(If Surgery)	No Operation	Operation
$a_1 = .333$ → RT	.02 ——(.95 X .30)——→	.007	.095
MC̄ ⟨ $a_2 = .552$ → RT̄	.02 ——(.95 X .02)——→	.011	.010
$a_3 = .115$ → R̄	.921 ——(.95 X .921)——→	.106	.101
		.124	.206

FIGURE 1. Contingencies for marker-positive, clinically negative (MC̄) patients.

The data on a_1, a_2, and a_3 come from a review of recent studies on the outcome of second-look operations in marker-positive, clinically negative disease patients (9-14). This review, which is similar to an analysis by Wanebo (9), is summarized in Table 2. Different criteria for marker positivity were used in the various studies, and different authors may use different definitions of "curative" resection (T). These differences, and chance variation, may explain the range of a_1 values (7% to 50%) seen in these studies. It seems reasonable to combine these data to obtain a_1=.333, a_2=.552, and a_3=.115 as in Figure 1.

The five-year survival rate, p_r=0.02, for untreated R patients is taken from Table 7 in Cochrane, et al. (15) for patients with unresectable disease. We are assuming that an untreated R patient has the same poor prognosis as a patient with initially unresectable disease. The five-year survival for R̄ patients is estimated as .921 (see next section). Perioperative mortality rates of 5% (ρ =0.95) are in line with recent reports for initial resections, though one might anticipate somewhat higher complication rates for second-look surgery. The most difficult and important survival parameter to estimate is p_s, the probability of surviving five years among re-resected RT patients who survive the perioperative period. Many re-resections involve metastases to local structures and, in more aggressive treatment settings, isolated metastases to the liver or lungs. Thus, it is unlikely that re-resected patients will have a five-year survival rate of 53%, which we take as the rate for originally resected disease patients. The value 30% on Figure 1 seems plausible to many surgeons. A range of values from 15% to 53% is studied in Table 3.

Table 2. Outcomes of Second-Look Surgery in Marker-Positive, Clinically Negative Patients

Reference	RT	$\overline{R}T$	$\overline{R}$	CEA Positivity Criterion
Minton and Martin (10)	4 (22)[*]	13 (72)	1 (6)	rising
Evans et al. (11)	1 (7)	10 (71)	3 (21)	rising
Steele et al. (12)	4 (25)	11 (69)	1 (6)	rising
Wanebo et al. (13)	7 (44)	7 (44)	2 (12)	elevated persistently
Attiyeh and Stearns (14)	16 (50)	12 (38)	4 (12)	elevated
TOTAL	32 (33.3)	53 (55.2)	11 (11.5)	

[*]   Numbers in parentheses are percentages

Table 3. Sample Sizes for a Clinical Trial Comparing Surgery with No Surgery in $M\overline{C}$ Patients

Assumptions[*]	Five Year Survival Rates (%)		Sample Size Needed[+]
	No Surgery	Surgery	
See Figure 1	12.4	20.6	850
10% operative mortality	12.4	19.5	1106
53% 5-year survival in RT patients with repeat resection	12.4	27.9	272
15% 5-year survival in RT patients with repeat resection	12.4	15.9	4156
$a_1=.25$, $a_2=.64$, $a_3=.11$	11.9	18.0	1424
100% 5-year survival in $\overline{R}$ patients	13.3	21.5	888
80% 5-year survival in $\overline{R}$ patients	11.0	19.3	772

[*]   The assumptions are the same as in Figure 1 except where otherwise indicated.

[+]   The sample sizes are based on a simple binomial comparison of the proportions surviving five years, assuming five-year potential follow-up on all patients. The total sample size required in both groups is calculated for a two-sided $\alpha=0.05$ level test with power 0.9 from equation (9) in Bacon and Berkeley (18).

In view of the uncertainties in some of these estimates, we have recalculated the survival rates of patients with and without surgery for several sets of assumptions

(Table 3). The benefits of surgery depend strongly on p_s, the five-year survival rate among re-resected RT patients, and on the proportion, a_1, with RT disease. If p_s is 0.53 instead of 0.30 as in Figure 1, five-year survival increases from 20.6% to 27.9% in the surgical group. If a_1 is only 0.25 instead of 0.333 as in Figure 1, the five-year survival drops to 18.0%. Changes in the estimate of the percentage of $\overline{R}$ patients surviving five years, p, have little impact on these results.

It appears from these analyses that second-look surgery benefits $M\overline{C}$ patients. However, the improvement in the five-year survival rate is modest. Over 12% would survive five years without the operation because 11.5% of people do not have recurrence (Figure 1). The five-year survival with surgery could be as low as 16% or as high as 28%, depending on the assumptions (Table 3). To demonstrate an improvement from 12.4% without surgery to 20.6% with surgery would require a clinical trial of 850 marker-positive, clinically negative patients (16) randomized either to immediate surgery or watchful waiting (Table 3). Such a trial is probably not feasible, because only about 15% of resected patients become marker-positive while clinically negative. Thus, one would need to resect and follow-up 850/.15=5667 patients just to obtain the required 850 $M\overline{C}$ patients for such a study, and, probably 50% more would be needed to compensate for failure to obtain patient consent and other losses.

It is feasible to obtain additional data on the percentage of re-resectable patients at second-look surgery (Table 2), and, as important, on the long-term survival of the patients having repeat resection. In such studies, careful description of the operational definition of "clinically negative" is essential. As diagnostic procedures improve, the proportion of $M\overline{C}$ patients without recurrence ($\overline{R}$) may rise, making surgery less attractive. Thus, the type of analysis in Figure 1 will need to be reviewed periodically to take into account new definitions of "clinically negative." Of course, as diagnostic procedures are perfected, one could hope to exclude $\overline{R}$ and $R\overline{T}$ patients reliably before operating.

CAN THE USE OF SERIAL MARKER DATA IN CONJUNCTION WITH SECOND-LOOK SURGERY IMPROVE OVERALL FIVE-YEAR SURVIVAL RATES OR OTHERWISE IMPROVE MANAGEMENT OF THE ENTIRE POPULATION OF INITIALLY RESECTED PATIENTS?

To gauge the impact and possible benefit of serial monitoring more broadly, various contingencies are elaborated for all four classes of patients, $M\overline{C}$, MC, $\overline{M}\overline{C}$, and $\overline{M}C$, in Figure 2. The proportions of patients in these four classes are assumed to be $e_1=.144$, $e_2=.113$, $e_3=.665$, and $e_4=.078$, as will be justified below, together with explanations of other estimates in Figure 2. The notation in Figure 2 is defined in Table 4. Notice that the $M\overline{C}RT$ population that would benefit from surgery in $M\overline{C}$ patients constitutes only

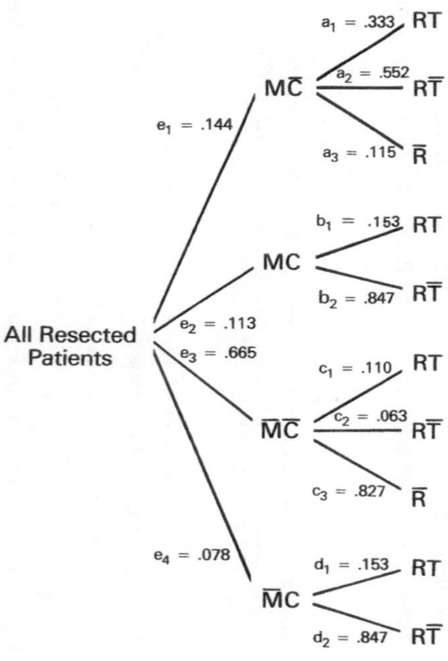

Figure 2 — Contingencies for all resected patients.

Tree structure:

All Resected Patients
- $e_1 = .144$ → M$\bar{\text{C}}$
  - $a_1 = .333$ RT
  - $a_2 = .552$ R$\bar{\text{T}}$
  - $a_3 = .115$ $\bar{\text{R}}$
- $e_2 = .113$ → MC
  - $b_1 = .153$ RT
  - $b_2 = .847$ R$\bar{\text{T}}$
- $e_3 = .665$ → $\bar{\text{M}}\bar{\text{C}}$
  - $c_1 = .110$ RT
  - $c_2 = .063$ R$\bar{\text{T}}$
  - $c_3 = .827$ $\bar{\text{R}}$
- $e_4 = .078$ → $\bar{\text{M}}$C
  - $d_1 = .153$ RT
  - $d_2 = .847$ R$\bar{\text{T}}$

	Percent of Total	(if surgery)	No Operation	Operate if M	Operate if C	Operate if M or C	Always Operate	Perfect Marker
a_1	4.8	$\dfrac{.02}{P_r}\ \dfrac{(.95 \times .30)}{\varrho \times P_s}$	.001	.014	.001	.014	.014	.014
a_2	7.9	$\dfrac{.02}{P_r}\ \dfrac{(.95 \times .02)}{\varrho \times P_r}$	.002	.002	.002	.002	.002	.002
a_3	1.7	$\dfrac{.921}{P}\ \dfrac{(.95 \times .921)}{\varrho \times P}$	.015	.014	.015	.014	.014	.015
b_1	1.7	$\dfrac{.02}{P_r}\ \dfrac{(.95 \times .30)}{\varrho \times P_s}$	.000	.005	.005	.005	.005	.005
b_2	9.6	$\dfrac{.02}{P_r}\ \dfrac{(.95 \times .02)}{\varrho \times P_r}$	.002	.002	.002	.002	.002	.002
c_1	7.3	$\dfrac{.02}{P_r}\ \dfrac{(.95 \times .30)}{\varrho \times P_s}$	.002	.002	.002	.002	.021	.021
c_2	4.2	$\dfrac{.02}{P_r}\ \dfrac{(.95 \times .02)}{\varrho \times P_r}$	.001	.001	.001	.001	.001	.001
c_3	55.0	$\dfrac{.921}{P}\ \dfrac{(.95 \times .921)}{\varrho \times P}$	.506	.506	.506	.506	.481	.506
d_1	1.2	$\dfrac{.02}{P_r}\ \dfrac{(.95 \times .30)}{\varrho \times P_s}$	.000	.000	.003	.003	.003	.003
d_2	6.6	$\dfrac{.02}{P_r}\ \dfrac{(.95 \times .02)}{\varrho \times P_r}$	.001	.001	.001	.001	.001	.001
	100.0		.530	.547	.538	.550	.544	.570

FIGURE 2. Contingencies for all resected patients.

.144 x .333=4.8% of the whole. The total percentage of potentially salvageable (RT) patients is only 4.8 + 1.7 + 7.3 + 1.2 = 15.0%. Most of the favorable survival experience derives from the $\overline{\text{MCR}}$ patients, who constitute 55.0%. If the assumptions in Figure 1 are correct, then the overall five-year survival rates are obtained by totaling the 10 rows, as shown. We compare these survival rates for five possible management strategies: Never operate, operate if the marker is positive (M), operate if clinical evidence for recurrence is found (C), operate if the marker is positive or if clinical evidence is found (M or C), and always operate. The results are also shown for a hypothetically "perfect marker" that could pick out all RT patients without error. To see how the corresponding columns in Figure 2 are constructed, consider the $\text{M}\overline{\text{C}}\text{RT}$ patient. If he has no operation, he contributes 0.144 x 0.333 x 0.02= 0.001 to overall five-year survival, whereas, if an operation takes place, the contribution is 0.144 x 0.333 x 0.95 x 0.30 = 0.014. Note that the RT patient benefits from surgery, because perioperative mortality is negligible compared to the gains of treatment. In contrast, $\overline{\text{RT}}$ and $\overline{\text{R}}$ patients are hurt by surgery because there are no therapeutic gains to balance against the risks of surgery. This phenomenon is illustrated by $\text{M}\overline{\text{CR}}$ patients, whose contributions drop from 0.015 to 0.014 with surgery.

Table 4. Definition of Probabilities in Figure 2[*]

$e_1 = P(M\overline{C})$	$e_3 = P(\overline{M}\overline{C})$
$e_2 = P(MC)$	$e_4 = P(\overline{M}C)$
$a_1 = P(RT\|M\overline{C})$	$c_1 = P(RT\|\overline{M}\overline{C})$
$a_2 = P(R\overline{T}\|M\overline{C})$	$c_2 = P(R\overline{T}\|\overline{M}\overline{C})$
$a_3 = P(\overline{R}\|M\overline{C})$	$c_3 = P(\overline{R}\|\overline{M}\overline{C})$
$b_1 = P(RT\|MC)$	$d_1 = P(RT\|\overline{M}C)$
$b_2 = P(R\overline{T}\|MC)$	$d_2 = P(R\overline{T}\|\overline{M}C)$

$\rho = P$ (survive surgery)

$P = P$ (survive 5 years$|\overline{R}$)

$P_r = P$ (survive 5 years$|R$)

$P_s = P$ (survive 5 years RT$|$and survive surgical resection)

---

[*] The notation $P(y|x)$ is the conditional probability of y given the event x. It is assumed that the probability of surviving surgery and an additional five years beyond surgery is ρP for an $\overline{R}$ patient, ρP_r for a nonresectable $R\overline{T}$ patient, and ρP_s for a resectable RT patient.

Even a perfect marker improves five-year survival rates only from 53.0% with no operation to 57.0% with operations solely on RT patients (Figure 2). This is because only the 15% of patients with RT disease benefit from surgery. Thus, no scheme of follow-up can promise great gains, given the present therapeutic options. Clinical follow-up alone (53.8%) is worse than CEA marker follow-up alone (54.7%). Combined follow-up with surgery either if the marker is positive or if disease is clinically detected yields 55.0% five-year survival. Thus, monitoring with CEA alone captures most of the gains that could be achieved by a combination of monitoring with CEA and clinical follow-up. This result suggests that one could achieve tremendous cost savings and reduce patient inconvenience, at very little loss in potential survival benefit, by simply monitoring laboratory CEA values and foregoing scheduled physical examinations and clinical studies. Perhaps periodic CEA measurements should be augmented by an educational program to inform patients of symptoms that would signal the need for a medical examination. Indeed, even before CEA had been fully evaluated, Cochrane, et al. (17) suggested that clinical follow-up was so unrewarding and anxiety provoking that it should be replaced by such an educational program. But the availability of a relatively inexpensive and harmless blood test for monitoring makes the idea of reducing or eliminating scheduled clinical follow-up even more attractive.

The strategy of operating on every patient (54.4%) is not as good as operating only on patients who are marker-positive (Figure 2). Moreover, these analyses ignore other adverse aspects of surgery, such as morbidity and cost. The $\overline{MC}$ patients have a 76.5% five-year survival rate without surgery and a 75.5% five-year survival rate with surgery and, even if the long-term survival were improved by surgery, many $\overline{MC}$ patients would be reluctant to face an immediate operative risk for only a possible slight improvement in five-year survival rates. This is not true for $M\overline{C}$, MC, or $\overline{M}C$ patients, who face a substantial short-term risk without surgery.

To see how sensitive these results are to the assumptions in Figure 2, the calculations were repeated under differing assumptions (Table 5). In every case, CEA monitoring alone was better than clinical monitoring alone, and in every case, CEA monitoring alone captured most of the gains that could be achieved by second-look surgery if either the marker turned positive or if clinical evidence of recurrence developed.

Since the validity of these analyses depends on the estimates in Figure 2, we now describe how the numbers in the figure were obtained. The quantities a_1, a_2, and a_3 were discussed above. We estimated b_1, b_2, d_1, and d_2 from earlier accounts of disease resectability in patients with clinical evidence of recurrence (C) (17-21). We are assuming that the chance of disease resectability (RT) in C patients is the same as that in MC and $\overline{M}C$ patients. The proportion of RT patients among C patients is estimated as 15.3% (Table 6). Data from Bacon and Berkeley (18) are excluded because the total number of patients examined was not given. The estimates e_1, e_2, e_3, and e_4 are derived from early publications on CEA monitoring (Table 7). The estimates of c_1, c_2, and c_3 cannot be obtained from the recent literature because there have been no recent studies of second-look surgery in $\overline{M}C$ patients. Instead, c_1, c_2, and c_3 were calculated indirectly from the laws of probability and from estimates of the probabilities of the states RT, $R\overline{T}$, and $\overline{R}$ in $\overline{C}$ patients. Wangensteen, et al. (26) who carried out second-look surgery in a group of 64 asymptomatic patients with resected colorectal cancer at about six months following the initial operation, found 9 (14%) RT, 20 (31%) $R\overline{T}$, and 35 (55%) $\overline{R}$ patients. However, all of their patients had nodes positive for disease initially , as did 90% of the patients studied by Gunderson and Sosin (27), who reported that 60% of asymptomatic patients with resected rectal carcinoma were disease free $(\overline{R})$ at second-look surgery. The data of Gerard (15) and recent adjuvant trials (28) show that roughly half of the resected patients are initially lymph node negative. For this reason, and because 78% are alive and free of clinical evidence of disease at two years (28), we assume that $P(\overline{R}|\overline{C})=.70$, $P(RT|\overline{C})=.15$, and P $(R\overline{T}|\overline{C})=.15$ for all patients who had initial resections. It turns out that these assumptions have no impact on the calculations in Table 5 because monitoring only alters therapy in the $M\overline{C}$, MC, and $\overline{M}C$ groups. From the relations $P(RT|\overline{C})$ (e_1+e_3) = $e_1 a_1 + e_3 c_1$, we solve for $c_1=.110$. Likewise, we obtain c_2 and c_3 from $P(R\overline{T}|\overline{C})$ $(e_1+e_3)=e_1 a_2 + e_3 c_2$ and $P(\overline{R}|\overline{C})$ $(e_1+e_3)=e_1 a_{3+} e_3 c_3$ respectively. Finally, to estimate p, the probability of survival in $\overline{R}$ patients, we decompose the overall five-year survival into P(5-year survival)=.53=P(R)p_r+P($\overline{R}$)p. But P($\overline{R}$)=.566=$e_1 a_3 + e_3 c_3$ (Figure 2) and P(R)=1-.566=.434. Hence, p=.921. Other plausible values of P($\overline{R}$ | $\overline{C}$) lead to values of p ranging from .8 to 1.0, but these variations have no effect on general conclusions (Table 3). The 53% five-year overall survival figure used in these analyses is found by taking a weighted average of the five-year survival rates in Gerard (15) for resectable node-negative colonic (68%), node-positive colonic (38%), node-negative rectal (59%), and node-positive rectal (31%) cancers. The weights are the expected proportions of these categories in a mixed population of 32% rectal and 68% colonic cancers. The breakdown into node-negative versus node-positive disease is given in Figures 3 and 4 of Gerard (15), and these calculations lead to five-year survival rates of 56% for colonic and 47% for rectal cancer, in line with recent literature. Table 5 also includes one example with 60% overall survival because very recent adjuvant trials are reporting slightly increased overall five-year survival rates (28).

247

Table 5. Overall Five-Year Survival Rates (%) for Various Management Strategies

Assumptions[*]	No Operation	Operate if M	Operate if C	Operate if M or C
As in Figure 2	53.0	54.6	53.8	54.9
10% operative mortality	53.0	54.4	53.7	54.7
53% 5-year survival in re-resected RT patients	53.0	56.1	54.4	56.6
15% 5-year survival in re-resected RT patients	53.0	53.7	53.3	53.8
a_1=.25, a_2=.64, a_3=.11	53.0	54.3	53.8	54.6
$P(RT|\bar{C})$=.12, $P(R\bar{T}|\bar{C})$=.23, $P(\bar{R}|\bar{C})$=.65	53.0	54.6	53.8	54.9
b_1=d_1-.1, b_2=d_2=.9	53.0	54.5	53.5	54.7
60% overall 5-year survival	60.0	61.6	60.8	61.9

[*] The assumptions are the same as in Figure 2 except where otherwise indicated.

Table 6. Numbers (and Percentages) of RT and $R\bar{T}$ Patients Among Those with Clinical Evidence of Recurrence (C)

Reference	RT	$R\bar{T}$
Ekmann et al. (19)	7 (19)	29 (81)
Spratt (20)	12 (17)	59 (83)
Tong et al. (21)	11 (17)	53 (83)
Cochrane et al. (17)	7 (10)	64 (90)
Total	37 (15.3)	205 (84.7)

Table 7. Numbers (and Percentages) of $M\bar{C}$, MC, $\bar{M}\bar{C}$ and $\bar{M}C$ Patients

Reference	$M\bar{C}$	MC	$\bar{M}\bar{C}$	$\bar{M}C$
MacKay et al. (22)	26 (12)	10 (4)	167 (76)	17 (8)
Mack et al. (23)	6 (27)	8 (36)	8 (36)	0 (0)
Sugarbaker et al. (24)	11 (33)	5 (15)	10 (30)	7 (21)
Beart et al. (25)	18 (12)	25 (17)	97 (65)	9 (6)
Total	61 (14.4)	48 (11.3)	282 (66.5)	33 (7.8)

DISCUSSION

In this chapter we reviewed some recent work on serial monitoring and emphasized that an assessment of the value of a marker could proceed by stages, first by demonstrating an association between marker profiles and risk of recurrence and then by studying the benefits for the patient who is marker-positive, clinically negative and for the entire population of patients with resected disease.

It appears that second-look surgery for $M\overline{C}$ patients improves five-year survival from about 12% to about 21%, but the data on which these conclusions depend are sparse, and very little long-term follow-up information for patients with repeat resections has been reported. More data of this type are needed because a clinical trial comparing surgery with watchful waiting in the marker-positive, clinically negative patients does not appear to be feasible.

The overall impact of monitoring and second-look surgery is limited because potentially treatable RT patients constitute but 15% of the whole. Even a perfect marker that detected all RT patients without error could only improve survival from 53% to 57% (Figure 2). The CEA marker detects only (4.8+1.7)/15=43% of all RT patients (Figure 2). Furthermore, from Figure 2, only .113/(.113+0.78)=59% of clinically positive patients are marker positive, and only .113/(.113+.144)=44% of marker-positive patients are clinically positive. These facts explain some of the pessimism expressed toward CEA monitoring (29).

Nonetheless, our analysis shows that CEA monitoring captures practically all of the survival benefit that a combination of CEA and clinical monitoring could achieve (Figure 2 and Table 5). Therefore, it appears that enormous expense and patient inconvenience could be avoided, at little risk, by reducing or eliminating scheduled clinical examinations and, instead, educating patients as to early symptoms of recurrence (17) and relying mainly on periodic CEA measurements. Presumably, a program of patient education plus CEA monitoring would yield results even closer to combined clinical follow-up and CEA monitoring than would CEA monitoring alone (Table 5). Against the benefits of reduced reliance on clinical follow-up must be weighed the needs of individual patients who may be reassured by careful clinical evaluation and the possibility, deemed remote (17), that clinical follow-up might detect a second primary tumor.

Analyses represented in Figure 2 could be refined by including other clinical contingencies and by developing statistical methods that take time of recurrence into account. However, if appreciable time is required for the marker to turn positive, one

249

would suppose that the potential improvements in five-year survival from monitoring would be even less than indicated in Table 5.

It is important to be cognizant of the rapid improvements in diagnostic radiology. Such methods are changing our definition of "clinically negative," and it will be worthwhile to review analyses, such as in Figure 2, in the future to take these advances into account. In the future it may be possible to identify marker-positive patients who have resectable disease and to avoid unavailing surgery.

Acknowledgments

I wish to thank Drs. David Byar, Martin Adson, Alfred Chang, Glenn Steele, Jr., and Paul Sugarbaker for helpful comments and Julie Paolella and Debbie Maloney for typing the manuscript.

References

1. Gail MH: Evaluating serial cancer marker studies in patients at risk of recurrent disease. Biometrics 37: 67-78, 1981.
2. Cox DR: Regression models and life tables (with discussion). J Royal Stat Soc 34: 187-220, 1972.
3. Schoenfeld D: The asymptotic properties of nonparametric tests for comparing survival distributions. Biometrika 68: 316-319, 1981.
4. Mantel N, Byar DP: Evaluation of response-time data involving transient states: An illustration using heart transplant data. J Am Stat Assoc 69: 81-86, 1974.
5. Mantel N, Haenszel W: Statistical aspects of the analysis of data from retrospective studies of disease. J Natl Cancer Inst 22: 719-748, 1959.
6. Gail MH, Eagan RT, Feld R, Ginsberg R, Goodell B, Hill L, Holmes EC, Lukeman JM, Mountain CF, Oldham RK, Pearson FG, Wright PW, and Lake WH: Prognostic factors in patients with resected stage I non-small cell lung cancer: A report from the Lung Cancer Study Group. Cancer 54: 1802-1813, 1984.
7 Lavin PT, Day J, Holyoke D, Mittelman A, Chu TM: Statistical evaluation of baseline and follow-up carcinoembryonic antigen in patients with resectable colorectal carcinoma. Cancer 47: 823-826, 1981.
8. Steele G Jr, Ellenberg S, Ramming K, O'Connell M, Moertel C, Lessner H, Bruckner H, Horton J, Schein P, Zamcheck N, Novak J, Holyoke ED: CEA monitoring among patients in multi-institutional adjuvant G.I. therapy protocols. Ann Surg 196: 162-169, 1982.
9. Wanebo HJ: Are carcinoembryonic antigen levels of value in the curative management of colorectal cancer. Surgery 89: 290-295, 1981.
10. Minton JP, Martin EW: The use of serial CEA determination to predict recurrence of colon cancer and when to do a second-look operation. Cancer 42: 1422-1427, 1978.
11. Evans JT, Mittelman, A, Chu M, Holyoke ED; Pre- and postoperative uses of CEA. Cancer 42: 1419-1422. 1978.
12. Steele G, Zamcheck N, Wilson RE, Mayer R, Lokich J, Rao P, Mattz J: Results of CEA-initiated "second-look" surgery for recurrent colorectal cancer. Am J Surg 139: 544-548, 1980.

13. Wanebo HJ, Stearns M, Schwartz MK: Use of CEA as an indicator of early recurrence and as a guide to a selected second-look procedure in patients with colorectal cancer. Ann Surg 188: 481-493, 1978.
14. Attiyeh FF, Stearns MW: Second-look laparotomy based on CEA elevations in colorectal cancer. Cancer 47: 2119-2125, 1981.
15. Gerard A: Carcinoma of the colon and rectum: prognostic factors and criteria of response. In: MJ Staquet (ed), Cancer therapy: Prognostic factors and criteria of response. Raven Press, New York, 1975, pp 199-227.
16. Gail M, Gart JJ: The determination of sample sizes for use with the exact conditional test in 2 x 2 comparative trials. Biometrics 29: 441-448, 1973.
17. Cochrane JPS, Williams JT, Faber RG, Slack WW: Value of outpatient follow-up after curative surgery for carcinoma of the large bowel. Br Med J 1: 593-595, 1980.
18. Bacon HE, Berkeley JL: The rationale of re-resection for recurrent cancer of the colon and rectum. Dis Colon Rectum 2: 549-554, 1959.
19. Ekmann C, Gustavson J, Henning A: Value of a follow-up study of recurrent carcinoma of the colon and rectum. Surg Gynecol Obstet 145: 895-897, 1977.
20. Polk HC, Spratt JS: Recurrent colorectal carcinoma: Detection, treatment, and other considerations. Surgery 69: 9-23, 1971.
21. Tong D, Russell AH, Dawson LE, Wisbeck W: Second laparotomy for proximal colon cancer. Am J Surg 145: 382-386, 1983.
22. MacKay AM, Patel S, Carter S, Stevens U, Laurence DJR, Cooper EH, Neville AM: Role of serial CEA assays in detection of recurrent and metastatic colorectal carcinoma. Br Med J 4: 382-385, 1974.
23. Mack J-P, Jaeger PH, Bertholet M-M, Ruegsegger CH, Loosli RM, Pettaval J: Detection of recurrence of large bowel carcinomas by radioimmunoassay or circulating carcinoembryonic antigen (CEA). Lancet ii: 535-540, 1974.
24. Sugarbaker PH, Zamcheck N, Moore FD: Assessment of serial carcinoembryonic antigen (CEA) assays in postoperative detection of recurrent colorectal cancer. Cancer 38: 2310-2315, 1976.
25. Beart RW, Metzger PP, O'Connell MJ, Schutt AJ: Postoperative screening of patients with carcinoma of the colon. Dis Colon Rectum 24: 585-588, 1981.
26. Wangensteen OH, Lewis FJ, Arhelger SW, Muller JJ, MacLean LD: An interim report upon the "second look" procedure for cancer of the stomach, colon and rectum and for "limited intraperitoneal carcinosis." Surg Gynecol Obstet 99: 257-267, 1954.
27. Gunderson LL, Sosin H: Areas of failure found at re-operation (second or symptomatic look) following curative surgery for adenocarcinoma of the rectum. Cancer 34: 1278-1292, 1974.
28. Gastrointestinal Tumor Study Group: Adjuvant therapy of colon cancer - results of a prospectively randomized trial. N Eng J Med 310 : 737-743, 1984.
29. Moertel CG, Schutt AJ, Go VJ: Carcinoembryonic antigen test for recurrent colorectal carcinoma: Inadequacy for early detection. J Am Med Assoc 239: 1065-1066, 1978.

21

PROGNOSTIC FACTORS FOR LIVER METASTASES FROM COLORECTAL CANCER

Daniel G. Haller

SUMMARY

Hepatic metastasis from colorectal cancer is a common problem in clinical oncology. Results of new operative and chemotherapeutic techniques suggest that some patients may benefit from therapeutic intervention. However, phase II studies of these therapies often cannot adequately evaluate the impact of the natural history of the disease on the survival of the treated patient population. A review of the literature demonstrates that patients with hepatic metastases from colorectal cancer may survive for more than two years if they have favorable prognostic variables. Those factors that seem to have significant prognostic influence include resection of the primary tumor, nodal involvement at the time of primary surgery, presence or absence of extrahepatic disease, extent of hepatic involvement, abnormalities of liver function tests, and performance status. Classification schema that utilize these known prognostic variables are necessary to improve communication among investigators and our ability to evaluate new therapies as they are reported.

INTRODUCTION

In the natural history of colorectal cancer, the most common site of distant metastatic disease is the liver. Ten to 25% of patients will present with hepatic metastases at the time of initial diagnosis, and the majority of patients with recurrent disease will develop liver metastases at some time (1-4). Recent increased interest in liver-directed therapies has stimulated much research into their technical and pharmacologic aspects, but has not often led to a better understanding of the natural history of hepatic metastases from colorectal cancer. The data provided from uncontrolled clinical trials of hepatic infusion therapies have suggested that improved survival times might be expected from such programs. However, retrospective control populations often demonstrate much shorter survival times than prospective treatment control populations, and wide variations between treated and untreated populations may be expected in trials with limited numbers of patients. Indeed, in 1978 Bengmark and

Hafstrom wrote that ". . . the natural history for patients with metastases in the liver might change as the attitude toward the . . . tumor changes . . . A consequence of this will be a desire to detect the secondary manifestations earlier, which in turn might change the 'natural course' " (5).

The purpose of this chapter is to review and identify significant prognostic variables in patients with hepatic metastases from colorectal cancer. The knowledge of such variables is important, not only for the definition of specific risks for groups and individuals, but also for the stratification of clinical trials and the evaluation of new therapies as they arise. A review of the literature suggests a number of possible prognostic variables in patients with metastatic colorectal cancer (Table 1). These variables relate not only to the nature of the primary tumor and hepatic involvement, but also to the potential impact on survival from host factors and treatment. Each of these variables will be examined and evaluated, and recommendations will be made concerning their use in the planning and analysis of results of clinical trials of patients with hepatic metastases from colorectal cancer.

Table 1. Possible Prognostic Variables of Hepatic Metastases from Colorectal Cancer

Variables	Nature of Variables
Primary Tumor	Site of Primary Nodal Involvement Histologic Grade
Hepatic Involvement	Synchronous versus Metachronous Disease-free Interval Extent of Hepatic Involvement Hepatic versus Extrahepatic Disease Laboratory Abnormalities
Host Factors	Age Sex Symptoms Performance Status
Therapy	Type of Primary Surgery Chemotherapy

THE PRIMARY TUMOR

In 1977, Silverman reported median survival times of patients with colorectal cancer based on a population of 9,745 patients (6). These data were selected from the End Results Group file at the National Cancer Institute. Median survival time for all patients with metastatic colon cancer was 10.5 months; for patients with rectal primary tumors, the survival time was 10.7 months. When only patients with hepatic metastases were considered, the median survival times for colon and rectal primary tumors were 10.0 and 10.4 months, respectively. Although reporting of the primary site was not uniformly done, no large differences in survival times were observed between patients with colon and rectal primary tumors once metastatic disease was diagnosed. Smaller studies have also failed to demonstrate that the site of the primary tumor has a significant impact on survival in such patients.

The extent of the primary tumor at the time of diagnosis has an impact on the survival of patients with observed hepatic metastases. In 1970, Cady reported that patients with direct extention of tumor into pericolonic tissues experienced a mean survival of 9.8 months, compared with 17.7 months for those without extension (7). In addition, patients without lymph node involvement survived longer than those with involvement of the regional nodes (17.8 versus 12.6 months). More recently, a retrospective review from the University of Alabama confirmed the negative prognostic impact of extracolonic extension of tumor and lymph node metastases on survival of patients with metastatic disease (8).

In many surgical intervention trials, the ability to perform a particular procedure may appear to confer a survival benefit. In most instances, more extensive procedures are associated with longer survival times, since these procedures are reserved for patients with less extensive, potentially curative disease. It is, therefore, no surprise that patients with colorectal cancer who have only exploratory or bypass procedures have distinctly inferior survival times (1.2 to 6.3 months) compared with those who are selected for resection (7 to 14 months) (7-12).

Although a prolonged disease-free interval may predict favorably for survival in some primary malignancies, the literature does not support this concept for hepatic metastases from colorectal cancer (1,8-10,13-16). In no published series is the survival time after diagnosis of metachronous hepatic--or extrahepatic--metastases significantly longer than after synchronously diagnosed metastatic disease. This suggests that, in patients considered for organ-directed management of hepatic metastases, disease-free survival need not be considered in the design and analysis of the clinical trial.

The impact of histologic grade on the survival of patients with metastatic colorectal cancer is unclear (Table 2) (2,8,9,11,13,17). There are a multitude of reasons why published studies do not agree on the significance of histologic grade in the natural history of this tumor, including size and selection of patient population and interpretation of available tissue specimens. For example, data from a series of patients from the Mayo Clinic appeared to demonstrate that patients with Broder's grades 1 and 2

255

tumors survived longer (32 months) than those patients with Broder's grades 3 and 4 tumors (20 months) (17). However, this comparison was based only on a small number of patients with unresected solitary liver metastases and no evidence of other residual disease. When all patients were considered regardless of disease extent, there appeared to be a negligible influence of histologic grade on survival.

Table 2. Impact of Histologic Grade on Survival

Source	Median Survival Time in Months		
	Poorly Differentiated (#)[*]	Moderately Differentiated (#)[*]	Well Differentiated (#)[*]
No impact on survival			
Morris (2)	11.2 (26)	11.8 (23)	---
Lahr (8)	5.4 (20)	6.9 (61)	5.8 (31)
Wagner (17)	8.0 (58)	---	12.0 (120)
Some impact on survival			
Pestana (9)	6.6 (181)	---	11.2 (389)
Jaffe (11)	3.0 (37)	5.7 (31)	6.3 (69)
Goslin (13)	6.0 (17)	17.0 (102)	30.0 (6)

[*] Number of patients reported.

The greatest range in median survival times relative to histologic grade has been reported by Goslin (13). Analysis of 125 patients referred to the Dana-Farber Cancer Institute revealed that patients with poorly differentiated tumors experienced a median survival time of 6.0 months (range, 2 to 10 months), whereas those with well-differentiated tumors survived 30 months. As noted in Table 2, however, the number of patients with poorly differentiated and well-differentiated tumors was small and accounted for less than 20% of all patients. Given the lack of agreement among investigators concerning the prognostic significance of histologic grade in patients with metastatic colorectal cancer, this variable should be addressed prospectively in clinical trials.

HEPATIC INVOLVEMENT

Patients with recurrent colorectal cancer rarely present with metastatic disease isolated in the liver. The recent interest in hepatic arterial infusion of fluoropyrimidines and hepatic resection for patients who develop liver metastases has led to the rediscovery of this observation. Newer diagnostic radiologic techniques and intraoperative staging, required for the placement of intra-arterial catheters, have reinforced the frequency of extrahepatic disease diagnoses, even in patients who present with hepatic metastases. Retrospective reviews of patients with hepatic metastases are frequently biased by nonuniform methods of diagnosing extrahepatic disease and by other conscious and unconscious selection criteria that may significantly affect survival time.

The precise impact, therefore, of the presence of extrahepatic disease is difficult to determine from retrospective reviews. Two recent studies have suggested that those patients with metastatic disease confined to the liver have a better prognosis than those with widespread metastases. In Goslin's review of 125 patients referred to the Dana-Farber Cancer Institute, 48 patients had extrahepatic disease; none of these patients showed symptoms of their extrahepatic tumors (13). Patients with hepatic involvement alone survived 18 months, compared with 9 months for those patients with more extensive disease. Similarly, in a study of 97 patients undergoing hepatic arterial ligation for hepatic metastases, 46 patients with disease confined to the liver survived 10.1 months. Those 51 patients who also had extrahepatic disease had a median survival time of 6.9 months (18).

Given the increased frequency of intraoperative staging and the availability of more precise radiographic techniques, it is likely that the true incidence of extrahepatic disease and its impact on survival will be better defined in the future. The early experience of investigators suggests that the survival time of patients with disease confined to the liver is superior to that of patients with more widespread disease, and that patients with extrahepatic involvement should either be excluded from studies or analyzed separately from patients with hepatic metastases alone.

Although there is disagreement about the best way to assess and report the extent of metastatic disease in the liver, the impact of disease extent on survival is clear (Table 3) (8,13,17,19-22). Utilizing techniques ranging from the surgeon's estimate in the operating room of the number and extent of metastases to sophisticated computed tomographic methods, investigators generally agree that patients with fewer than four metastases in the liver or those with tumor confined to a single lobe in the liver experience a surprisingly long survival time (10.5 to 24 months). Patients with solitary metastases have the best survival rates. In Wagner's series of patients from the Mayo Clinic with potentially resectable--but unresected--liver metastases, 39 patients with isolated metastases survived a median of 20 months. The two-year survival rate was 44% (17). However, patients with widespread involvement survived a median of 11 months, and only 14% of patients were alive at two years. These data suggest that the extent of hepatic involvement should be accurately assessed and reported in analyses of natural history and of treatment results.

Table 3. Extent of Hepatic Involvement: Median Survival, Months

Source	Unilobar*	Bilobar
Wood (20)	10.6-16.7	3.1
Pettavel (19)	10.7-21.5	1.4-4.7
Lahr (8)	10.5-11.3	4.5
Wagner (17)	15.0-20.0	11.0
Wanebo (22)	12.0-18.0	3.0-8.0
	1-3 Metastases	>4 Metastases
Nielsen (21)	18.0	5.0
Goslin (13)	24.0	10.0
Lahr (8)	11.0	4.1
Wagner (17)	20.0	11.0

* The higher number reflects survival time of patients with solitary lesions.

Simple, noninvasive and reproducible laboratory tests would be of value in the diagnosis and management of hepatic metastases. Studies have demonstrated that alkaline phosphatase, 5'-nucleotidase, and other liver function tests have an acceptable predictive value for the diagnosis of liver involvement (23). More important, recent reports have also demonstrated that elevated liver function studies at the time of diagnosis correlate with poor survival rates (1,8,12,13,18,24). Two extensive multivariate analyses of prognostic factors in metastatic colorectal cancer with liver involvement have demonstrated that the median survival time of patients with normal to fewer than two times normal levels of alkaline phosphatase was 8.0 to 9.2 months, whereas more significant elevations were associated with survival times of 2.5 to 3.0 months (8,12). In addition, Kemeny has demonstrated in patients with liver metastases that lactate dehydrogenase (LDH) levels appeared to have prognostic significance; the median survival time of patients with a normal LDH was 18 months, compared with 9 months for those with moderate elevations and 6 months for those with gross elevations (>1000 U/l) (24).

Although it may be presumed that abnormalities in liver function test levels generally reflect the extent of tumor within the liver, it is also apparent that their prognostic significance and their reproducibility merit their inclusion in the classification schema of hepatic metastases.

HOST FACTORS

The response of the host to the metastatic tumor appears to have a strong predictive value for the duration of survival. Some studies have analyzed patients relative to the presence or absence of symptoms, although they have not defined the nature of those symptoms (7,8). Generally, patients without symptoms survive longer than patients with symptoms, although this may merely reflect the extent of both intra- and extrahepatic disease. Weight loss prior to the diagnosis of metastatic disease is a more quantifiable measure of the impact of the tumor on the host. Patients without weight loss appear to survive significantly longer (8.0 to 17.4 mo) compared with those patients having any degree of weight loss (5.0 to 9.9 mo) (7,12,13,25).

The performance status (PS) of the patient, as typically measured by the Eastern Cooperative Oncology Group (ECOG) scale, is considered to be an important factor in patient survival and is a stratification criterion in many randomized treatment studies. In 1980, Lavin reported the survival characteristics of 1,314 patients treated with various chemotherapeutic programs entered into ECOG trials (25). The ambulatory (PS 0-1) patients survived significantly longer than non-ambulatory (PS 2-3) patients (9.5 versus 4.3 mo). Other studies have confirmed these findings (12,13,18, 26).

Some measurement of host response to the tumor should also be included in prospective or retrospective analyses of patients with hepatic metastases. The ECOG performance status scale is widely accepted and may be successfully utilized in any study situation.

MULTIFACTORIAL SURVIVAL ANALYSES

In order to assist in identifying dominant prognostic factors for patients with liver metastases from colorectal carcinoma, a number of investigators have retrospectively reviewed large series of patients from their institutions. They have subsequently performed multifactorial analyses to identify those factors with the most powerful significance. Lahr et al. reviewed and analyzed the survival times of 175 patients from the University of Alabama who had hepatic metastases (8). Twenty-two single factors were analyzed and ranked, the most significant of which are presented in Table 4. Multifactorial analysis identified a number of important factors relating to disease extent and two that were possibly related to patient selection (resection of primary tumor and chemotherapeutic treatment).

Bedikian analyzed 232 untreated patients from The University of Texas System Cancer Center, M. D. Anderson Hospital and Tumor Institute at Houston who had metastatic colorectal cancer (12). In Table 4, the single factors that had the most impact on survival are ranked. Not all patients had liver metastases, and those who did have liver involvement lived shorter times than those who did not (5.0 versus 8.0 months). The most important factors according to stepwise regression analysis were alkaline phosphatase and albumin levels, duration of symptoms prior to the diagnosis of incurable metastatic disease, and resection of the primary tumor.

Table 4. Survival Analyses of Significant Prognostic Variables

Source	Single-Factor Analysis	Multifactorial Analysis
Lahr (8)	Bilirubin Primary tumor resected Alkaline phosphatase Lactate dehydrogenase (LDH) Number of metastases Location of metastases Albumin Prothrombin time Extracolonic extension Sex Symptoms Nodal involvement Chemotherapy	Alkaline phosphatase Bilirubin Primary tumor resected Location of metastases Nodal involvement Albumin Chemotherapy
Bedikian (12)	Primary tumor resected Alkaline phosphatase Weight loss Liver metastases (present) Abdominal mass Hemoglobin Albumin Lymphocyte and monocyte counts Performance status Disease-free interval	Alkaline phosphatase Albumin Symptom duration Primary tumor resected

Taken together, these data suggest that a number of prognostic variables are important in the prediction of survival of patients with metastatic colon cancer. If patient selection factors, such as the initial surgical approach and the administration of chemotherapy, are excluded, the variables that best correlate with survival time include: laboratory tests (alkaline phosphatase, bilirubin, and albumin levels), extent of tumor involvement (nodal and hepatic), and host factors. Given the limitations of these retrospective analyses, these data support the conclusions from earlier reports and form the basis for a classification schema for patients with metastatic colorectal cancer.

CLASSIFICATION SCHEMA

A number of classification schema have evolved as the need to predict for individual and group survival increased. Early systems utilized single variables and typically correlated survival with extent of hepatic involvement (20,21). Recently, Wanebo presented a staging system based on the surgeon's description of extent of liver metastases at laparotomy (22). In this system, the median survival time for patients with stage I disease (< 25%) was 18 months; for patients with stage II disease (26-75%), 8 to 9 months; and for patients with stage III disease (> 75%), 3 months.

Other systems have included different variables, such as abnormalities in the liver function tests. The Lausanne System stages disease by presence or absence of hepatomegaly and by an elevated alkaline phosphatase level (19). A classification system has been proposed by Petrelli that includes four factors: percentage of liver involvement, abnormalities in liver function tests, performance status, and presence or absence of extrahepatic disease (18). This system utilizes the major variables suggested by other studies and deserves prospective validation.

Recently, a group of investigators met in Leyden, The Netherlands, to formulate a working staging system for hepatic metastases (27). This system has not yet been published, but it would be valuable to establish a common mechanism by which treatment research on this clinical problem could progress. The need for this is emphasized by the fact that, of five large randomized protocols in the United States comparing hepatic arterial infusions of floxuridine and intravenous therapy, no two utilize the same stratification criteria.

CONCLUSIONS

Recent advances in the delivery of chemotherapeutic agents directed to the liver had led to controversy concerning the survival advantages of such therapy compared with historical controls. The limitations of this approach are well-known, and the selection of proper controls is often very difficult. In the review of the literature, there are few retrospective analyses that approach the available data comparably, and the patient populations often appear hopelessly dissimilar. The intent of this review is to bring together such data as currently exist and to encourage their inclusion in clinical trials for prospective evaluation.

What is apparent from the literature is the extraordinary range of median survival times demonstrated in patients with hepatic metastases from colorectal cancer. Although the commonly accepted median survival times for such patients is six months, the actual time of survival may be somewhat shorter or very much longer, depending on major prognostic variables for that individual or that group of patients. In most recent series, patients with limited hepatic involvement, no extrahepatic disease, and a normal performance status can be expected to have a median survival time of two years. However, inclusion in a phase II study of a large number of patients with such favorable prognostic characteristics could imply treatment advantages when none may exist. Proper analyses of such trials, therefore, mandates inclusion of known patient characteristics. Although current randomized trials evaluating the role of hepatic intra-arterial infusion of fluoropyrimidines utilize these characteristics as stratification criteria, no uniform classification system exists. Systems that incorporate known prognostic variables should be developed and agreed upon. They should then be implemented in future trials to improve communication among investigators interested in therapy for hepatic metastases.

References

1. Bergtsson G, Carlsson G, Hafstrom L, Jonsson PE: Natural history of patients with untreated liver metastases from colorectal cancer. Am J Surg 141: 586-589, 1981.
2. Morris MJ, Newland RC, Pherls MT, MacPherson JG: Hepatic metastases from colorectal carcinoma: An analysis of survival rates and histopathology. Aust NZ J Surg 47: 365-368, 1977.
3. Bengmark S, Hafstrom L: The natural history of primary and secondary malignant tumors of the liver. Cancer 23: 198-202, 1969.
4. Oxley EM, Ellis H: Prognosis of carcinoma of the large bowel in the presence of liver metastases. Br J Surg 56: 149-152, 1969.
5. Bengmark S, Hafstrom L: The natural course for liver cancer. In: IM Ariel (ed), Progress in clinical cancer (VII). Grune & Stratton, New York, 1978, pp 195-199.
6. Silverman DT, Murray JL, Smart CR, Brown CC, Myers MH: Estimated median survival times of patients with colorectal cancer based on experience with 9,745 patients. Am J Surg 133: 289-293, 1977.
7. Cady B, Monson DO, Swinton NW: Survival of patients after colonic resection for carcinoma with simultaneous liver metastases. Surg Gynecol Obstet 131: 697-700, 1970.
8. Lahr CJ, Soong SJ, Cloud G, Smith JW, Urist MM, Balch CM: A multifactorial analysis of prognostic factors in patients with liver metastases from colorectal cancer. J Clin Oncol 1: 720-726, 1983.
9. Pestana C, Reitemeier RJ, Moertel CG, Judd ES, Dockerty MB: The natural history of carcinoma of the colon and rectum. Am J Surg 108: 826-829, 1964.
10. Abrahms MS, Lerner HJ: Survival of patients at Pennsylvania Hospital with hepatic metastases from carcinoma of the colon and rectum. Dis Colon Rectum 14: 431-434, 1971.
11. Jaffe BM, Donegan WL, Watson F, Spratt JS: Factors influencing survival in patients with untreated hepatic metastases. Surg Gynecol Obstet 127: 1-11, 1968.
12. Bedikian AY, Chen TT, Malahy MA, Patt YZ, Bodey GP: Prognostic factors influencing survival of patients with advanced colorectal cancer: Hepatic-artery infusion versus systemic intravenous chemotherapy for liver metastases. J Clin Oncol 2: 174-179, 1984.

13. Goslin R, Steck G, Zamcheck N, Mayer R, MacIntyre J: Factors influencing survival in patients with hepatic metastases from adenocarcinoma of the colon or rectum. Dis Colon Rectum 25: 749-754, 1982.
14. Rapoport AH, Burleson RL: Survival of patients treated with systemic fluorouracil for hepatic metastases. Surg Gynecol Obstet 130: 773-777, 1970.
15. Flanagan L, Foster JH: Hepatic resection for metastatic cancer. Am J Surg 113: 551-557, 1967.
16. Foster JH, Berman MH: Resection of metastatic tumors. In: Solid liver tumors: Major problems in clinical surgery, Vol 22. WB Saunders, Philadelphia, 1977, pp 209-234.
17. Wagner JS, Adson MA, VanHeerden JA, Ilstrup DM: The natural history of hepatic metastases from colorectal cancer. Ann Surg 199: 502-507, 1984.
18. Petrelli NJ, Bonnheim DC, Herrera LO, Mittelman A: A proposed classification system for liver metastases from colorectal carcinoma. Dis Colon Rectum 27: 249-252, 1984.
19. Pettavel J, Morgenthaler F: Protracted arterial chemotherapy of liver tumors: An experience of 107 cases over a 12-year period. In: IM Ariel (ed). Progress in clinical cancer (VII). Grune & Stratton, New York, 1978, pp 217-233.
20. Wood CB, Gillis CR, Blumgart LH: A retrospective review of the natural history of patients with liver metastases from colorectal cancer. Clin Oncol 2: 285-288, 1976.
21. Nielsen J, Balslev I, Jensen HE: Carcinoma of the colon with liver metastases. Acta Chir Scand 137: 463-465, 1971.
22. Wanebo H: A staging system for liver metastases from colorectal cancer. (Abstract) Proc Am Soc Clin Oncol 2: 646, 1984.
23. Kim NK, Yasmineh WG, Freier EF, Goldman AI, Theologides A: Value of alkaline phosphatase, 5'-nucleotidase, γ-'glutamyltransferase, and glutamate dehydrogenase activity measurements (single and combined) in serum in diagnosis of metastasis to the liver. Clin Chem 23: 2034-2038, 1977.
24. Kemeny N, Braun D: Advanced colorectal carcinoma: Clinical and laboratory parameters as indicators of response and survival (Abstract). Proc Am Soc Clin Oncol 22: 336, 1981.
25. Lavin P, Mittelman A, Douglass H, Engstrom P, Klassen D: Survival and response to chemotherapy for advanced colorectal carcinoma. Cancer 46: 1536-1543, 1980.
26. Bonomi PD, Rossoff AH, Raynor WJ, Quadeer M: Prediction of survival duration in patients with metastatic measurable colorectal adenocarcinoma (Abstract). Proc Am Soc Clin Oncol 21: 161, 1980.
27. Van de Velde CJL, Sugarbaker PH: Liver Metastasis: Basic Aspects, Detection, and Management. In: Developments in Oncology, vol 24. Martinus Nijhoff, Boston, 1984, pp 383.

SECTION V.

ANALYSIS OF FAILURE

22

CLINICAL PATTERNS OF FAILURE AFTER RESECTION OF COLON AND RECTUM CARCINOMA METASTASES TO THE LIVER

Glenn D. Steele, Jr.

SUMMARY

Data are presented on 43 patients from Brigham and Women's Hospital who underwent major hepatic resections for cure of primary and secondary liver tumors. These included 30 asymptomatic colorectal cancer patients with single or multiple resectable hepatic metastases. The results of this series of patients were analyzed by carefully documenting the clinical patterns of failure of the surgical procedures. The results reinforce the value of serial elevation of carcinoembryonic antigen as the best indicator of recurrence in predominantly asymptomatic patients. Not surprising based on the natural history of the disease is the observation that the majority of unresected patients die from liver failure whereas following hepatic resection, death results predominantly from failure outside of the liver. Thus, the pattern of failure after resection of hepatic metastases suggests that the proximate cause of death in these patients has been changed. Although the data confirm the safety of major hepatic resection performed properly on selected patients, the single most important predictor of local hepatic recurrence in patients with metastatic disease was the lack of clean margins at the time of the initial hepatic resection. Hence, while failure due to hepatic involvement may be prevented surgically, initiation of systemic adjuvant therapy protocols after liver resection should be our treatment goal. To accomplish this objective, however, more effective systemic therapy for large bowel cancer must be developed.

INTRODUCTION

We have reviewed the outcome of all major hepatic resections performed during a seven-year period at the Brigham & Women's Hospital for cure of primary and secondary liver tumors. Immediate and long-term outcome in 43 patients were reviewed. Patients ranged in age from 21 to 85 years, with a median age of 57 years. The predominant primary tumor diagnosis was hepatoma, but miscellaneous diagnoses included gallbladder cancers, isolated metastatic lesions with unknown primary sites, and occasional rupturing adenomas. By far, however, the largest group of patients who underwent resection at this time were those with single or multiple resectable hepatic metastases from colorectal cancers (30 patients). All of these patients were asymptomatic and, therefore, cure was the goal, not palliation. Since no prospective, controlled series comparing surgery to no treatment will ever be performed once patients are found to have resectable liver tumors, we have attempted to analyze the outcome of our surgical procedures by examining how we failed.

PATIENT REFERRAL PATTERN

The referral pattern is important to know when considering a patient population such as this that is automatically highly biologically selected. Most of our patients with colorectal cancer metastases were referred because of serial increases in carcinoembryonic antigen values as their only or first indication of suspected colorectal cancer recurrence after primary tumor resection (1,2). A number of other patients were referred for implantation of continuous-infusion drug delivery systems and were found at surgery to have resectable metastases and therefore underwent curative resection (3). Several patients were referred because previously unsuspected liver metastases noted at the time of primary colon or rectum cancer resection were thought to necessitate major hepatic surgery that would be better performed after recovery from the initial colorectal procedure.

CLINICAL EVALUATION AND MANAGEMENT

Details of each patient's diagnosis, presenting complaints, and important preoperative studies, as well as the surgery performed and the outcome is presented in Table 1. All of these patients underwent a battery of tests to exclude the possibility of extrahepatic tumor. Interestingly, computed tomographic (CT) scans of the chest were positive in approximately 15% of the colorectal cancer patients who had negative chest roentgenograms for extrahepatic pulmonary spread. Desite abdominal CT scans in all patients, approximately one third who were operated on were found at lapatoromy either to have previously unsuspected extrahepatic metastases or isolated liver metastases that were not anatomically resectable. Only patients with laparotomy-proven liver-only resectable metastases underwent resection. No debulking was done, since it is completely unjustified in patients with adenocarcinoma of the gastrointestinal tract. Hepatic angiography was performed on all patients, not to confirm the presence of liver tumor, since in our experience the majority of patients with colorectal cancer and liver metastases did not show any vascular blush, but simply to define the arterial anatomy.

268

Table 1. Details of All Major Liver Resections

Case#	Diagnosis	Presenting Symptoms	Positive Preoperative Tests	Resection Performed	Lesion Site and Size (Diameter)	Outcome
1	colon cancer	asymptomatic	liver scan	left lobectomy	single left lobe met*	NED – 91 mo
2	colon cancer	asymptomatic	liver scan, elevated CEA	trisegmentectomy/ resection right hemidiaphragm	single right lobe met extending into diaphragm	dead of systemic disease – 61 mo
3	colon cancer	asymptomatic	liver scan, elevated CEA	trisegmentectomy	single right lobe met 22 cm	NED – 48 mo
4	sarcoma	pain	CT scan	right lobectomy	single right lobe lesion	dead of systemic disease – 37 mo
5	rectal cancer	asymptomatic	noted at surgery for primary	right lobectomy/ left wedge (after decreased CEA on 5-FU)	multiple bilobar mets	NED – 36 mo
6	colon cancer	asymptomatic	CT scan, elevated CEA	trisegmentectomy	single right lobe met 24 cm	alive with systemic disease – 36 mo
7	colon cancer	asymptomatic	liver scan, CT scan, elevated CEA	extended left lobectomy	single left lobe met 24 cm	alive with systemic disease – 30 mo
8	colon cancer	asymptomatic	liver scan	right lobectomy	single right lobe met	NED – 30 mo (lost to follow-up)

269

Case#	Diagnosis	Presenting Symptoms	Positive Preoperative Tests	Resection Performed	Lesion Site and Size (Diameter)	Outcome
9	colon cancer	asymptomatic	elevated CEA	right lobectomy/ left wedge	multiple bilobar mets	NED – 21 mo (received 5-FU postop for CEA elevation)
10	colon cancer	asymptomatic	liver scan, CT scan, elevated CEA	right lobectomy	multiple right lobe mets	alive with systemic disease – 21 mo
11	hepatoma	pain, FUO	CT scan, liver scan	right lobectomy	right lobe primary 8 cm	NED – 20 mo
12	colon cancer	asymptomatic	liver scan, slightly elevated CEA	left lobectomy	single left lobe met	alive with recurrent liver met – 26 mo
13	hepatoma	pain, mass	CT scan	trisegmentectomy	single right lobe resection at junction with left lobe	NED – 23 mo
14	gallbladder cancer	incidental finding at cholecystectomy	-------	major hilar wedge	contiguous extension into gallbladder fossa	alive with local recurrence – 21 mos
15	colon cancer	asymptomatic	CT scan elevated CEA	right lobectomy	multiple right lobe mets	NED – 19 mo
16	colon cancer	asymptomatic	noted at surgery for primary	right lobectomy	single right lobe met	alive with systemic disease – 17 mo (received 5-FU postop for CEA elevation)

Case#	Diagnosis	Presenting Symptoms	Positive Preoperative Tests	Resection Performed	Lesion Site and Size (Diameter)	Outcome
17	rectal cancer	asymptomatic	CT scan, elevated CEA	right lobectomy	single right lobe met 8 cm	dead of systemic disease – 17 mo
18	hepatoma	intraperito- neal bleeding	CT scan	right lobectomy	right lobe primary - dome 6 cm	NED – 16 mo
19	diffuse histiocytic lymphoma	pain, leth- argy, hyper- calcemia	CT scan	trisegmentectomy	single right lobe lesion at junction of left 22 cm	NED – 15 mo (postop combina- tion chemo- therapy)
20	colon cancer	asymptomatic	CT scan elevated CEA	left lobectomy/ implant drug infusion device	multiple bi- lobar mets	alive with un- resectable right lobe mets – 12 mo
21	colon cancer	asymptomatic	liver scan, CT scan, elevated CEA	extended left lobectomy	single left lobe met - 20 cm	NED at death - 12 mo
22	rectal cancer	asymptomatic	liver scan, elevated CEA	right lobectomy	single right lobe met	dead of regional pelvic recur- rence - 15 mo
23	colon cancer	asymptomatic	liver scan, CT scan elevated CEA	right lobectomy	single right lobe met	NED – 7 mo
24	colon cancer	asymptomatic	liver scan, CT scan elevated CEA	right lobectomy	single right lobe met 12 cm	alive with sys- temic disease - 14 mo

271

Case#	Diagnosis	Presenting Symptoms	Positive Preoperative Tests	Resection Performed	Lesion Site and Size (Diameter)	Outcome
25	colon cancer	asymptomatic	liver scan, CT scan, elevated CEA	extended left lobectomy/removal of right hemi-diaphragm	single left lobe met with extension to diaphragm 20 cm	alive with regional disease - 16 mo
26	rectal cancer	asymptomatic	liver scan, CT scan elevated CEA	trisegmentectomy	single right lobe met at junction with left 12 cm	NED - 9 mo
27	nonseminoma embryonic tumor	asymptomatic	CT scan, elevated AFP elevated HCG	right lobectomy	single right lobe met 6 cm	NED - 6 mo
28	gallbladder cancer	incidental finding at cholecystectomy	————	right lobectomy	contiguous extension into gallbladder fossa	alive with wide-spread abdominal disease - 11 mo
29	colon cancer	asymptomatic	CT scan, elevated CEA	trisegmentectomy	single right lobe met 16 cm	NED - 6 mo
30	colon cancer	asymptomatic	elevated CEA	right lobectomy	multiple right lobe mets	alive with systemic disease - 6 mo
31	colon cancer	asymptomatic	noted at surgery for primary	right lobectomy	multiple right lobe mets	NED - 9 mo (CEA elevation)
32	colon cancer	asymptomatic	elevated CEA	right lobectomy/left wedge after FUdR regional infusion	multiple bilobar mets	postoperative death at day 60 from hepatic failure

Case#	Diagnosis	Presenting Symptoms	Positive Preoperative Tests	Resection Performed	Lesion Site and Size (Diameter)	Outcome
33	rectal cancer	asymptomatic	liver scan, CT scan	extended left lobectomy	single left lobe met 16 cm	NED – 10 mo
34	acute myelogenous leukemia with abscess right lobe	FUO, sepsis	CT scan	right lobectomy	right lobe abscess 10 cm	NED – 4 mo
35	colon cancer	pain	liver scan, CT scan, elevated CEA	trisegmentectomy/ removal of right hemidiaphragm	multiple right lobe mets with extension into diaphragm	dead with recurrent left lobe mets – 9 mo
36	colon cancer	asymptomatic	noted at surgery for primary	trisegmentectomy	single right lobe met 15 cm	postoperative death at day 35 from hepatic failure (left lateral segment met at autopsy)
37	rectal cancer	asymptomatic	CT scan, elevated CEA	right lobectomy	multiple right lobe mets responded to infusion chemotherapy	NED – 3 mo
38	colon cancer	asymptomatic	noted at surgery for primary	right lobectomy/ left lateral segmentectomy	multiple bilobar mets	NED – 4 mo
39	colon cancer	asymptomatic	liver scan, CT scan elevated CEA	right lobectomy	single right lobe met	NED – 4 mo

Case#	Diagnosis	Presenting Symptoms	Positive Preoperative Tests	Resection Performed	Lesion Site and Size (Diameter)	Outcome
40	colon cancer	asymptomatic	elevated CEA	left lobectomy	single left lobe met 8 cm	NED – 4 mo
41	nonseminoma embryonic tumor	asymptomatic	CT scan, elevated AFP elevated HCG	extended left lobectomy	single left lobe met	NED – 2 mo
42	colon cancer	asymptomatic	elevated CEA	left lobectomy	single left lobe met 8 cm	NED – 2 mo
43	adenoma	intraperito-neal bleed-ing	————	right lobectomy	right lobe lesion at dome	NED – 1 mo

* abbreviations used: met/mets – metastasis, metastases; 5-FU – 5-fluorouracil; NED – no evidence of disease; CEA – carcinoembryonic antigen; CT – computed tomographic; FUO – fever of unknown origin; AFP – alpha fetoprotein; HCG – human chorionic gonadotropin; FUdR – 5 – fluorouridine deoxyribonucleotide.

This was particularly important in patients who had undergone regional chemotherapeutic infusion after which obliteration of major hepatic arterial inflow was quite common.

Operations

Nineteen patients underwent right hepatic lobectomy, nine underwent trisegmentectomy (formal right hepatic lobectomy and medial left hepatic segmentectomy), five underwent left hepatic lobectomy, five underwent extended left lobectomy (formal left hepatic lobectomy and anterior right hepatic segmentectomy, the so-called left trisegmentectomy of Starzl et al.) (4), five underwent right lobectomy plus left lobe wedge resection or lateral segmentectomy, and one patient underwent a major hilar wedge resection.

Results

Two of these 43 patients died during their postoperative convalescence. Both were operated on for resection of large metastatic tumors of the right lobe of the liver from colon cancer, and both died after complicated episodes of recurrent infection in the hepatic bed, intermittent bouts of sepsis, rebleeding from the raw liver surface, and finally hepatic failure.

Morbidity in our 41 surviving patients was minimal. Average hospitalization was 15 days.

Other workers have attempted to evaluate the results by comparing survival curves of patients with surgically resected tumors to historical or retrospective series of patients with unresected tumors. Our own natural history studies of patients with liver tumors, predominantly colorectal cancer metastases, have revealed a much better than expected survival time regardless of the therapy offered and regardless of the response to therapy (5). We believe, therefore, that any attempt to compare survival of operated and unoperated liver tumor patients is most likely an exercise in selection and nothing more. We have simply presented our survival curve for both the total patient population and those whose colorectal metastases were resected (Figure 1). Survival after hepatic resection of single or multiple colorectal cancer metastases in our series compares favorably with most recent single institutional series (6-12). Thirty-four of the 43 patients are still alive at a median of 12 months after liver resection. Expected survival one year after surgery is 90%; two years after surgery, 75%; and three years after surgery, 65%. One patient with no evidence of recurrent colorectal cancer was lost to follow-up 2.5 years after liver resection. One patient died 12 months after left hepatic lobectomy for colon cancer metastases. Although clinically free of disease, no autopsy was performed after a fatal stroke.

275

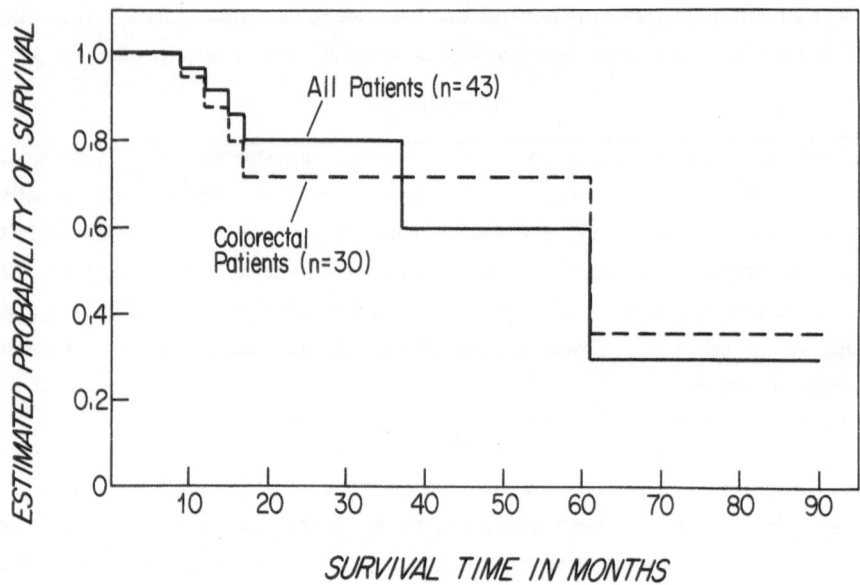

FIGURE 1.   Cumulative survival (Kaplan-Meier) after major curative liver resection.

In the 30 patients whose colorectal cancer metastases were resected, death from hepatic failure was prevented in marked contrast to our natural history experience (5). Despite the unexpectedly long survival time in our first series of treated and untreated patients who presented with liver-only or liver-predominant metastases from colorectal cancer, when they died, 90% died from liver failure. The surgically treated patients in our present series have either been selected to include those who could not have died from liver failure under any circumstances or their proximate cause of death was changed because of our successful removal of liver metastases.

Of the 13 patients with recurrence, eight are still alive. Details of all patients who had recurrence after resection are summarized in Table 2. Surprisingly, ten recurrences were outside of the residual or regenerated liver. One patient had recurrence in the right hemidiaphragm at a site contiguous to the previously resected tumor. Undoubtedly, residual local tumor was present despite pathologically free margins ater the initial operation. The predominant sites of failure in these patients were lung and bone, usually with multiple lesions occurring simultaneously.

Table 2. Details of Therapeutic Failures After Liver Resection For Colorectal Cancer Metastases

Case#	Initial Liver Resection Performed	Time Until Recurrence After Resection	Presenting Symptoms At Recurrence After Resection	Site of Failure	Status and Treatment
1	trisegmentectomy/ removal right hemidiaphragm	21 mo	asymptomatic, elevated CEA	lung and bone	dead at 61 mo after multiple resections of mets* – Irradiation and 5-FU
2	trisegmentectomy	30 mo	asymptomatic, elevated CEA	lung	alive with disease 36 mo – 5-FU
3	extended left lobectomy	24 mo	asymptomatic, elevated CEA	lung	alive with disease 30 mo – 5-FU
4	right lobectomy (multiple mets)	9 mo	asymptomatic, elevated CEA	lung/intra-abdominal	alive with disease 21 mo – 5-FU
5	left lobectomy (single met, "dirty" margin)	20 mo	asymptomatic, liver scan	right lobe met	alive with disease 26 mo – No treatment
6	right lobectomy	15 mo	asymptomatic, elevated CEA	lung and bone	alive with disease 17 mo – 5-FU
7	right lobectomy	6 mo	asymptomatic, elevated CEA	lung	dead of widespread disease at 17 mo – 5-FU
8	left lobectomy/infusion chemotherapy for bilobar mets	12 mo	asymptomatic, re-exploration to "stage"	continued unresectable liver met at re-exploration	alive with disease 18 mo – 5-FU
9	right lobectomy	12 mo	rectal pain, tumor at low anterior resection suture line	pelvic recurrence	dead after resection of local recurrence 15 mo – 5-FU

277

Case#	Initial Liver Resection Performed	Time Until Recurrence After Resection	Presenting Symptoms At Recurrence After Resection	Site of Failure	Status and Treatment
10	right lobectomy	12 mo	asymptomatic, elevated CEA	lung	alive with disease 14 mo – 5-FU
11	extended left lobectomy/removal of right hemidiaphragm	10 mo	elevated CEA, FUO	right diaphragm/ bed of left lobectomy	alive with disease 16 mo – Irradiation
12	right lobectomy (multiple mets)	6 mo	asymptomatic, elevated CEA	lung	alive with disease 10 mo – 5-FU
13	trisegmentectomy/ right hemidiaphragm removal	6 mo	asymptomatic, elevated CEA	left lobe liver mets	dead at 9 mo

* abbreviations used: met/mets – metastasis, metastases; 5-FU – 5-fluorouracil; CEA – carcinoembryonic antigen; FUO – fever of unknown origin

The only solid predictor of local liver recurrence in the patients with metastatic disease was inadequate tumor margin at the time of initial hepatic resection. Two of the three patients with colorectal cancer metastases who had recurrence in the residual or regenerated liver had pathologically inadequate margins of resection at their initial liver operation. Unfortunately, clean margins did not guarantee the absence of subsequent systemic failure.

DISCUSSION

Our data confirm the safety of major hepatic resection when performed properly for appropriate indications. Mortality greater than 10% is not to be accepted. The question of whether or not this procedure should be performed, even though it can be performed, is less easily decided. Certainly in the setting of primary hepatocellular tumors that are resectable, surgery is generally the only available therapy and can provide long-term survival. The results from resected colorectal cancer metastases when confined to the liver, even when metastases are large or multiple, are interesting. Our own data are similar to those of the other current series and imply that perhaps 50% of patients may have benefited from surgery. Long-term survival rates in these patients, however, cannot automatically be ascribed to successful surgery. Almost a quarter of all patients with colorectal cancer will have hepatic metastases, but probably only 5% will have resectable hepatic metastases. Selection of such a small subset of patients may be the key to the better-than-expected survival, quite unrelated to the surgery performed. Nevertheless, the pattern of failure in our patients after resection of hepatic metastases implies that we may have changed the proximate cause of death. More important, the data reveal that at least 50% of patients with successfully resected tumors still have recurrence, with most patients failing outside the liver. The next treatment goal in these patients should be the initiation of experimental systemic adjuvant therapy protocols after liver resection. Obviously, this still is predicated on the weakest link in the entire disease attack -- discovering effective systemic therapy for colon or rectal cancer.

ACKNOWLEDGEMENT

Supported in part by the National Cancer Institute, grant CA 04486 and the National Cancer Institute award 5T32 CA05280-05.

References

1. Steele G Jr, Zamcheck N, Wilson RE, Mayer RJ, Loklch J, Maltz J: Results of CEA-initiated "second-look" surgery. Am J Surg 139: 544-548, 1980.

2. Steele G Jr, Ellenberg S, Ramming K, O'Connell M, Moertel C, Lessner H, Bruckner H, Horton J, Schein P, Zamcheck N, Novak J, Holyoke ED: CEA monitoring among patients in multi-institutional adjuvant GI therapy trials. Ann Surg 196: 162-169, 1982.
3. Weis GR, Garnick MB, Osteen RT, Steele GD Jr, Wilson RE, Schade D, Kaplan WD, Boxt LM, Kandarpa K, Mayer RJ, Frei ET III: Long-term hepatic arterial infusion of 5-fluorodeoxyuridine for liver metastases using an implantable pump. J Clin Oncol 1: 337-344, 1983.
4. Starzl TE, Iwatsuki S, Shaw BW Jr, Waterman PM, Van Thiel D, Diliz HS, Dekker A, Bron KM: Left hepatic trisegmentectomy. Surg Gynecol Obstet 155: 21-27, 1982.
5. Goslin R, Steele G Jr, Zamcheck N, Mayer R, Macintyre J: Factors influencing survival in patients with hepatic metastases from adenocarcinoma of the colon or rectum. Dis Colon Rectum 25: 749-754, 1982.
6. Wilson SM, Adson MA. Surgical treatment of hepatic metastases from colorectal cancers. Arch Surg 111; 330-334, 1976.
7. Adson MA, van Heerden A: Major hepatic resections for metastatic colorectal cancer. Ann Surg 191: 576-583, 1980.
8. Foster JH, Berman MM: Solid liver tumors. Major Probl Clin Surg 22: 1-342, 1977.
9. Fortner JG, Kim DK, MacLean BJ: Major hepatic resection for neoplasia: personal experience in 108 patients. Ann Surg 188: 363-370, 1978.
10. Thompson HH, Tompkins RK, Longmire WP: Major hepatic resection: a 25 year experience. Ann Surg 197: 375-388, 1983.
11. Iwatsuki F, Shaw BW, Starzl TE: Experience with 150 liver resections. Ann Surg 197: 247-253, 1983.
12. Rajpal S, Dasmahapatera KS, Ledesma EJ, Mittelman A: Extensive resections of isolated metastasis from carcinoma of the colon and rectum. Surg Gynecol Obstet 155: 813-816, 1982.

23

DRUG RESISTANCE IN COLON CANCER

Gregory A. Curt and Bruce A. Chabner

SUMMARY

Colon cancer cells demonstrate broad resistance to anticancer drugs, both in vitro and in vivo. The pattern of cross-resistance to natural compounds, such as doxorubicin and the Vinca alkaloids suggests a pattern of pleiotropic drug resistance. However, whether defective drug accumulation, specific membrane markers, or reversibility of resistance by calcium channel blockers, as described in tumors with pleiotropic drug resistance, pertains in colon carcinoma cells as well remains to be determined.

The 5-fluoropyrimidines are the best-studied agents in the treatment of colorectal carcinoma. This chapter outlines the mechanisms of 5-fluoropyrimidine resistance that have been specifically described in colon carcinoma and suggests strategies for the reversal of de novo drug resistance.

INTRODUCTION

Colon cancer cells demonstrate broad, though poorly characterized, resistance to chemotherapeutic agents. As shown in Table 1, both murine colon carcinoma cells (colon 38) and a human colon carcinoma xenograft (CX-1) exhibit resistance to most clinically useful anticancer drugs. From this preclinical sensitivity profile, only 5-fluorouracil (5-FU), actinomycin-D, alkylating agents, and cisplatin would merit clinical trials in colon cancer.

The pattern of de novo resistance to "natural compounds," such as antitumor antibiotics and the Vinca alkaloids, suggests the phenomenon of pleiotropic drug resistance. In both murine and human tumor models, it has been consistently demonstrated that resistance to a natural compound may confer cross-resistance to structurally unrelated drugs with dissimilar mechanisms of action (1). It has been suggested that tumor cells with pleiotropic drug resistance are defective in their ability to accumulate or retain the drug, although the precise mechanism of "altered permeability" remains to be elucidated. Particularly intriguing is the ability of calcium channel blockers, such as verapamil, to reverse the resistant phenotype (2,3) and the presence of specific cell membrane glycoprotein changes that may serve as a marker of the resistant phenotype (4). However, whether the pleiotropic drug-resistant model is applicable to human colorectal cancer remains to be determined.

These in vitro data find their in vivo parallel in the poor response rates of patients with metastatic colon cancer to chemotherapy. Although over 40 single agents have been used to treat patients with colorectal cancer (5), only three classes of drugs have demonstrated reproducible clinical activity. 5-FU, the most extensively studied drug in this disease (over 2000 patients evaluated on studies), is capable of inducing disease regression in approximately 20% of patients (6). In a series of 179 patients with large bowel cancer, the nitrosoureas have demonstrated objective responses, including bis-chloroethyl nitrosourea (BCNU) (12.5% response rate), chloroethyl cyclohexyl nitrosourea (CCNU) (10% response rate), and methyl-CCNU (17.5% response rate) (7). In a randomized trial of 40 patients, the activity of methyl-CCNU appeared equal to or better than 5-FU (8). Finally, the bioreductive alkylating agent, mitomycin C, also has reproducible activity in this disease. Although the initial Japanese data suggested a 32% response rate in 154 patients with gastrointestinal malignancy (9), objective response rates in 12-16% of patients with colorectal cancer are generally accepted (5,10,11). Combination chemotherapy with 5-FU, nitrosoureas, mitomycin C, actinomycin D, and cyclophosphamide offer no therapeutic advantage over single agents (11).

Table 1. Clinical Compounds - Spectrum of DN 2 Activity

Drug	Murine Tumors Colon L1210	(38)	Lung (Lewis)	Mammary (CDBF1)	Melanoma (B16)	Human Tumor Xenografts Colon (CX-1)	Lung (LX-1)	Mammary (MX-1)
Methotrexate	+	-	-	-	-	-	-	-
Actinomycin-D	-	-	-	+	+	+	-	+
Melphalan	+	-	-	+	+	+	+	+
5-Fluorouracil	+	+	-	+	-	-	-	-
Cyclophosphamide	+	-	+	+	-	-	-	+
Vincristine	-	-	-	-	+	-	+	+
Doxorubicin	+	-	-	+	+	-	+	+
BCNU*	+	-	+	+	+	-	+	+
Cisplatin	+	-	-	+	+	+	-	+

* BCNU - bis-chloroethyl nitrosourea

This report summarizes the mechanisms of drug resistance in colon cancer to 5-FU and suggests rational initiatives that offer hope of improved therapeutic results.

MECHANISMS OF RESISTANCE

5-Fluorouracil (5-FU)

As shown in Figure 1, the general mechanisms of the development of tumor cell resistance to 5-FU has been a subject of long and intensive investigation (12-25). To understand precisely how colon tumors in particular develop 5-FU resistance, it is important to review the drug's mechanism of action.

As shown in Figure 2, 5-FU is a prodrug that must be metabolized intracellularly to kill cells. Cytotoxicity occurs through three distinct mechanisms:

1. Conversion to the deoxynucleotide by thymidine phosphorylase and subsequent phosphorylation to fluorodeoxyuridine monophosphate (FdUMP) by thymidine kinase. In the presence of sufficient intracellular folate cofactors (in particular 5,10-methylene tetrahydrofolate), FdUMP complexes with and directly inhibits thymidylate synthetase, resulting in "thymineless death."

2. 5-FdUMP can be further phosphorylated to 5-fluorodeoxyuridine triphosphate (5-FdUTP), which can be incorporated directly into deoxyribonucleic acid (DNA). Although it was reported in 1981 that 5-FU can be incorporated into the DNA of a bacteriophage that utilizes uracil rather than thymidine and that 5-FdUTP functions as a substrate for calf thymus DNA polymerase (26), this pathway is just now beginning to be studied as a potentially important determinant of cytotoxicity in tumor cells. To date, this phenomenon has been reported only in HeLa cells (27), murine L1210, and human leukemia cell lines (28), although it may be important to the recently reported clinical synergism of 5-FU and cisplatin (vide infra).

3. 5-FU can be anabolized to 5-fluorouridine monophosphate (5-FUMP) either by direct conversion by orotic acid phosphoribosyl transferase (OPRTase) in the presence of 5-phosphoribosyl-1-pyrophosphate (PRPP) or conversion to the ribonucleotide 5-fluorouridine (5-FUR) by uridine phosphorylase, followed by formation of 5-fluorouridine monophosphate (5-FUMP) by uridine kinase. The phosphorylated product, 5-fluorouridine triphosphate (5-FUTP), is incorporated into ribonucleic acid (RNA) and alters RNA maturation.

Since 5-FU must be anabolized to active species to cause cytotoxicity, studies of tumor cells with either de novo or acquired drug resistance have concentrated on deletion of activation enzymes, as well as amplification or altered drug affinity of the target enzyme, thymidylate synthetase. Cells in which 5-FU resistance is due to decreased activity of OPRTase, uridine kinase, and thymidine kinase or decreased pools of PRPP have been well documented (Figure 1).

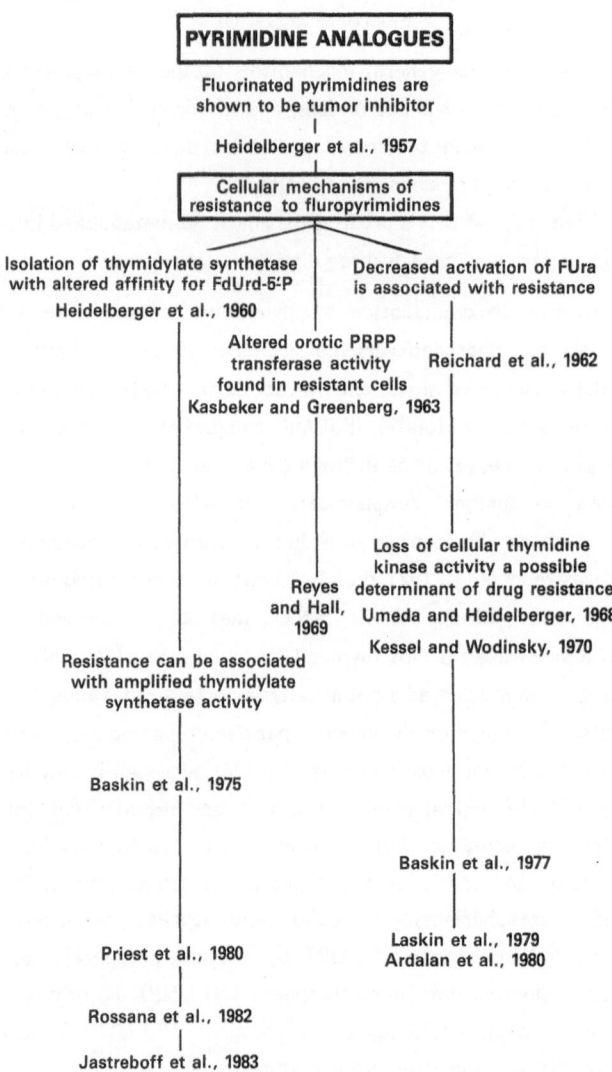

FIGURE 1. Historical overview of studies on fluoropyrimidine resistance. (From McLellan W, McAllister PR, Woodman PW: "Development of Drug Resistance in Cancer Cells." A bibliographic tracing developed by CHI Research and Dynamac Corp. under NCI Contract N01-CO-33933.) (References 12-25)

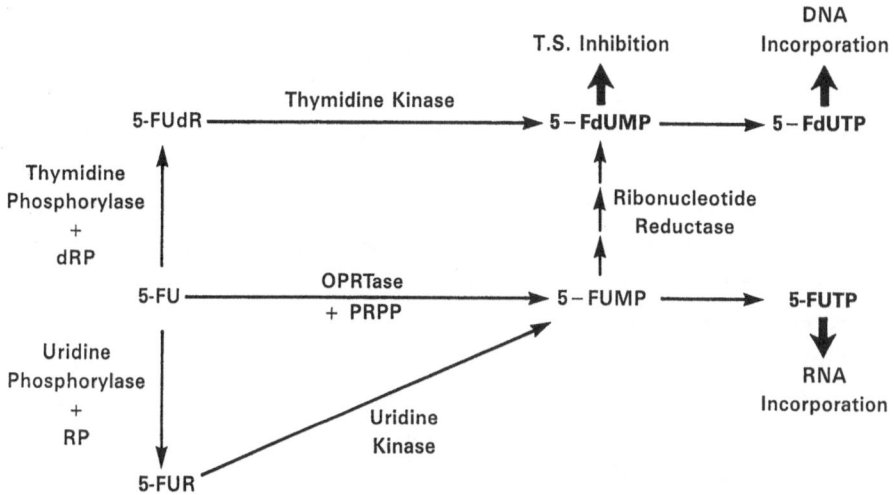

FIGURE 2. Activation pathways of 5-fluorouracil. RP, ribose phosphate; dRP, deoxy-ribose phosphate; TS, thymidylate synthetase; 5-FU, 5-fluorouracil; 5-FUdR, 5-fluoro-deoxyuridine; 5-FdUMP, 5-fluorodeoxyuridine monophosphate; 5-FdUTP, 5-fluorodeoxy-uridine triphosphate; 5-FUR, 5-fluorouridine; 5-FUMP, 5-fluorouridine monophosphate; 5-FUTP, 5-fluorouridine triphosphate; OPRTase, orotic acid phosphoribosyl transferase; PRPP, phosphoribosyl pyrophosphate.

While focusing on the mechanisms of drug cytotoxicity and resistance in colon cancer in particular, it was determined that human colorectal xenografts differ in the pathways by which they activate 5-FU. Some colon carcinoma cells specifically activate 5-FU to ribonucleotides predominantly by OPRTase, while others utilize the uridine phosphorylase and kinase pathway (29). The ratio of intracellular ribose-1-phosphate to PRPP and the relative specific activity of uridine phosphorylase and OPRTase were critical determinants of the pathway utilized. This is important in determining the modulating effects of exogenous purines. Since exogenous purines deplete intracellular PRPP pools, 5-FU-ribonucleotide formation (and cytotoxicity) is decreased in those cells utilizing the OPRTase pathway, but not in the xenograft utilizing the uridine phosphorylase-kinase pathway. Thus, human colon carcinoma cells are heterogeneous in their metabolism of 5-FU, and these differences may be important to drug resistance and its potential reversibility.

These in vitro findings may have a clinical parallel. Dexter and co-workers described the isolation and characterization of cell line DLD-1 established from a patient with adenocarcinoma of the sigmoid colon (30). Cytogenetically and histologically, the original isolate consisted of two distinct clones. Although drug metabolism studies were not performed, as much as a 50-fold difference in sensitivity was observed between the parent line and individual subclones. Thus, colon carcinoma in patients may become heterogeneous through mutation, even though monoclonal in origin, or may be polyclonal in origin; in either case, the heterogeneity has attendant implications for the emergence of drug-resistant subclones.

Studies of the mechanism of fluoropyrimidine resistance in colon cancer have been few. In detailed studies of 5-FU resistance of four murine carcinoma cell lines, drug activity was best correlated with intracellular pools of PRPP, the cofactor used by OPRTase to anabolize 5-FU to 5-FUMP (31). In two 5-FU-sensitive cell lines, intracellular pools of PRPP were two- to fourfold greater than in cells with de novo resistance and correlated with higher PRPP synthetase levels in sensitive cells.

Cellular resistance to 5-fluorodeoxyuridine (5-FUdR), which is predominantly anabolized to 5-FdUMP, is dependent on levels of the target enzyme thymidylate synthetase. In five human gastrointestinal tumor cell lines, in vitro sensitivity was inversely proportional to thymidylate synthetase levels (32).

Since inhibition of thymidylate synthetase by FdUMP requires the presence of 5,10-methylene tetrahydrofolate as a cofactor, the availability of intracellular folates may be an important determinant of enzyme inhibition. In a study of six human colon carcinoma xenografts, it was reported that exogenous folate cofactor must be added to cytosol preparations of four 5-FU-resistant lines to achieve maximum binding of FdUMP to thymidylate synthetase (33). However, in two sensitive xenografts, target enzyme binding to FdUMP was initially maximal, suggesting that inadequate intracellular concentration of reduced folates may be important to de novo 5-FU resistance in colon cancer. These data serve as the rationale for combining 5-FU with leucovorin in ongoing pilot studies (vide infra).

While incorporation of 5-FUTP into RNA appears to be critical for drug cytotoxicity in some human tumors, particularly MCF-7 breast cancer (34), the importance of this pathway in human colon cancer cells remains uncertain. While fluoropyrimidines appear to kill LoVo human colon cancer lines by incorporation into RNA (35), this mechanism seems of lesser importance in human colon carcinoma xenografts. Houghton and Houghton studied four human xenografts passaged in nude mice, and they determined that intracellular formation of FdUMP and inhibition of thymidylate synthetase were most critical for tumor cell kill (36). No correlation was found between tumor response and 5-FU incorporation into RNA in these xenograft systems.

In more recent studies using 5-FU-sensitive human colon carcinoma cell line HT29, Glazer and Hartman were able to detect 5-FU-substituted messenger RNA (mRNA) following drug treatment (37). However, there was no detectable difference in the ability of a drug-substituted message to translate polypeptides. Although there was no impairment of ribosomal RNA processing or DNA/RNA synthesis, there was a direct correlation between specific incorporation of 5-FUTP into nuclear RNA and cell death (38). Thus, 5-FU substitution into small nuclear RNA species, which contain large amounts of uridylic acid and are important to exon recognition during mRNA splicing (39), may be important to 5-FU toxicity in colon cancer.

NEW TREATMENT STRATEGIES

The biochemical pharmacology of drug resistance in colon cancer has suggested several strategies to improve therapeutic results in this disease (Table 2). The rationale for exposing tumor cells to the highest achievable drug concentration is based on the linear relationship between dose and fractional cell kill for many antitumor agents (40). The pharmacologic rationale for 5-FU infusion directly into the hepatic artery of patients with colon cancer that has metastasized to the liver is predicated on the rapid clearance of drug (41). The intra-arterial route achieves the best therapeutic advantage for organs with low blood flow or high clearance rates (42). For intra-arterial 5-FU, gradients of up to 1000-fold can be achieved between the hepatic artery and the systemic circulation. A controlled multi-institutional trial has recently been funded by the National Cancer Institute to compare intravenous versus intra-arterial 5-FU infusion in patients with colon cancer who are at high risk for hepatic metastasis.

Table 2. Strategies to Overcome 5-FU Resistance

	Mechanism of Resistance	Treatment Strategy
1.	Inadequate local drug concentration	Regional perfusion (hepatic artery)
2.	Defective drug activation	Biochemical modulation Methotrexate PALA
3.	Decreased intracellular folate pools	High-dose leucovorin
4.	Increased DNA repair	Inhibition of repair Cisplatin

Since defective drug activation has been demonstrated in colon cancer cells with low intracellular pools of PRPP, drugs that modulate PRPP pool size have been used to increase fluoropyrimidine anabolism. Agents such as methotrexate and phosphono-N-acetyl-L-aspartic acid (PALA) greatly increase intracellular pools of PRPP and augment 5-FU cytotoxicity in culture by inhibiting de novo nucleotide synthesis. However, the issue of methotrexate-5-FU synergy is complex and dependent on methotrexate's antipurine effect, which inhibits RNA synthesis and secondarily decreases 5-FUTP incorporation into RNA, the importance of de novo and salvage pathways for nucleic acid synthesis, cell population kinetics, and intracellular PRPP levels. In the six most recent trials of methotrexate and 5-FU for advanced colorectal cancer, response rates varied from 6-53% (43-48), although the overall response rate in 133 evaluable patients was 32%. The toxicity of the combination may be severe, as four drug-related deaths were reported in these trials. Superiority of sequential regimens has not been established in randomized trials.

Similarly, the coadministration of PALA and 5-FU produces greater toxicity and response rates no better than 5-FU alone (49-53). In these trials, PALA limited the total dose of 5-FU that could be administered. However, because low doses of PALA are sufficient to inhibit low tumor levels of aspartate carbamoyl transferase, low-dose PALA/full-dose 5-FU is empirically logical (54) and awaits clinical evaluation.

Because decreased intracellular folate pools may impair binding of FdUMP to thymidylate synthetase, 5-FU has been administered with concomitant high-dose leucovorin in patients with advanced colorectal cancer. Leucovorin can be converted intracellularly to reduced folates and may, in fact, augment clinical response. Preliminary results of 5-FU and high-dose leucovorin are encouraging. In one study of 30 patients, response rates were 56% in previously untreated patients and 21% in patients who had previously received 5-FU (55). Recently, responses in previously treated patients have been confirmed (56).

Since increased DNA repair appears to be an important factor in colon cancer's resistance to nitrosoureas (57,58) and 5-FU can be incorporated into DNA as FUTP, 5-FU has recently been combined with cisplatin, a potent inhibitor of DNA repair, in treating metastatic colorectal cancer (59). Of 38 evaluable patients, 32% responded to treatment. Again, treatment was toxic with two episodes of gram-negative sepsis and one drug-related death.

Phase II Single-Agent Studies

While biochemical modulation would appear to have real potential in improving the chemotherapy of colon cancer, none of these sequential or combination regimens have been compared to single-agent 5-FU in randomized clinical trials. In addition, the toxicity of these regimens may be considerable. Therefore, patients with metastatic colon cancer may be considered appropriate for entry into phase II studies of new agents.

Unfortunately, results of these studies have been unimpressive to date. Table 3 shows the single-agent response rates in 11 of the most active phase II drugs from a total of 57 most recently studied agents. In no case does response exceed that achievable with 5-FU alone.

Table 3. Phase II Drug Activity in Colon Cancer

Drug	Evaluable Patients	Response (%)
4'-Epidoxorubicin	14	21
Ftorafur	222	14
Triazinate	97	13
ICRF-187	98	8
Methyl-G	196	8
Streptozotocin	78	8
Thioguanine	222	5
VP-16	162	4
Vindesine	129	4
PCNU[*]	127	4
Procarbazine	38	3

[*]   PCNU - N-(2-chloroethyl)-N-2'-(2,6-dioxo-3-piperidyl)-N-nitrosourea

In summary, the chemotherapy of colon cancer remains unimpressive. Colon cancer in vitro and in vivo is broadly resistant to most known drugs. Improvement in current treatment options is likely to result from early intervention with regimens (perhaps involving biochemical modulation) with greater activity than those currently available. Further characterization of pleiotropic drug resistance and its reversibility may have real application in sensitizing colon cancer cells to natural compounds such as antitumor antibiotics and the Vinca alkaloids. Effective new drugs may be discovered by preclinical screening using the panel of 19 well-characterized human colon cancer cell lines and targeted treatment using monoclonal antibodies, which holds as yet untested promise. Certainly the magnitude of the clinical problem justifies redoubled efforts in this disease.

References

1. Curt GA, Clendeninn NJ, Chabner BA: Drug resistance in cancer. Cancer Treat Rep 68: 87-99, 1984.
2. Tsuruo T, Iida H, Tsukagoshi S: Overcoming of Vincristine resistance in P388 leukemia in vivo and in vitro through enhanced cytotoxicity of Vincristine and Vinblastine by verapamil. Cancer Res 41: 1967-1972, 1981.
3. Tsuruo T, Iida H, Tsukagoshi S: Increased accumulation of Vincristine and Adriamycin in drug-resistant P388 tumor cells following incubation with calcium antagonists and calmodulin inhibitors. Cancer Res 42: 4730-4733, 1982.
4. Juliano RL, Ling V: A surface glycoprotein modulating drug permeability in Chinese hamster ovary cell mutants. Biochim Biophys Acta 455: 152-162, 1976.
5. Heal JM, Schein PS: Management of gastrointestinal cancer. Med Clin North Am 61: 991-999, 1977.
6. Wasserman TH, Comis RL, Goldsmith M, Handelsman H, Penta JS, Slavik M, Soper WT, Carter SK: Tabular analysis of the clinical chemotherapy of solid tumors. Cancer Chemother Rep 6: 399-419, 1975.
7. Moertel CG: Therapy of advanced gastrointestinal cancer with the nitrosoureas. Cancer Chemother Rep 4: 27, 1973.
8. Frank W, Osterberg AE: Mitomycin C (NSC-26980) -- an evaluation of the Japanese reports. Cancer Chemother Rep 9: 114-119, 1960.
9. Moertel CG: Clinical management of advanced gastrointestinal cancer. Cancer 36: 675, 1975.
10. Moertel CG: Chemotherapy of gastrointestinal cancer. N Engl J Med 299: 1049-1052, 1978.
11. Moertel CG, Reitemier RJ, Hahn RG: Combination chemotherapy in advanced gastrointestinal cancer. Cancer Res 30: 1425-1428, 1970.
12. Heidelberger C, Chaudhari NK, Danneberg P, Mooren D, Griesbach L, Duschinsky R, Schnitzer RJ, Pleven E, Scheiner J: Fluorinated pyrimidines. A new class of tumour inhibitory compounds. Nature 179: 663-666, 1957.
13. Heidelberger C, Kaldor G, Mukherjee KL, Danenberg PB: Studies on fluorinated pyrimidines. XI. In vitro studies on tumor resistance. Cancer Res 20: 903-909, 1960.
14. Reichard P, Skold O, Klein G, Revesz L, Magnusson P-H: Studies on resistance against 5-fluorouracil. I. Enzymes of uracil pathway during development of resistance. Cancer Res 22: 235-243, 1962.
15. Kasbeker DK, Greenberg DM: Studies on tumor resistance to 5-fluorouracil. Cancer Res 23: 818-825, 1983.
16. Umeda M, Heidelberger C: Comparative studies of fluorinated pyrimidines with various cell lines. Cancer Res 28: 2529-2538, 1968.
17. Reyes P, Hall TC: Synthesis of 5-fluorouridine-5'-phosphate by a pyrimidine phosphoribosyl transferase of mammalian origin. II. Correlation between the tumor levels of the enzymic and 5-fluorouracil-promoted increase in survival of tumor-bearing mice. Biochem Pharmacol 18: 2587-2590, 1969.
18. Kessel D, Wodinsky I: Thymidine kinase as a determinant of the response to 5-fluoro-2'-deoxyuridine in transplantable murine leukemias. Mol Pharmacol 6: 251-254, 1970.

19. Baskin F, Carlin SC, Kraus P, Freidkin M, Rosenberg RN: Experimental chemotherapy of neuroblastoma. II. Increased thymidylate synthetase activity in a 5-fluorodeoxyuridine-resistant variant of mouse neuroblastoma. Mol Pharmacol 11: 105-117, 1975.
20. Baskin F, Davis R, Rosenberg RN: Altered thymidine kinase or thymidylate activities in 5-fluorodeoxyuridine-resistant variants of neuroblastoma. J Neuro Chem 29: 1031-1037, 1977.
21. Laskin JD, Evans RM, Slocum HK, Burke D, Hakala MT: Basis for natural variation in sensitivity to 5-fluorouracil in mouse and human cells in culture. Cancer Res 39: 383-390, 1979.
22. Ardalan B, Cooney DA, Jayaram HN, Carrico CK, Glazer RI, Macdonald J, Schein PS: Mechanisms of sensitivity and resistance of murine tumors to 5-fluorouracil. Cancer Res 49: 1431-1437, 1980.
23. Priest DG, Ledford BE, Doig MT: Increased thymidylate synthetase in 5-fluorodeoxyuridine-resistant cultured hepatoma cells. Biochem Pharmacol 29: 1549-1553, 1980.
24. Rossana C, Rao LG, Johnson LF: Thymidylate synthetase overproduction in 5-fluorodeoxyuridine-resistant mouse fibroblasts. Mol Cell Biol 2: 1118-1125, 1982.
25. Jastreboff MM, Kedzierska B, Rode W: Altered thymidylate synthetase in 5-fluorodeoxyuridine-resistant Ehrlich ascites carcinoma cells. Biochem Pharmacol 32: 2259-2267, 1983.
26. Tanaka M, Yoshida S, Saneyoshi M, Yamaguchi T: Utilization of 5-fluoro-2'-deoxycytidine triphosphate in DNA synthesis and from calf thymus. Cancer Res 41: 4132-4135, 1981.
27. Cheng YC, Nakayama K: Effects of 5-fluoro-2'-deoxyuridine on DNA metabolism in HeLa cells. Mol Pharmacol 23: 171-174, 1983.
28. Tanaka M, Kimura K, Yoshida S: Enhancement of the incorporation of 5-fluorodeoxyuridylate into DNA of HL-60 cells by metabolic modulations. Cancer Res 43: 5145-5150, 1983.
29. Houghton JA, Houghton PJ: Elucidation of pathways of 5-fluorouracil metabolism in xenografts of human colorectal adenocarcinoma. Eur J Cancer Clin Oncol 19: 807-815, 1983.
30. Dexter DL, Spremulli EN, Fligiel Z, Barbosa BS, Vogel R, Van Voorhees A, Calabresi P: Heterogeneity of cancer cells from a single human colon carcinoma. Am J Med 71: 949-955, 1981.
31. Ardalan B, Villacote D, Heck D, Corbett T: Phosphoribosyl pyrophosphate, pool size and tissue levels as a determinant of 5-fluorouracil response in murine colonic adenocarcinomas. Biochem Pharmacol 31: 1989-1992, 1982.
32. Washtien WL: Thymidylate synthetase levels as a factor in 5-fluorodeoxyuridine and methotrexate cytotoxicity in gastrointestinal tumor cell lines. Mol Pharmacol 21: 723-729, 1982.
33. Houghton JA, Maroda SJ, Phillips JO, Houghton PJ: Biochemical determinants of responsiveness to 5-fluorouracil and its derivatives in xenografts of human colorectal adenocarcinomas in mice. Cancer Res 41: 144-151, 1981.
34. Kufe DW, Major PP: 5-Fluorouracil incorporation into human breast cancer RNA correlates with cytotoxicity. J Biol Chem 256: 9802-9806, 1981.
35. Drewinko B, Yang LY, Ho DHW, Benvenuto J, Loo TL, Freireich EJ: Treatment of cultured human colon carcinoma cells with fluorinated pyrimidines. Cancer 45: 1144-1148, 1980.
36. Houghton JA, Houghton PJ: On the mechanism of cytotoxicity of fluorinated pyrimidines in four human colon adenocarcinoma xenografts maintained in immunodeprived mice. Cancer 45: 1159-1163, 1980.

37. Glazer RL, Hartman KD: In vitro translation of messenger RNA following exposure of human colon carcinoma cells in culture to 5-fluorouracil and 5-fluorouridine. Mol Pharmacol 23: 540-546, 1983.
38. Glazer RL, Lloyd LS: Association of cell lethality with incorporation of 5-fluorouracil and 5-fluorouridine into nuclear RNA in human colon carcinoma cells in culture. Mol Pharmacol 21: 468-471, 1982.
39. Ohshima Y, Itoh M, Okada N, Miyata T: Novel models for RNA splicing that involves small nuclear RNA. Proc Natl Acad Sci USA 78: 4471-4474, 1981.
40. Skipper HE, Schabel FM Jr, Lloyd HH: Dose-response and tumor cell repopulation rate in chemotherapeutic trials. In: A Rosowsky (ed), Advances in Cancer Chemotherapy, Vol. I. Marcel Dekker, New York, 1979, pp 297.
41. Ensminger WD, Rosowsky A, Raso VO, Levin DC, Glode M, Come S, Steele G, Frei E III: A clinical pharmacological evaluation of hepatic arterial infusion of 5-fluoro-2'-deoxyuridine and 5-fluorouracil. Cancer Res 38: 3784-3792, 1978.
42. Collins JM, Dedrick RL: Pharmacokinetics of anticancer drugs. In: BA Chabner (ed), Pharmacologic principles of cancer treatment. WB Saunders, Philadelphia, 1982, pp 77-99.
43. Kemeny N, Michaelson R: Phase II trial of low-dose methotrexate and sequential 5-fluorouracil in the treatment of metastatic colorectal carcinoma (Abstract). Proc Am Soc Clin Oncol 1: 95, 1982.
44. Solan A, Vogel SE, Kaplan BH, Berenzweig M, Richard J, Lanham R: Sequential chemotherapy of advanced colorectal cancer with standard or high dose methotrexate followed by 5-fluorouracil. Med Pediatr Oncol 10: 145-148, 1982.
45. Cantrell JE, Brunet R, Lagarde C, Schein PS, Smith FP: Phase II study of sequential methotrexate-5-FU in advanced measurable colorectal cancer. Cancer Treat Rep 66: 1563-1564, 1982.
46. Hermann R, Mangold C, Holtzmann K, Fritz D: Sequentielle verabreichung von methotrexat und fluorouracil bei metastasierenden kolorektalen karzinomen. Dtsh Med Wochenschr 107: 491-493, 1982.
47. Mehrotra S, Rosenthal CJ, Gartner B: Biochemical modulation of antineoplastic response in colorectal carcinoma (Abstract). Proc Am Soc Clin Oncol 1: 100, 1982.
48. Weinerman B, Schacter B, Schippen H, Bowman D, Levitt M: Sequential methotrexate and 5-FU in the treatment of colorectal cancer. Cancer Treat Rep 66: 1553-1557, 1982.
49. Camancho FJ, Muggia FM, Kaplan BH: A trial of N-(phosphonacetyl)-L-aspartate and 5-fluorouracil in patients with metastatic colorectal cancer (Abstract). Proc Am Soc Clin Oncol 1: 457, 1981.
50. Bedikian AY, Stroehlein JR, Karlin DA, Bennetts RW, Bodey GP, Valdivieso M: Chemotherapy for colorectal cancer with combination of PALA and 5-FU. Cancer Treat Rep 65: 747-753, 1981.
51. Presant CA, Ardalan B, Multhauf P, Chan C, Staples R, Green L, Browning S, Carr BI, Chang FF, Thayer W: Continuous five-day infusion of PALA and 5-FU: A pilot phase II trial. Med Pediatr Oncol 11: 162-165, 1983.
52. Weiss GR, Ervin TJ, Mushad MW, Kufe DW: Phase I trial of combination therapy with continuous infusion PALA and bolus injection of 5-FU. Cancer Treat Rep 66: 277-303, 1982.
53. Weiss GR, Erwin TJ, Meshad MW, Schade D, Branfman AR, Bruni RJ, Chadwick M, Kufe DW: A phase I trial of combination therapy with continuous infusion PALA and continuous infusion 5-FU. Cancer Chemother Pharmacol 8: 301-304, 1982.
54. Casper ES, Vale K, Williams LS, Martin DS, Young CW: Phase I and clinical pharmacologic evaluation of biochemical modulator of 5-fluorouracil with N-(phosphonacetyl)-L-aspartic acid. Cancer Res 43: 2324-2329, 1983.

55. Machover D, Schwartzenberg L, Goldschmidt E, Tourani JM, Michalski B, Hayat M, Dorval T, Misset JL, Jasmin C, Maral R, Mathe G: Treatment of advanced colorectal and gastric adenocarcinomas with 5-FU combined with high dose folinic acid: A pilot study. Cancer Treat Rep 66: 1803-1807, 1982.

56. Rustum Y, Petrelli P: A phase I-II study of combination 5-fluorouracil and high-dose leucovorin in advanced colorectal carcinoma. Minutes of the Biological Modulators Advisory Group, National Cancer Institute, NIH, Bethesda, Maryland, January 1983, pp 14-21.

57. Erickson LC, Oseika R, Kohn K: Differential repair of 1-(2-chloroethyl)-3-(4-methylcyclohexyl)-1-nitrosourea-induced DNA damage in two human colon tumor cell lines. Cancer Res 38: 802-808, 1978.

58. Thomas CB, Oseika R, Kohn K: DNA cross-linking by in vivo treatment with 1-(2-chloroethyl)-3-(4-methylcyclohexyl)-1-nitrosourea of sensitive and resistant human colon carcinoma xenografts in nude mice. Cancer Res 38: 2448-2454, 1978.

59. Einhorn LH, Williams SD, Lochner PJ: Combination chemotherapy with platinum plus 5-FU in metastatic colorectal carcinoma (Abstract). Proc Am Soc Clin Oncol 1: 93, 1984.

293

24

BIOLOGY OF COLON CANCER RESISTANCE TO TREATMENT

Paul V. Woolley III, Daniel D. Von Hoff, Gregg W. Kyle, Shailendra Kumar,
Robert A. Nagourney, Thu-Trang P. Luc, and Kenneth L. Mossman

SUMMARY

We have asked whether there is objective laboratory evidence to demonstrate the resistance of clinically observed colon cancer to treatment. A review of data from 14 drugs tested in the human tumor stem cell assay showed that, for at least 10 of these drugs, colon tumor stem cells were less sensitive than breast, ovary, or lymphoma cells. These results were corroborated by studies with cultured cells in vitro and by studies of human tumor samples using a Fast green dye-exclusion technique. The resistance of HT-29 colon cancer cells correlated with stability of its chromatin against breakage by radiation. Interferon resistance was also studied, but was not mediated at the chromatin level. Colon cancer cells are inherently resistant to drugs and radiation. This resistance is probably multifactorial and includes effects at the membrane, the chromatin complex, and other sites not yet fully characterized.

INTRODUCTION

Carcinoma of the large bowel is a common disease in our society; over 130,000 new cases are reported each year. Clinically, there is a need for systemic therapies that can be used as an adjuvant following surgery or can be used for advanced disease. However, despite intensive efforts over the past 25 years, progress in the development of effective drug therapy for large bowel cancer has been slow. An accumulating body of clinical and biologic data indicates that this tumor is inherently resistant to drugs with different mechanisms of action. A detailed investigation of the existence and nature of this resistance is germane to continued efforts toward the development of effective therapy.

The most widely used drug for treatment of large bowel cancer is 5-fluorouracil (5-FU), and extensive literature on this drug has accumulated. Intravenous 5-FU produces objective clinical responses in about 20% of patients with advanced measurable large bowel cancer. This response rate is largely independent of the schedule of drug administration, although there is some evidence that a five-day loading course or prolonged intravenous infusion will improve response rates (1). Nonetheless, treatment with 5-FU alone falls far short of being either reliable or curative therapy for large bowel cancer. During the 1970's, there was hope that combining 5-FU with other active agents would produce combinations having a greater activity than the individual components. Initial therapeutic trials with combinations of 5-FU, nitrosoureas, vincristine, and ditriazenoimidazole carboxamide (DTIC) suggested that the response rate to these combinations would exceed 40% (2,3). With greater experience, these hopes have not prevailed and recent randomized trials have produced discouraging results on the use of drug combinations in advanced colon cancer (4,5).

These results hold true not only for the treatment of advanced disease, but also for the management of patients receiving adjuvant therapy. Although there have been many well-designed prospective randomized trials of 5-FU used alone or in combination with other agents in the management of postoperative patients at high risk of relapse, the results have either been disappointingly negative or have demonstrated at best a marginal effect upon recurrence rates (6,7).

Other areas of active research in the use of fluorinated pyrimidines have included modulating the toxicity or therapeutic effect of these drugs by scheduling them with other agents, such as methotrexate (8), leucovorin (9), allopurinol (10), thymidine (11), or phosphonacetyl-L-aspartate (PALA) (12). While the use of these agents are founded on biochemical rationale and have taught us much about interactions among chemotherapeutic agents, these approaches have not yet markedly improved the therapeutic effectiveness of drugs for large bowel cancer.

Because of this lack of dependable and effective drug combinations for routine clinical use, it is currently regarded as scientifically and ethically appropriate for research centers to employ investigational drugs as initial therapy in patients with advanced large bowel cancer. However, empiric phase II testing has also had a disappointing history in terms of identification of active new agents. Table 1 presents a list of some drugs that have been tested over the past few years. These include alkylating agents, antimetabolites, anthracyclines, and other agents with diverse mechanisms of action. The results indicate that empiric drug testing has been a very inefficient mechanism of identifying new agents for large bowel cancer. They further suggest a profound biologic problem (13), namely that colon cancer cells are intrinsically more resistant to drugs with a wide variety of mechanisms of action than are cells of other lineages. It is essential at this point in our approach to this disease to ask whether such resistance can be demonstrated by techniques other than clinical observation, whether it is possible to characterize the biochemical components of this resistance, and whether we can identify mechanisms for circumventing it.

Table 1. Phase II Studies of Drugs for Colon Cancer

Drug	No. Patients	No. Response
4-Epidoxorubicin	14	3 (21%)
3-Deazauridine	15	0 (0%)
Ftorafur	222	32 (14%)
Hexamethylmelamine	83	11 (13%)
ICRF-159	98	8 (8%)
ICRF-187	47	0 (0%)
Ifosfamide	33	1 (3%)
Indicine-N-oxide	30	0 (0%)
Methotrexate	57	3 (5%)
Methyl-CCNU*	342	29 (8%)
Mitoxantrone	13	0 (0%)
PCNU	127	5 (4%)
Piperazinedione	29	0 (0%)
Procarbazine	38	1 (3%)
Rubidizone	25	1 (4%)
Spirogermanium	80	0 (0%)
Thioguanine	222	12 (5%)
VM-26	83	2 (2%)
VP-16	162	7 (4%)

* CCNU - chloroethyl cyclohexyl nitrosourea; PCNU - chloroethyl dioxo-piperidyl nitrosourea

Source: National Cancer Institute, Cancer Treatment Evaluation Program Protocol Information System.

Some of the possible mechanisms of tumor resistance to drugs include poor vascularity and limited diffusion of the drug into the tumor and a small or slowly proliferating stem cell pool. The inherent properties of the tumor cell, including membrane transport, pleiotropic resistance, efficient DNA repair mechanisms, and high chromatin stability should be considered. In addition, the role of tumor heterogeneity, including genetic drift and gene amplification, must be evaluated. In this discussion we are concerned with the inherent biology of tumor cells and not the diffusion and vascular access of drugs to bulky tumors, although these considerations may be important in the overall delivery of drugs to their sites of action. However, the failure of combination drug regimens to demonstrate significant activity in minimal or microscopic disease indicates that drug delivery to bulky tumors is not the only limiting factor in the treatment of colon cancer. There is evidence that some of the resistance may be overcome by increasing drug dosage. Current results with direct intra-arterial infusion of fluorinated pyrimidines to the liver indicate that this improves response rates (14), as do preliminary data showing responses of colon cancer to high doses of melphalan infused into the peritoneal cavity (15).

COLONY-FORMING ASSAYS

A direct demonstration of the relative resistance of colon cancer cells to drugs can be made from studies of the colony-forming ability of human tumors cloned in soft agar in the presence of various concentrations of different drugs. A summary of the data derived by Dr. Daniel Von Hoff at the University of Texas, San Antonio is presented in Tables 2 and 3. These tables were compiled from a summary of over 11,000 tumor samples studied at that institution. They compare data for colon cancer with similar data at the same drug concentration and duration of exposure for breast and ovarian carcinoma and lymphoma. The criterion for inclusion of these 14 drugs was simply that there were sufficient values for comparison among the four cell lines. In this protocol, drugs are tested at concentrations that approximate clinically achievable levels and at various periods of exposure, one-hour, two-hour, or continuous exposure. Table 2 summarizes the data for 14 drugs using a one-hour exposure time. For the first 11 drugs listed, the colon tumor cells were less sensitive to inhibition than were breast, ovarian, or lymphoma cells, for at least one of the concentrations studied. The lymphoma cells were the most sensitive, while breast and ovarian tumor cells were intermediate in their sensitivity and colon tumor cells were the lowest. For the last three drugs listed, the colon tumors showed somewhat more sensitivity than the other cell lines. Thus, while the relationship was not absolute, the colon tumor cells were less sensitive than the other cell lines for the majority of drugs studied.

Table 3 shows another representation of the same data. In this case, all results at each drug concentration have been pooled and the periods of exposure, one hour, two hours, and continuous, have been grouped as a single number. The relationship is still maintained, and the colon cancer lines are less sensitive than the other cells for almost all drugs studied. Breast and ovarian tumor cells lack the high sensitivity of the lymphomas to drugs, but in most cases are more sensitive than colon tumor cells.

Additional information in this regard has been obtained from studies of the viability of samples of human colon tumors with exposure to various drugs. In this case the assay for cytotoxicity has been the Fast green dye-exclusion assay, recently employed by Weisenthal and co-workers (16). Representative data for a surgical tumor sample are shown in Table 4. The data once again document the inherent resistance of colon tumors to a variety of commonly used cytotoxic agents at clinically achievable concentrations.

Table 2. Drugs Tested in the Human Tumor Stem Cell Assay[*]

Drug	Concentration (μg/ml)	% Colonies Sensitive			
		Colon	Breast	Ovary	Lymphoma
[†]Fludarabine	1.0	14	28	25	100
[†]5-Fluorouracil	6.0	13	15	15	60
[†]Doxorubicin	0.04	11	11	17	20
	0.4	25	16	8	25
[†]BCNU	0.1	10	36	25	33
[†]Bisantrene	0.5	9	16	17	22
	10.0	15	28	31	50
[†]Dihydroxy-anthracine-dione	0.05	15	19	20	26
[†]Melphalan	0.1	15	20	22	42
	1.0	14	0	27	-
	10.0	14	0	21	-
[†]Mitomycin-C	0.1	15	18	16	60
[†]Cisplatin	0.2	16	19	17	50
[†]Vincristine	0.1	10	9	27	100
Vinblastine	0.05	25	25	17	62
Methylglyoxal-bis-guanyl-hydrazone	10.0	23	0	15	26
Echinomycin	0.01	22	25	9	0
Tiazofurin	1.0	21	19	10	0
	10.0	41	6	11	-

[*]   University of Texas Health Sciences Center, San Antonio

[†]   All points represent one hour exposure at the indicated drug concentration. For the ten drugs marked with dagger (†), the colon colonies were less sensitive than all other lines tested for at least one concentration.

[‡]   BCNU - bis-chloroethyl nitrosourea.

Table 3. Drugs Tested in the Human Tumor Stem Cell Assay[*]

		Cumulative Results			
		% Colonies Sensitive			
Drug	Concentration (μg/ml)	Colon	Breast	Ovary	Lymphoma
[†]Fludarabine	1.0	14	27	16	44
	10.0	40	44	20	78
[†]5-Fluorouracil	6.0	13	15	15	60
	10.0	11	6	14	0
[†]Doxorubicin	0.04	11	12	15	22
	0.40	27	20	11	25
[†]BCNU	0.1	10	40	25	33
[†]Bisantrene	10.0	16	28	31	72 (5 μg/ml)
[†]Dihydroxy-anthracenedione	0.05	10	20	18	29
[†]Melphalan	0.1	16	20	22	43
[†]Mitomycin-C	0.1	14	18	15	60
[†]Cisplatin	0.2	14	20	17	50
[†]Vincristine	0.01	10	9	27	44
[†]Vinblastine	0.05	26	19	16	66
	10.0	18	35	27	33
Methylglyoxal-bis-guanyl-hydrazone	10.0	17	7	11	24
Tiazofurin	1.0	19	15	14	22
	10.0	31	10	11	33
Echinomycin	0.01	22	26	9	0

[*]   University of Texas Health Sciences Center, San Antonio

[†]   Each point is the cumulative result of all tests at the given drug concentration conducted either for 1 or 2 hours of exposure or for continuous exposure. For the eleven drugs marked with a dagger (†), the colon colonies were less sensitive than all other lines tested, at least at one drug concentration.

[‡]   BCNU - bis-chloroethyl nitrosourea

IN VITRO STUDIES OF CYTOTOXICITY AND DNA DAMAGE

In vitro studies comparing the sensitivity of colon cancer cells in culture to those of other types also support these conclusions. Several current studies at Georgetown University are directed at identifying the responsiveness of cells to drugs, radiation, or interferon alone or in combination and at identifying possible synergistic interaction between these modalities in producing cytotoxicity. Figure 1 shows the responses of several cell lines to radiation, nitrogen mustard, and 5-FU. In each case, the HT-29 cells are less sensitive than the leukemia and lymphoma cell lines. While the resistance of the HT-29 cells is relative and not absolute, the disparity between them and the leukemia and lymphoma lines is clear.

Table 4. Fast Green Dye-Exclusion Assay of Drug Effects Upon a Sample of Colon Tumor Obtained at Laparotomy

Drug	Concentration (mcg/ml)	Interpretation
Nitrogen Mustard	3.5	+
	1.7	-
Doxorubicin	1.2	-
Mitomycin-C	10	-
Cisplatin	1.0	-
5-Fluorouracil	50	-
Methotrexate	500	-
5-Fluorouracil/Nitrogen Mustard	50/3.5	+
	5/0.35	-

+ = tumor sensitive to drug

- = tumor resistant to drug

Further studies at Georgetown may suggest a biologic basis for this resistance. Using the alkaline elution assay developed by Kohn (17), we have examined the ability of radiation to produce single- and double-strand breaks in the DNA of the cell lines mentioned in Figure 1. Figure 2 shows the rate of production of single-strand breaks in these cells as a function of the radiation dose. In this Figure, an increased rate of single-strand break formation is reflected by an increased slope of the curve. There is a distinct difference between the lymphoma-leukemia cell lines and the colon cell line. The wide disparity between the radiation survival of HT-29 colon cells and a group of leukemia and lymphoma lines is paralleled by a resistance of the colon HT-29 line to formation of single-strand breaks by radiation. A similar phenomenon is shown in Figure 3, which presents double-strand break formation as a function of radiation dose in six cell lines. The line most resistant to double-strand breakage is colon HT-29, while the most sensitive is the Molt 3 lymphoma line. The Molt 4 and Daudi lymphoma lines are intermediate. Thus, there is once again a close correlation between sensitivity to radiation as measured by colony formation and induction of double-strand breaks by

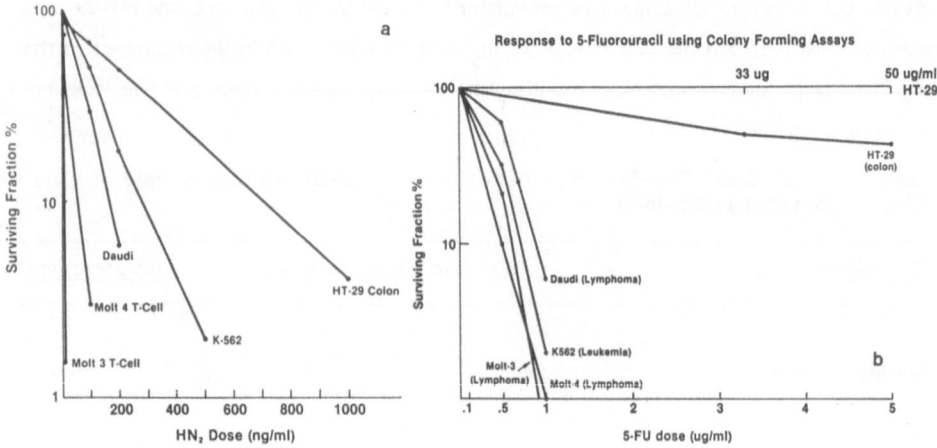

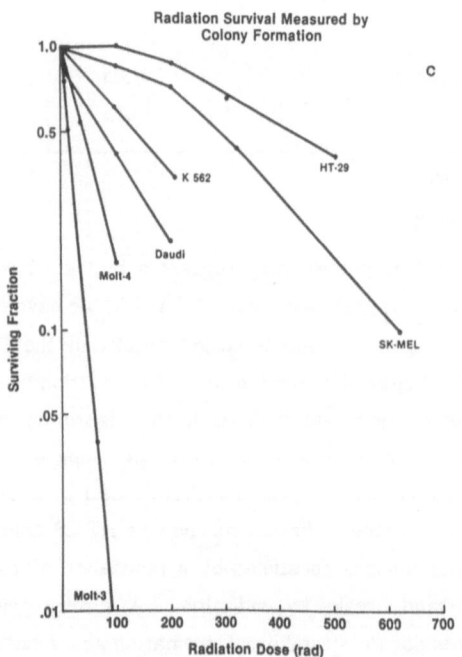

FIGURE 1. The response of several cell lines to nitrogen mustard (HN₂) (1a), 5-fluorouracil (5-FU) (1b), and radiation (1c), as determined by formation of colonies in soft agar. Note that the scale for the HT-29 cell line in Figure 1b is given at the top and is not identical to the scale for the leukemia and lymphoma cells.

302

external radiation. These data demonstrate the relative stability of the chromatin complex of colon tumor cells (HT-29) to radiation damage as compared to leukemia and lymphoma cells. The basis of this resistance is not evident from these experiments, but it deserves further investigation. It is also noteworthy that other investigators have shown a correlation between the DNA repair capacity of colon cancer cells and their sensitivity to cytotoxic drugs. Erickson and Kohn (18,19) have demonstrated that cell lines capable of excising 0^6-ethylguanine residues produced by bis-chloroethyl nitrosourea (BCNU) (Mer$^+$) are less sensitive to the cytotoxic effects of BCNU than are cells that cannot excise such damage (Mer$^-$). It seems likely that the biologic resistance of colon cancer to drugs and radiation is a multifactorial phenomenon that depends both upon resistance to DNA damage and the repair of that damage once it occurs.

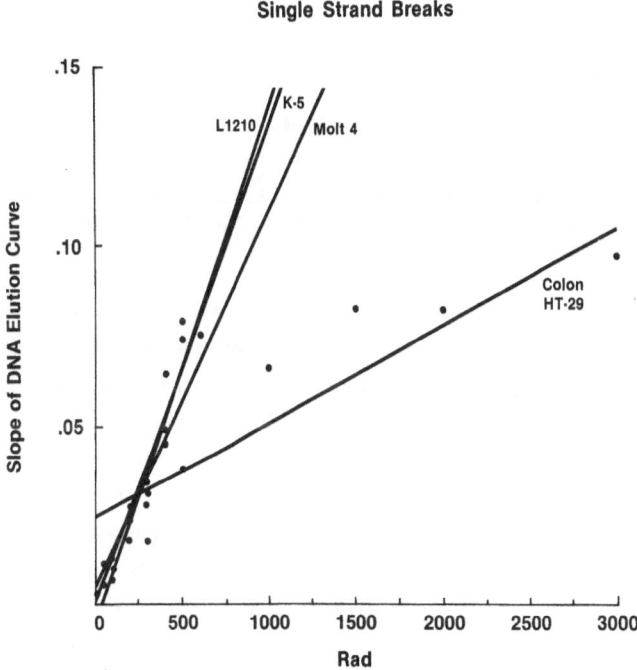

FIGURE 2. The production of single-strand breaks in the DNA of several cell types by radiation. Those curves with the greater slopes represent more DNA damage than those with the lesser slopes. Thus, HT-29 is the least susceptible to DNA strand breaks caused by radiation.

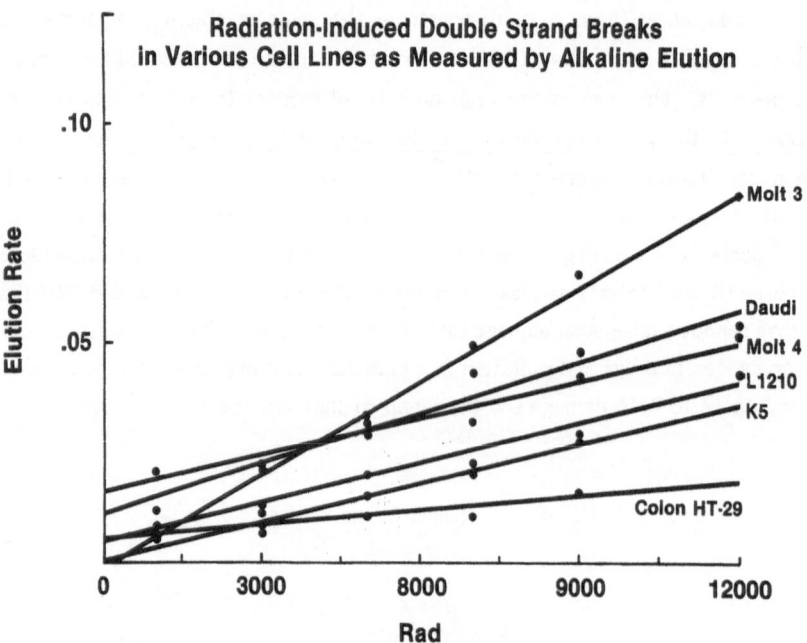

FIGURE 3. Double-strand breaks in the DNA of several cell types caused by radiation. As was the case in the single-strand break assay, the HT-29 colon cells are the least sensitive to double-strand breaks by radiation.

However, not all resistance to cytotoxic agents is mediated at the chromatin level. Data to demonstrate this come from our studies of alpha interferon and its effects upon HT-29 colon cancer cells and other cell lines. Alpha interferon is currently undergoing extensive evaluation as a therapeutic modality in cancer. It is directly cytotoxic to some cancer cells and also participates in cell-mediated tumor growth inhibition by stimulating certain natural killer (NK) cell populations. Recent clinical trials of alpha interferon have shown it to be ineffective in colon cancer (20). The effect of alpha interferon upon colony formation of HT-29 cells (Figure 4) is biphasic, suggesting a heterogenous cell population, part of which is responsive to interferon. Furthermore, alpha interferon shows synergy with other agents in its cytotoxic effects upon some cell lines, e.g., K562 leukemia cells. This cell line is responsive to alpha interferon, to 5-FU, and to nitrogen mustard as single agents. When combinations of

5-FU and interferon are examined for cytotoxic effects on K562 cells and the results are plotted on an isobologram, a synergistic interaction between the two drugs is seen. These results are illustrated in Figure 5, which displays 45% survival of K562 cells at combinations of interferon and 5-FU far below the 45% isoeffect lines. Other studies have demonstrated synergy between interferon and nitrogen mustard and interferon and radiation in killing this leukemia cell line. However interferon is not synergistic with radiation or nitrogen mustard in its effects upon HT-29 cells. Thus another feature of the resistance of HT-29 cells to treatment is a lack of synergy between interferon and either nitrogen mustard or radiation. In the case of interferon and 5-FU, however, some evidence of synergy has been noted.

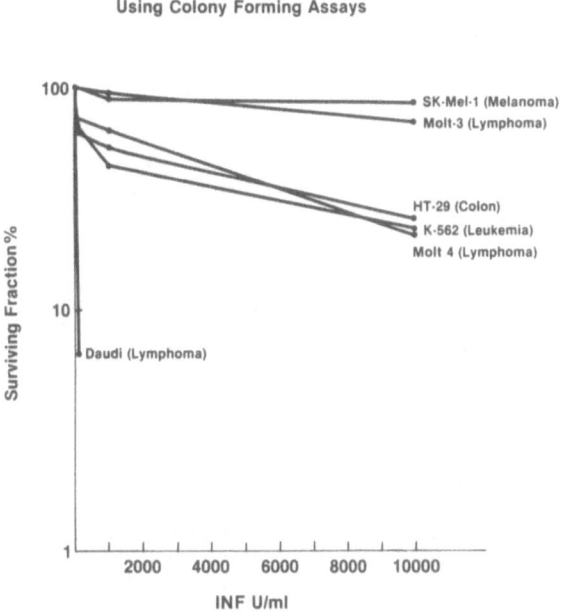

FIGURE 4. The inhibition of colony formation in several cell types by purified alpha interferon.

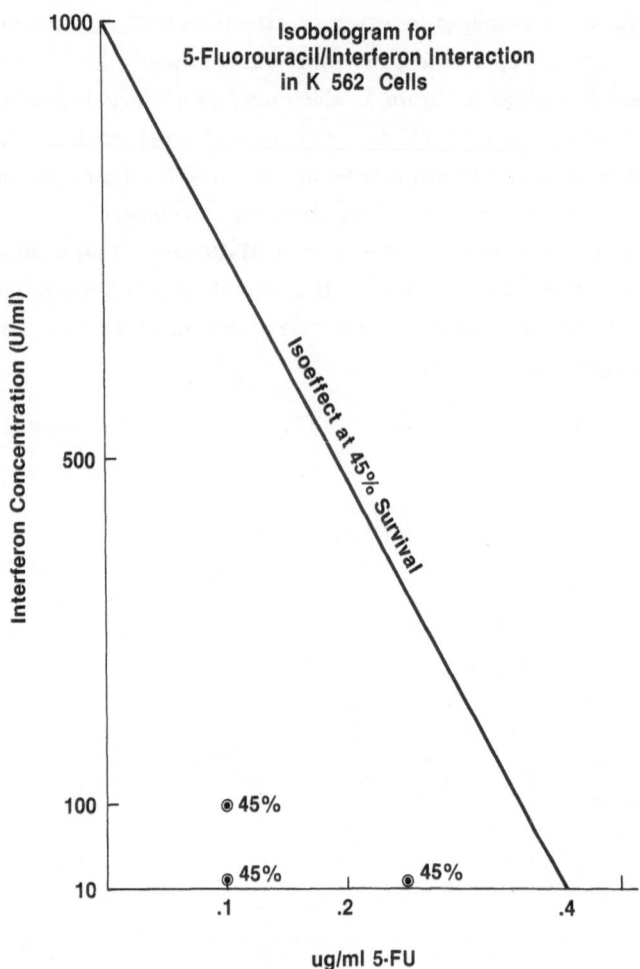

FIGURE 5. Studies with combinations of interferon and 5-fluorouracil, showing that at the 45% isoeffect level, these agents produce combined effects other than would be predicted by simple addition of their separate cytotoxic capabilities.

As part of these studies, we have asked whether synergistic effects between interferon and alkylating agents or radiation are the results of the potentiation by interferon of the effects of these agents upon DNA. Thus, since radiation produces strand breaks in DNA, it is of interest to know whether interferon increases that effect. Likewise it could be asked whether interferon interferes with the DNA repair that follows radiation damage. Finally, since nitrogen mustard and other chloroethyl alkylating agents induce cross-links between both DNA strands and between DNA and protein, we wondered whether interferon potentiates this cross-linking process in cells treated with nitrogen mustard. We have examined these questions using alkaline elution analysis, both in cell lines resistant to interferon and in lines for which interferon and nitrogen mustard or radiation have synergistic effects. In all cases, interferon as a single agent does not induce single- or double-strand breaks in cellular DNA. This result is independent of whether the cells are sensitive or resistant to the cytotoxic effects of interferon. Furthermore, interferon neither potentiates the rate of strand break formation by radiation in cells nor inhibits the repair of these lesions following radiation exposure. Finally, interferon does not potentiate the formation of cross-links in the chromatin complex by nitrogen mustard. While these experiments do not define the mechanism of resistance of HT-29 cells to interferon alone or to the synergy between interferon and other agents, they do say what this resistance is not. Sensitivity to the combined effects of interferon and radiation or alkylating agents is not the result of increased DNA damage or inhibition of DNA repair caused by interferon exposure or the potentiation of the cross-linking effects of nitrogen mustard.

CONCLUSION

Thus, we can make the following general statements about the biology of colon cancer resistance to treatment. First, on the basis of both clinical observation and laboratory evidence, this disease possesses demonstrable resistance to many drugs and to radiation. This resistance is probably multifactorial. For example, broad resistance to drugs of diverse mechanisms of action has been termed pleiotropic resistance (for review, see 21,22). This may be a membrane-mediated phenomenon that is dependent upon the synthesis of specific glycoproteins or other substances. However, another facet of this phenomenon is the relative stability of the chromatin of HT-29 cells to radiation damage. Presumably this could be mediated by chromatin proteins that stabilize the DNA. This is an area that deserves further research. Since other workers have shown that efficient repair of DNA confers resistance to alkylating agents, both induction of damage and repair of this damage are active processes that may vary between resistant and sensitive cells. Finally, colon cancer is relatively resistant to interferon, but this resistance is not mediated at the chromatin level. Given our lack of success with empiric drug trials in this disease, it is imperative at this point to undertake an intensive

307

investigation of the biology of the multiple factors that contribute to the resistance of colon tumor cells to treatment and to develop rational approaches to overcome this resistance in an effort to introduce effective therapeutic modalities into the clinical arena.

ACKNOWLEDGMENT

This research is supported in part by funds from Hoffman-LaRoche Corporation (KLM,PVW), NCI grant CA 27733 (DDVH), and American Cancer Society grant CH162C (DDVH).

References

1. Ansfield F, Klotz J, Nealon T, Ramirez G, Minton J, Hill G, Wilson W, Davis H, Cornell G: A phase III study comparing the clinical utility of four regimens of 5-fluorouracil. Cancer 39: 34-40, 1977.
2. Moertel CG, Schutt AJ, Hahn RG, Reitemeier RJ: Therapy of advanced colorectal cancer with a combination of 5-fluorouracil, methyl-1-3-(2-chloroethyl)-1-nitrosourea, and vincristine. J Natl Cancer Inst 54: 69-71, 1975.
3. Macdonald JS, Kisner DF, Smythe T, Woolley PV, Smith L, Schein PS: 5-Fluorouracil, methyl-CCNU and vincristine in treatment of advanced colorectal cancer: A phase II study utilizing weekly 5-fluorouracil. Cancer Treat Rep 60: 1597-1600, 1976.
4. Engstrom PF, MacIntyre JM, Douglass HO Jr, Muggia F, Mittelman A: Combination chemotherapy of advanced colorectal cancer utilizing 5-fluorouracil, semustine, dacarbazine, vincristine, and hydroxyurea: A phase III trial by the Eastern Cooperative Oncology Group (EST: 4275). Cancer 49: 1555-1560, 1982.
5. Windschitl H, Scott M, Schutt A, McCormack G, Everson L, Cullinan S, Gerstner J, Krook J, Laurie J, Shreck R, Marschke R, Pfeifle D: Randomized phase II studies in advanced colorectal carcinoma: A North Central Cancer Treatment Group study. Cancer Treat Rep 67: 1001-1008, 1983.
6. Gastrointestinal Tumor Study Group: Adjuvant therapy of colon cancer. Results of a prospectively randomized trial. N Engl J Med 310: 737-743, 1984.
7. Higgins FA, Lee LE, Dwight RW, Keehn RJ: The case for adjuvant 5-fluorouracil in colorectal cancer. Cancer Clin Trials 1: 35-41, 1978.
8. Bertino JR, Sawicki WL, Lindquist CA, Gupta VS: Schedule-dependent antitumor effects of methotrexate and 5-fluorouracil. Cancer Res 37: 327-328, 1977.
9. Machover D, Schwarzenberg L, Goldschmidt E, Tourani JM, Michalski B, Hayat M, Dorval T, Misset JL, Jasmin C, Maral R, Mathe G: Treatment of advanced colorectal and gastric adenocarcinomas with 5-FU combined with high-dose folinic acid: A pilot study. Cancer Treat Rep 66: 1803-1807, 1982.
10. Howell SB, Wung WE, Taetle R, Hussain F, Romine JS: Modulation of 5-fluorouracil toxicity by allopurinol in man. Cancer 48: 1281-1289, 1981.
11. Spiegelman S, Nayak R, Sawyer R, Stolfi R, Martin D: Potentiation of the antitumor activity of 5-FU by thymidine and its correlation with the formation of (5-FU) RNA. Cancer 45: 1129-1134, 1980.

12. Weiss GR, Ervin TJ, Meshad MW, Kufe DW: Phase II trial of combination therapy with continuous-infusion PALA and bolus-injection 5-FU. Cancer Treat Rep 66: 299-303, 1982.

13. Van Putten CM, Sluijter EA, Smink T, Mulder JH: Why do colon tumors respond poorly to chemotherapeutic agents? Recent Results Cancer Res 79: 10-18, 1981.

14. Ensminger WD, Gyves JW: Regional chemotherapy of neoplastic diseases. Pharmacol Ther 21: 277-293, 1983.

15. Howell SB, Pfeifle CE, Olshen RA: Intraperitoneal chemotherapy with melphalan. Ann Intern Med 101: 14-18, 1984.

16. Weisenthal LM, Marsden JA, Dill PL, Macaluso CK: A novel dye exclusion method for testing in vitro chemosensitivity of human tumors. Cancer Res 43: 749-757, 1983.

17. Kohn KW, Ewig RAG, Erickson LC, Zwelling LA: Measurement of strand-breaks and cross-links by alkaline elution. In: EC Friedberg and PC Hanawalt (eds), DNA repair, A laboratory manual of research procedures. Marcel Dekker, New York, 1981, pp 379-401.

18. Zlotgorski C, Erickson LC: Pretreatment of normal human fibroblasts and human colon carcinoma cells with MNNG allows chloroethylnitrosourea to produce DNA interstrand cross-links not observed in cells treated with chloroethylnitrosourea alone. Carcinogenesis 4: 759-763, 1983.

19. Erickson LC, Bradley MO, Ducore JM, Ewig RAG, Kohn KW: DNA cross-linking and cytotoxicity in normal and transformed human cells treated with antitumor nitrosoureas. Proc Natl Acad Sci USA 77: 467-471, 1980

20. Silgals RM, Ahlgren JD, Neefe JR, Rothman J, Rudnick S, Galicky FP, Schein PS: A phase II trial of high-dose intravenous interferon alpha-2 in advanced colorectal cancer. Cancer 54: 2257-2261, 1984.

21. Curt GA, Clendininn NJ, Chabner BA: Drug resistance in cancer. Cancer Treat Rep 68: 87-99, 1984.

22. Goldie JH, Coldman AJ: The genetic origin of drug resistance in neoplasms: Implications for sytemic therapy. Cancer Res 44: 3643-3653, 1984.

25

CIRCUMVENTION OF NEOPLASTIC HETEROGENEITY BY SYSTEMICALLY ACTIVATED MACROPHAGES

Isaiah J. Fidler, J. Milburn Jessup, Eugenie S. Kleinerman,
William E. Fogler and Amitabha Mazumder

SUMMARY

The continuous growth of metastases that are resistant to conventional therapies is the major cause of death from colorectal carcinoma. Recent data indicate that metastases can arise from the nonrandom spread of specialized subpopulations of cells that preexist within the primary tumor, that metastases can be clonal in their origin, that different metastases can originate from different progenitor cells, and that metastatic cells can have an increased rate of spontaneous mutation as compared with benign, nonmetastatic cells. Therefore, the successful therapy of disseminated metastases will have to circumvent the problems of cancer heterogeneity and the development of tumor cell resistance to therapy.

Appropriately activated macrophages can fulfill these demanding criteria. Macrophages obtained from normal donors or from patients with colorectal carcinoma can be activated to become tumoricidal subsequent to endocytosis of phospholipid vesicles (liposomes) containing specific immunomodulators. Macrophages thus activated can recognize and destroy neoplastic cells in vitro or in vivo, while leaving nonneoplastic cells unharmed. Moreover, macrophage destruction of tumor cells is not associated with the development of tumor cell resistance.

The major limitations of many cancer therapies are their lack of selectivity against cancer cells. The ability of tumoricidal human monocytes to distinguish neoplastic from bystander nonneoplastic cells, therefore, presents an attractive possibility for treatment of disseminated cancer.

INTRODUCTION

The treatment of colorectal cancer metastases poses the most formidable problem to the clinical oncologists treating this dreadful disease. By the time many colorectal cancers are diagnosed, micrometastases are already present in visceral organs, such as the liver, making surgical removal impossible. Exacerbating the problem of treating metastases is the fact that cancer cells in different metastases, and within a single metastasis, may respond differently to radiotherapy or chemotherapy. The rapid emergence of metastases that are resistant to conventional therapeutics is due in part to the heterogeneous nature of malignant neoplasms (1,2). The cellular heterogeneity of neoplasms has been appreciated since the 1800s, when histologic observations of malignant neoplasms characterized them as pleomorphic. More recently, cells obtained from animal and human neoplasms are phenotypically diverse with regard to virtually all biologic characteristics, including immunogenic properties, cell surface receptors and products, response to a variety of cytotoxic agents, invasion, and metastatic potential (1,2). Recent data from our laboratory and many others indicate that metastases can arise from the nonrandom spread of specialized subpopulations of cells that preexist with the primary tumor (3), that metastases can be clonal in their origin, and that different metastases can originate from different progenitor cells (4). Such data provide an explanation for the clinical observations that even within the same patient, different metastases can exhibit different susceptibilities to therapeutic modalities, such as chemotherapy (1). The implication of the varied responses of tumor cells to conventional treatment modalities, is that the successful therapy of disseminated metastases will have to circumvent the problems of biologic heterogeneity and the development of resistance by tumor cells.

There is a growing body of evidence suggesting that macrophages activated to the tumoricidal state can fulfill these demanding tasks (5). In this chapter, we review some of the evidence to support this suggestion as well as summarize work from our laboratories that deals with the in vitro properties of activated human monocytes, as well as with methods to achieve the in situ activation of macrophages and the destruction of established metastases in experimental animals.

Although macrophages can play a prominent role in host defense against neoplasia, in reality this is but a minor function of these versatile cells. Cells of the macrophage-histiocyte series are important components of the host system responsible for homeostasis. A primary function of macrophages in the body is the clearance and catabolism of aged cells, cellular debris, and serum proteins. The removal of effete red blood cells is a continuous process that requires that macrophages distinguish old from young cells, as well as damaged from healthy cells (6). Macrophages are also involved in the controlled metabolism of lipids and iron, in host response to injury and inflammation, and in the defense against microbial and parasitic infestations. Macrophages are also an important component of both the afferent and efferent arms of the immune system, and finally, these cells can be important in the defense against neoplasms (reviewed in 5).

ACTIVATION OF HUMAN BLOOD MONOCYTES BY IMMUNOMODULATORS ENTRAPPED IN LIPOSOMES

Continuous functions of macrophages (removal of aged red blood cells) do not require that the phagocytes receive activation stimuli. In contrast, rare functions, such as antitumor properties, are not carried out by normal macrophages. Rather, macrophages must receive activation signals to acquire appreciable antitumor properties. There are two major pathways to achieve macrophage activation in vivo. Frequently, macrophages are activated as a consequence of their interaction with micro-organisms or their products, for example, endotoxins, the bacterial cell wall skeleton, and small components of the bacterial cell wall skeleton such as muramyl dipeptide (MDP) (7,8). In vivo activation of macrophages can also take place after their interaction with soluble mediators released by sensitized lymphocytes. The soluble lymphokine that induces macrophage activation is referred to as macrophage-activating factor (MAF) (9,10). MAF specifically interacts with monocytes or macrophages bearing appropriate surface receptors (10). Macrophages rendered tumoricidal in vitro by MAF or MDP acquire the ability to recognize and destroy neoplastic cells both in vitro and in vivo by a mechanism that requires cell-to-cell contact (11). The ability of tumoricidal macrophages to recognize and selectively destroy neoplastic cells while leaving non-neoplastic cells unharmed has been demonstrated in a wide range of experimental systems (5,9,12).

Because macrophages from tumor-bearing animals can respond to activating stimuli and become tumoricidal (reviewed in 5), finding a means to activate macrophages in situ becomes desirable. Early attempts to activate macrophages by the systemic administration of crude preparations of lymphokines have not been successful. Although intratumoral inoculation of lymphokine preparations containing MAF induced partial regression of human skin tumors (13-15), the in vivo administration of lymphokines to bring about systemic activation of macrophages has not been accomplished. After injection into the circulation, lymphokines have short half-lives, because they rapidly bind to serum proteins (9). Moreover, many crude lymphokine preparations are antigenic, and therefore, their repeated administration may not be feasible. Another serious obstacle to therapeutic activation of macrophages in situ by crude lymphokines may be the fact that macrophages are susceptible to lymphokine activation for only three to four days after their emigration from the circulation into tissues (16,17). Once activated, macrophages are tumoricidal for only three-to-four days, and with the decay of their tumoricidal properties, they are refractory to reactivation by soluble MAF (17). The therapeutic use of synthetic MDP has also been hindered because, after parenteral administration, this agent is cleared from the circulation within 60 minutes and excreted

313

in the urine (18). This brief period of availability is insufficient to render macrophages tumoricidal even under ideal in vitro conditions (19,20).

Advances in liposome technology have provided a mechanism for activating macrophages in situ with soluble MAF, MDP, or both. Liposomes can be used to carry agents to cells of the reticuloendothelial system, since these cells are responsible for the rapid clearance of particulate material from the circulation. There are several advantages to using liposome-encapsulated materials to activate cells of the macrophage-histiocyte series in vivo. Liposomes are nonimmunogenic, and thus elicitation of allergic reactions commonly associated with the systemic administration of other immune adjuvants may be avoided (21). In several rodent systems, the encapsulation into liposomes of MDP alone, MAF alone, or both agents has been highly effective in activating macrophages' antitumor properties in vitro (5,16,22-27) and in vivo (25-32). Furthermore, as discussed below, multiple intravenous (i.v.) injections of liposomes containing immunomodulators into mice with well-established spontaneous lung and lymph node metastases resulted in the activation of tumoricidal properties of lung macrophages and the eradication of the metastases (27-32).

In the first set of experiments, we set out to determine whether the in vitro incubation of human blood monocytes with liposomes containing the lymphokine MAF (33,34) or a lipophilic analog of MDP, muramyl tripeptide phosphatidylethanolamine (MTP-PE, 35) would result in the monocytes' activation to the tumoricidal state. Peripheral blood mononuclear cells were obtained from normal donors by separation on a Percoll gradient. The adherent monocytes were incubated with free or liposome-entrapped MAF produced from concanavalin-A-stimulated allogeneic lymphocytes and with free or liposome-entrapped MDP. The control and treated monocytes were tested for cytotoxic activity against radiolabeled (^{125}IUdR) allogeneic tumor cells. The activated monocytes lysed tumorigenic melanoma target cells, but not normal cells. The endocytosis of liposomes containing immunomodulators, but not of those containing control compounds, led to the activation of cytotoxic properties in the monocytes. Activation by liposome-encapsulated MDP or MAF was very efficient and required less than 1/800 of the amount of free agents necessary to achieve the same levels of cytotoxicity (33-35). Control studies concluded that the activation of monocytes to become tumoricidal was caused by either MDP or by MAF and was not attributed to contamination with endotoxins, concanavalin-A, or gamma interferon.

The phagocytosis of multilamellar vesicles (MLV) by human monocytes was influenced by the chemical composition and the surface charge of the liposomes. Essentially, negatively charged MLV consisting of phosphatidylcholine-phosphatidylserine

(PC/PS) (7:3 molar ratio) bound to and were more rapidly endocytosed by blood monocytes than neutral MLV consisting of PC alone (27). PC/PS MLV are therefore better suited to deliver agents intracellularly to the human monocytes. The in vitro interaction of MLV-containing immunomodulators with monocytes resulted in the activation of the monocytes to lyse allogeneic tumor cells, but not of normal cells (33-36). Monocyte activation by liposome-encapsulated MAF or MDP was not caused by free material released from leaky liposomes. We base this conclusion on data of experiments in which the incubation of monocytes with liposomes containing medium and suspended in the same amount of free MAF or MDP as contained within the liposomes did not activate monocyte tumoricidal activity. This finding also demonstrates that the mere binding of MLV to the monocyte surface did not render the cells responsive to lower amounts of activators leaking out of the liposomes. In addition, our studies show that liposome-encapsulated MAF or MDP activated tumoricidal activity of normal monocytes, thus supporting the hypothesis that monocyte-mediated cytotoxicity can be induced by the interaction of immunomodulators with intracellular sites (5).

These data show that at least in vitro, human monocytes respond well to allogeneic MAF or muramylpeptides entrapped within liposomes to become cytotoxic against tumorigenic targets.

THE INTERACTION OF TUMORICIDAL HUMAN MONOCYTES WITH HETEROGENEOUS NEOPLASMS

Rodent macrophages activated by liposome-entrapped MAF, MDP, or both acquire the ability to recognize and lyse neoplastic cells by a mechanism that requires cell-to-cell contact (11, 37-39). In the next set of studies, we investigated whether human blood monocytes activated to the tumoricidal state by interaction with liposomes containing MAF or MDP could also discriminate between tumorigenic and nontumorigenic human target cells under conditions of cocultivation that more closely resemble in vivo conditions (36). We used highly purified preparations (> 98%) of human blood monocytes devoid of spontaneous cytotoxicity. Monocytes incubated with liposomes containing control substances did not lyse the allogeneic A375 melanoma, HT-29 colon carcinoma, or glioblastoma targets. In contrast, the incubation of the blood monocytes with liposomes containing immunomodulators generated cytotoxic properties against the three tumorigenic target cells, but not against three nontumorigenic target cells.

To assess whether tumoricidal human blood monocytes could selectively lyse neoplastic cells, we examined their ability to discriminate between tumorigenic and normal cells under cocultivation conditions. This experiment was repeated several times with monocytes from different donors. Tumorigenic A375 melanoma, HT-29 colon carcinoma, or NAT-glioblastoma and nontumorigenic lung cells, dermal fibroblasts, or kidney cells were prelabeled with either ^{3}H-thymidine or ^{14}C-thymidine. Various combinations of tumor and normal cells were cultured alone, with control monocytes, or with tumoricidal monocytes for 72 hours. Control monocytes were not cytotoxic against any of the tumorigenic or nontumorigenic targets. Monocytes preincubated with liposomes containing immunomodulators (MAF or MDP) lysed tumorigenic A375 melanoma, HT-29 colon carcinoma, and glioblastoma cells, but left the lung cells, dermal fibroblasts, or kidney cells unharmed. The ability of tumoricidal monocytes to lyse allogeneic tumor cells was independent of the radiolabel used. In all the combinations, activated monocytes lysed neoplastic cells but not nonneoplastic cells. Moreover, when two different tumorigenic target cells were cocultivated with activated monocytes, release of both ^{3}H and ^{14}C was detected. In contrast, neither radiolabel was released from cocultivated cultures of nontumorigenic target cells (36).

IN VITRO ACTIVATION OF BLOOD MONOCYTES OBTAINED FROM PATIENTS WITH COLORECTAL CARCINOMAS

These data raise the possibility that similar to rodent macrophages, human monocytes-macrophages could be activated in situ to the tumoricidal state by systemically administered immunomodulators encapsulated in liposomes and that this could provide a potential therapeutic modality for enhancing host-mediated destruction of metastases. Prior to embarking on such an ambitious project, it is necessary to examine whether blood monocytes of patients with colorectal carcinoma can respond to activation stimuli delivered via liposomes. Several questions require answers. (1) Can blood monocytes obtained from colorectal carcinoma patients be rendered cytotoxic in vitro against allogeneic tumor targets such as colon carcinoma cells? (2) Does the stage of disease influence the responsiveness of blood monocytes to activation? (3) Do different patients' monocytes respond differently to various activators? (4) Will monocytes of colorectal carcinoma patients be rendered tumoricidal, i.e. destroy tumor cells, but not normal cells?

We studied these questions with blood monocytes obtained from 11 patients with colorectal carcinomas (Dukes' A, 1; Dukes' B, 5; Dukes' C, 4; Dukes' D,1) and from 8 normal donors. The monocytes were used in parallel studies on the same day as positive controls. All blood monocytes were incubated for 24 hours in vitro with the following immunomodulators: free and liposome-encapsulated lymphokines (MAF), free and lipo-some-encapsulated muramyl peptides (MDP, MTP-PE, or both). Monocytes incubated in medium alone served as negative controls. Monocytes incubated with endotoxins (LPS) served as positive controls. The cytotoxic properties of each patient's monocytes were tested against several allogeneic tumorigenic (A375 melanoma, HT-29 colon carcinoma, and glioblastoma) and nontumorigenic targets (embryonic skin cells or embryonic lung cells).

Control blood monocytes (medium treated) were not spontaneously cytotoxic against the neoplastic cells. Those monocytes activated in vitro with any of the free or the liposome-entrapped agents became tumoricidal, i.e. they lysed neoplastic cells, but not normal cells. Moreover, the level of monocyte-mediated tumor lysis was comparable to that observed with blood monocytes obtained from normal donors.

The data therefore show that blood monocytes of patients with local or disseminated colorectal carcinoma can be activated to become tumoricidal by interaction with various immunomodulators (MAF, MDP, MTP-PE) encapsulated in liposomes. All such activating agents produced the tumoricidal state in the blood monocytes.

IN SITU STIMULATION OF MOUSE MACROPHAGES TO BECOME TUMORICIDAL

The possibility of stimulating monocyte-macrophages in situ by the administration of immunomodulators encapsulated within liposomes could be an attractive approach for augmenting the host's natural defense mechanism. The passive localization of liposomes to phagocytic cells in vivo could provide a highly effective mechanism for directing liposome-encapsulated materials to macrophages (40).

We examined whether the in situ activation of macrophages by i.v. administration of liposomes containing MDP resulted from the direct interaction of MDP and macrophages or whether it occurred indirectly by the action of lymphokines released by sensitized T-cells. We used three groups of mice with impaired T-cell function: mice exposed to ultraviolet radiation, adult thymectomized X-irradiated mice, and athymic nude mice. Mice were given i.v. injections of multilamellar liposomes containing MDP or placebo preparations. Their alveolar macrophages were harvested 24 hr later and assessed for cytotoxic properties against syngeneic tumor targets. Macrophages harvested from all groups of mice became tumoricidal in response to liposome-encapsulated MDP, demonstrating that liposome-MDP activation of macrophages occurred directly and is a thymus-independent process (41).

TREATMENT OF MURINE MELANOMA METASTASES BY SYSTEMICALLY ADMINISTERED IMMUNOMODULATORS ENCAPSULATED IN LIPOSOMES

These data raised the possibility that macrophages activated in situ to the tumoricidal state by systemically administered immunomodulators encapsulated in

317

liposomes could provide a potential therapeutic modality for enhancing host destruction of metastases. To test this possibility, we treated mice bearing spontaneous metastases with i.v. injections of PC/PS-MLV that contained either MAF or MDP or both. We used PC/PS-MLV as carriers because they are not toxic at the dose used here (42) and because they are arrested efficiently in the lungs as well as organs of the reticuloendothelial system following i.v. injections (25,27,40). The B16-BL6 melanoma cell line, which is syngeneic to C57BL/6 mice, was used to determine the effectiveness of liposome-encapsulated immunomodulators in the treatment of metastases. After implantation into the footpad, this tumor metastasizes to lymph nodes and to the lungs in over 90% of the mice (41). The footpad of each C57BL/6 mouse was injected with syngeneic B16-BL6 melanoma cells. Four weeks later, when the implants were 10-12 mm, the leg bearing the tumor, including the popliteal lymph node, was amputated. Three days later, animals were injected intravenously with liposomes containing immunomodulators or placebo preparations. Both test and control groups were treated twice weekly for four weeks. The mice were monitored daily and moribund animals were killed and autopsied to determine the presence of melanoma. Spontaneous metastases in the lung and lymph nodes were well established at the time liposome treatment began. Many individual metastases could be seen microscopically. Nearly all of the mice treated with i.v. injections of control substances or with liposomes containing control substances died by day 90 of the experiment, i.e. 60 days after the resection of the primary tumor. In marked contrast, about 70% of mice injected i.v. with liposome-encapsulated immunomodulators were alive when the experiments were terminated at day 200. In this tumor system, the lymph node and lung metastases contained an estimated 10^7 cells at the time of the first liposome treatment. Since the median survival time of mice injected with as few as 10 viable B16 cells (admixed with 10^6 dead cells) is about 40 days (43), we speculate that the tumor burden in the mice surviving on day 200 must have been reduced to fewer than 10 viable cells. Similar data on the successful treatment of several different mouse cancer metastases systems have now been published (44,45). Studies on mice treated with liposome-encapsulated MDP that have residual metastatic disease (albeit reduced compared with untreated control mice) have revealed that the tumor cells present in the lesions are still fully susceptible to destruction by activated macrophages. This is consistent with the evidence discussed earlier, which suggests that tumor cell resistance to killing by activated macrophages is not likely to be a rate-limiting factor in the effectiveness of liposome-encapsulated macrophage activators. The more challenging problem will be the extent of the tumor burden that can be handled by activated macrophages at the time therapy is initiated.

THE INVOLVEMENT OF ACTIVATED MACROPHAGES IN THE
DESTRUCTION OF MELANOMA METASTASES

The regression of established metastases after the systemic administration of liposomes containing immunomodulators was due to the activation of macrophages to the tumoricidal state. This conclusion is based upon the following: first, administration of macrophage-activating agents encapsulated within liposomes that are not retained in the lung microvasculature failed to activate lung macrophages and no regression of lung metastases was observed. Second, the pretreatment of tumor-bearing animals with agents that are toxic for macrophages (silica, carageenan, hyperchlorinated drinking water) before systemic therapy with liposome-encapsulated immunomodulators abrogated the response to liposome therapy and such animals soon died of metastatic disease. Third, i.v. injection of macrophages activated in vitro by incubation with liposomes containing MAF effects a reduction in the metastatic burden comparable to that achieved by systemic administration of liposome-encapsulated activators (46). Fourth, morphologic and functional analysis of macrophages isolated from pulmonary metastases of mice given i.v. injections of liposomes containing lipophilic MDP revealed that macrophages containing phagocytosed liposomes infiltrate and localize within pulmonary metastases. Furthermore, once localized, macrophages that have engulfed liposomes containing MDP, but not those macrophages that have engulfed liposomes containing control substances, were tumoricidal against the melanoma cells (47).

CONCLUSIONS

Human blood monocytes from normal donors or patients with colorectal carcinomas can be activated in vitro to the tumoricidal state by various immunomodulators entrapped within liposomes. Subsequent to activation, the monocytes acquire the ability to recognize and lyse tumorigenic cells while leaving nontumorigenic cells unharmed, even under conditions of cocultivation. Systemic administration of liposomes containing immunomodulators, such as lymphokines or MDP activate rodent macrophages in situ and thereby augment host resistance against spontaneous metastases. The stimulation of host antitumor responses by liposome-encapsulated lymphokines or MDP does not require the participation of functional T-lymphocytes or natural killer (NK) cells. Rather, the destruction of established metastases after the multiple systemic administration of liposome-encapsulated immunomodulators is directly mediated by activated macrophages.

319

Although the initial results reported from our laboratory regarding the use of macrophages for the destruction of metastases are encouraging, it is unlikely that this therapeutic approach could serve for treatment of large tumor burdens. For this reason, potential therapeutic regimens designed to stimulate host immunity must be used in combination with other treatment modalities, such as chemotherapy, which is used to reduce the tumor burden first; the activated macrophages can then lyse tumor cells that are resistant to the chemotherapy. Colorectal carcinoma metastasizes early and primarily to the liver, an organ rich in reticuloendothelial cells. Directing of liposomes to fixed phagocytes of the liver (Kupffer cells) or to free monocytes can now be achieved with ease. Whether activated liver Kupffer cells or free blood monocytes can destroy hepatic carcinoma micrometastases awaits investigation.

References

1. Fidler IJ, Hart IR: Biological diversity in metastatic neoplasms: Origins and implications. Science 217: 998-1003, 1982.
2. Poste G, Fidler IJ: The pathogenesis of cancer metastasis. Nature 283: 139-146, 1979.
3. Fidler IJ, Kripke ML: Metastasis results from preexisting variant cells within a malignant tumor. Science 197: 893-895, 1977.
4. Talmadge JE, Wolman SR, Fidler IJ: Evidence for the clonal origin of spontaneous metastases. Science 217: 361-363, 1982.
5. Fidler IJ, Poste G: Macrophage-mediated destruction of malignant tumor cells and new strategies for the therapy of metastatic disease. Springer Semin Immunopathol 5: 161-174, 1982.
6. Tanaka Y, Schroit A: Insertion of fluorescent phosphatidylserine into the plasma membrane of red blood cells: Recognition by autologous macrophages. J Biol Chem 258: 11335-11343, 1983.
7. Chedid L, Carelli L, Audibert F: Recent developments concerning muramyl dipeptide, a synthetic immunoregulating molecule. J Reticuloendothel Soc 26: 631-641, 1979.
8. Lederer E: Synthetic immunostimulants derived from the bacterial cell wall. J Med Chem 23: 819-825, 1980.
9. Fidler IJ, Raz A: The induction of tumoricidal capacities in mouse and rat macrophages by lymphokines. In: E Pick (ed) Lymphokines. Academic Press, New York, 1981, pp. 345-363.
10. Poste G, Kirsh R, Fidler IJ: Cell surface receptors for lymphokines. Cell Immunol 44: 71-88, 1979.
11. Bucana C, Hoyer LL, Hobbs B, Breesman S, McDaniel M, Hanna MG Jr: Morphological evidence for the translocation of lysosomal organelles from cytotoxic macrophages into the cytoplasm of tumor target cells. Cancer Res 36: 4444-4458, 1976.
12. Hibbs JB Jr: Discrimination between neoplastic and non-neoplastic cells in vitro by activated macrophages. J Natl Cancer Inst 53: 1487-1492, 1974.
13. Papermaster BW, Gilliand CD, McEntire JE, Rodes ND, Dunn PA: In vivo biological studies with lymphoblastoid lymphokines. In: AL Goldstein and MA Chirigos (eds) Lymphokines and Thymic Hormones: Their Potential Utilization in Cancer Therapeutics. Raven Press, New York, 1981, pp. 289-299.

14. Papermaster BW, Holtermann OA, Rosner D, Klein E, Dao T, Djerassi I: Regressions produced in breast cancer lesions by a lymphokine fraction from a human lymphoid cell line. Res Commun Pathol Pharmacol 8: 413-416, 1974.
15. Salvin SB, Youngner JS, Nishio J, Neta R: Tumor suppression by a lymphokine released into the circulation of mice with delayed hypersensitivity. J Natl Cancer Inst 55: 1233-1236, 1975.
16. Poste G, Kirsh R, Fogler W, Fidler IJ: Activation of tumoricidal properties in mouse macrophages by lymphokines encapsulated in liposomes. Cancer Res 39: 881-892, 1979.
17. Poste G, Kirsh R: Rapid decay of tumoricidal activity and loss of responsiveness to lymphokines in inflammatory macrophages. Cancer Res 39: 2582-2590, 1979.
18. Parant M, Parant F, Chedid L, Yapo A, Petit JF, Lederer E: Fate of the synthetic immunoadjuvant, muramyl dipeptide (^{14}C-labeled) in the mouse. Int J Immunopharmacol 1: 35-41, 1979.
19. Sone S, Fidler IJ: In vitro activation of tumoricidal properties in rat alveolar macrophages by synthetic muramyl dipeptide encapsulated in liposomes. Cell Immunol 57: 42-50, 1981.
20. Sone S, Fidler IJ: Synergistic activation by lymphokines and muramyl dipeptide of tumoricidal properties in rat alveolar macrophages. J Immunol 125: 2454-2460, 1980.
21. Allison AC: Mode of action of immunological adjuvants. J Reticuloendothel Soc 26: 61-630, 1979.
22. Fidler IJ, Raz A, Fogler WE, Hoyer LC, Poste G: The role of plasma membrane receptors and the kinetics of macrophage activation by lymphokines encapsulated in liposomes. Cancer Res 41: 495-504, 1981.
23. Fogler WE, Raz A, Fidler IJ: In situ activation of murine macrophages by liposomes containing lymphokines. Cell Immunol 53: 214-219, 1980.
24. Sone S, Poste G, Fidler IJ: Rat alveolar macrophages are susceptible to activation by free and liposome-encapsulated lymphokines. J Immunol 124: 2197-2201, 1980.
25. Fidler IJ, Raz A, Fogler WE, Kirsh R, Bugelski P, Poste G: Design of liposomes to improve delivery of macrophage-augmenting agents to alveolar macrophages. Cancer Res 40: 4460-4466, 1980.
26. Fidler IJ, Raz A, Fogler WE, Hoyer LC, Poste G. The role of plasma membrane receptors and the kinetics of macrophage activation by lymphokines encapsulated in liposomes. Cancer Res 41: 495-504, 1980.
27. Schroit AJ, Fidler IJ: Effects of liposome structure and lipid composition on the activation of the tumoricidal properties of macrophages by liposomes containing muramyl dipeptide. Cancer Res 42: 161-167, 1982.
28. Fidler IJ: Therapy of spontaneous metastases by intravenous injection of liposomes containing lymphokines. Science 208: 1469-1471, 1980.
29. Fidler IJ, Sone S, Fogler WE, Barnes ZL: Eradication of spontaneous metastases and activation of alveolar macrophages by intravenous injection of liposomes containing muramyl dipeptide. Proc Natl Acad Sci USA 78: 1680-1684, 1981.
30. Fidler IJ, Fogler WE: Activation of tumoricidal properties in macrophages by lymphokines encapsulated in liposomes. Lymphokine Research 1: 73-77, 1982.
31. Fidler IJ: The in situ induction of tumoricidal activity in alveolar macrophages by liposomes containing muramyl dipeptide is a thymus-independent process. J Immunol 127: 1719-1720, 1981.
32. Fidler IJ, Schroit AJ: Synergism between lymphokines and muramyl dipeptide encapsulated in liposomes: In situ activation of macrophages and therapy of spontaneous cancer metastases. J Immunol 133: 515-518, 1984.
33. Kleinerman ES, Schroit AJ, Fogler WE, Fidler IJ: Tumoricidal activity of human monocytes activated in vitro by free and liposome-encapsulated human lymphokines. J Clin Invest 72: 1-12, 1983.

34. Kleinerman ES, Fidler IJ: Production and utilization of human lymphokines containing macrophage-activating factor (MAF) activity. Lymphokine Research 2: 7-12, 1983.

35. Kleinerman, ES, Erickson KL, Schroit AJ, Foler WE, Fidler IJ: Activation of tumoricidal properties in human blood monocytes by liposomes containing lipophilic muramyl tripeptide. Cancer Res 43: 2010-2014, 1983.

36. Fidler IJ, Kleinerman ES: Lymphokine-activated human blood monocytes destroy tumor cells but not normal cells under cocultivation conditions. J Clin Oncol 2: 937-943, 1984.

37. Bucana CD, Hoyer LC, Schroit AJ, Kleinerman E, Fidler IJ: Ultrastructural studies of the interaction between liposome-activated human blood monocytes and allogeneic tumor cells in vitro. Am J Pathol 112: 101-111, 1983.

38. Hibbs JB Jr: Heterocytolysis by macrophages activated by Bacillus Calmette-Guerin: Lysosome exocytosis into tumor cells. Science 184: 468-471, 1974.

39. Fidler IJ: Recognition and destruction of target cells by tumoricidal macrophages. Isr J Med Sci 14: 177-191, 1978.

40. Schroit AJ, Hart IR, Madsen J, Fidler IJ: Selective delivery of drugs encapsulated in liposomes: Natural targeting to macrophages involved in various disease states. J Biol Response Mod 2: 97-100, 1983.

41. Fidler IJ: The in situ induction of tumoricidal activity in alveolar macrophages by liposomes containing muramyl dipeptide is a thymus-independent process. J Immunol 127: 1719-1720, 1981.

42. Hart IR, Fogler WE, Poste G, Fidler IJ: Toxicity studies of liposome-enapsulated immunomodulators administered intravenously into dogs and mice. Cancer Immunol Immunother 10: 157-166, 1981.

43. Griswold DP Jr: Consideration of the subcutaneously implanted B16 melanoma as a screening model for potential anticancer agents. Cancer Chemotherapy Reports 3: 315-323, 1972.

44. Deodhar SD, Barna BP, Edinger M, Chiang T: Inhibition of lung metastases by liposomal immunotherapy in a murine fibrosarcoma model. J Biol Response Mod 1: 27-34, 1982.

45. Lopez-Berestein G, Milas L, Hunter N, Mehta K, Eppstein D, VanderPas MA, Mathews TR, Hersh EM: Prophylaxis and treatment of experimental lung metastases in mice after treatment with liposome encapsulated 6-O-steroyl-N-acetyl muramyl-L-aminobutyryl-D-isoglutamine. Clin Exp Metastasis 2: 366-367, 1984.

46. Fidler IJ, Barnes Z, Fogler WE, Kirsh R, Bugelski P, Poste G: Involvement of macrophages in the eradication of established metastases following intravenous injection of liposomes containing macrophage activators. Cancer Res 42: 496-501, 1982.

47. Key ME, Talmadge JE, Fogler WE, Bucana C, Fidler IJ: Isolation of tumoricidal macrophages from lung melanoma metastases of mice treated systemically with liposomes containing a lipophilic derivative of muramyl dipeptide. J Natl Cancer Inst 69: 1189-1198, 1982.

INDEX

Actinomycin-D, 281, 282
Activated macrophages, in neoplastic
  heterogeneity, 311–320
Adenocarcinomas, colonic
  laser therapy for, 132
  peritoneovenous shunting with, 45
Adjuvant chemotherapy
  liver metastases survival rates and, 12–13
  liver resection with, 160, 164, 176
  quality of life issues with, 93
Adjuvant radiation therapy
  chemotherapy combined with, 151
  colon cancer with, 153–156
  extramural tumor extension and, 146
  failure patterns with, 153
  location of tumor and, 146
  lymph node involvement and, 146
  preoperative use of, 149–150
  rectal cancer with, 146–149
  sandwich technique using, 151
  stage of disease and, 146, 147, 150–151
  strip technique using, 155–156
  surgical extirpation combined with,
    147–149
  treatment techniques with, 149–153
  tumor size and, 153–155
Adrenal gland metastasis, 37
Angiography, computed tomographic,
  183–185
Animal model of colorectal cancer metastasis,
  31–38
Antibodies, radiolabeled, *see* Radiolabeled
  antibodies
Argon laser, 129
  mechanism of, 129–130
  methods using, 130–131
  results with, 131–132
  variables in treatment with, 131
Ascites, malignant
  cellular immune response in, 49
  complications of peritoneovenous shunting
    in, 49–51
  indications for peritoneovenous shunting
    in, 42
  metastatic tumor diversity in, 43
  organ inhibitory effects on, 47–48
  paracentesis in, 41–42
  peritoneovenous shunting for, 41 51
  sites of metastatic cell colonization in,
    43–48

Assays, in clinical response prediction,
  187–195
A375-M cell line, in metastatic capacity
  study, 25, 26, 27
A375-P cell line, in metastatic capacity study,
  25, 26, 27

BCNU
  collateral sensitivity of, 193
  dose response effects of, 194
  soft agar sensitivity testing of, 190
  starch microspheres in hepatic arterial
    chemotherapy (HAC) with, 143
Biliary cancer, intrahepatic, 197, 204
Bone cancer
  computed tomography for, 227
  liver metastases resection and, 276
Brain
  effects of cancer and its treatment on,
    75–76
  quality of life studies of, 76–77, 78
Breast cancer, with 5-fluorouracil (5-FU)
  therapy, 286
5-bromodeoxyuridine (BUdR)
  hepatic arterial chemotherapy (HAC)
    with, 137
  yttrium-90 starch microspheres study with,
    141–142
B16 melanoma cell line, in lectin-reactive
  glycoprotein studies, 58–61

Calcium channel blockers, 281–282
Carafate, in hepatic artery chemotherapy, 110
Carcinoembryonic antigen (CEA)
  response criteria for, 21
  second-look surgery following, 235
  as serial marker, 239–240, 246, 249
CCNU, *see* Methyl chloroethyl cyclohexyl
  nitrosourea (CCNU)
Chemotherapy
  adjuvant, *see* Adjuvant chemotherapy
  adjuvant radiation therapy combined with,
    151
  collateral sensitivity of, 193
  dose response effects in, 194
  drug resistance in, 281–290
  hepatic artery, *see* Hepatic arterial
    chemotherapy (HAC)

quality of life issues with, 91–92, 94
regional, *see* Regional infusion
  chemotherapy
response in, *see* Response criteria
soft agar drug sensitivity testing in,
  190–192
systemic versus regional, 110–114
see also specific drugs
Cimetidine, in hepatic artery chemotherapy,
  110
Cisplatin, resistance to, 281, 282
Cloning, *see* Soft agar cloning technique
Cognitive deficits in head and neck cancer,
  76–77
Collateral sensitivity, 193
Colloid cell tumors, 54, 153
Colon cancer
  drug resistance in, 281–290
  nude mice in study of, 23–29
Combination chemotherapy, drug resistance
  in, 282, 288, 297–298
Computed tomographic angiography,
  183–185
Computed tomography (CT), 179–180
  delayed iodine imaging in, 180
  hepatic-specific agents in, 180
  recurrent disease on, 225–227
  therapeutic response evaluation with,
    227–230
Continuous hepatic arterial chemotherapy,
  104–110
  operative technique in, 106–107
  patients in study of, 105–106
  response of tumor in, 108–109
  results of therapy with, 107–108
  systemic chemotherapy compared with,
    110–114
  toxicity in, 109–110
Cost factors
  medical reimbursement system and, 94–95
  quality of life issues and, 87–88, 93
Cotton-top tamarin model
  biology of cancer in, 32–34
  characteristics of cancer in, 32–38
  frequency of cancer in, 32, 33
  hereditary component in, 34
  histology of cancer in, 34–36
  mean colony ages at death in, 32, 33
  metastatic site in, 31, 37
  potential for metastasis in, 36–38
  primary carcinoma location in, 32, 33

Delayed iodine imaging, 180
Depressive disorder, 76

Dose response effects, 194
Doxorubicin, with radiolabeled antibodies,
  203
Drug resistance, 281–290
  biology of, 295–308
  colony-forming assays for, 298–299
  cytotoxicity and DNA damage in, 300–307
  Phase II single-agent studies in, 288–290,
    296–297
  strategies to overcome, 287–290
Drugs, *see* Chemotherapy *and specific drugs*
DU145 cell line, in metastatic capacity study,
  25, 26, 27
DX-3 cell line, in metastatic capacity study,
  25, 26. 27

Electrocautery, 129
Endoscopic laser surgery, *see* Laser surgery
EOE-13 (emulsion), 180
Esophageal cancer, 134

Fab fragment of IgG, 198, 201
Ferritin, with radiolabeled antibodies,
  199, 200
Floxuridine, 261
5-fluorodeoxyuridine (FUdR)
  continuous hepatic artery infusion with,
    109, 111
  hepatic arterial chemotherapy (HAC) with,
    138
  liver resection with intra-arterial, 176
  quality of life issues in use of, 91, 92
  starch microspheres in arterial
    chemotherapy with, 139, 143
  toxicity with, 109, 114
5-fluorouracil (5-FU)
  adjuvant radiation therapy combined with,
    151
  collateral sensitivity of, 193
  combination chemotherapy with, 102–103
  cytotoxicity with, 109, 283, 284
  dose response effects of, 194
  hepatic arterial chemotherapy (HAC) with,
    138
  liver resection with adjuvant, 160, 176
  mean response time for, 102
  nonlinear pharmacokinetics of, 139–140
  prevention of hepatic metastases with,
    176–177
  quality of life issues in use of, 91, 93
  radiolabeled antibodies with, 203
  resistance to, 281, 282, 283–287, 295–296
  response criteria for, 216–217

soft agar sensitivity testing of, 190, 192
systemic chemotherapy using, 102–103
Functional Living Index for Cancer (FLIC), 97

Gardner's syndrome, 130–133
Gastric cancer, and laser treatment, 134
Gastrointestinal malignancies, with radiolabeled antibodies, 197–206
Goblet cell colorectal carcinoma, 54, 64
Grade of tumor
liver metastases survival time and, 13
metastatic colorectal carcinoma and, 53, 54
primary tumor survival time and, 255–256

Hepatic arterial chemotherapy (HAC)
dog model study of, 141–142
drug resistance and, 287
general principles of, 138–140
limitations of, 139
microcirculation and, 140
pharmacokinetics of, 137–143
starch microspheres with, 140–141
Hepatic metastases, see Liver metastases
Hepatoma, with radiolabeled antibodies,
197, 204
Hodgkin's disease, with radiolabeled antibodies, 204, 205
HT29 cell line
5-fluorouracil (5-FU) resistance and, 287
metastatic capacity study with, 25, 26, 27

Immune response, with peritoneovenous
shunting, 49
Immunoglobulin G(IgG), Fab fragment of,
198, 201
Implantable infusion pump
local surgical treatment of hepatic
metastases compared with, 124, 125
regional hepatic arterial chemotherapy
with, 104
Infusion therapy
advantages and disadvantages of, 95–96
asymptomatic patients and treatment issues
with, 90–91
cost issues in, 87–88
disruption of patient lifestyle with, 87
patient desire for treatment with, 86–87
patient role in selection of, 89–90
quality of life issues with, 83–97
regional, see Regional infusion
chemotherapy
response criteria and, 214, 215

Intraperitoneal chemotherapy, with liver
resection, 160–161, 164, 176

Karnofsky scale, 97

Lactate dehydrogenase (LDH), in liver
metastases, 258
Large bowel cancer, 6
Large cell lymphoma/lymphosarcoma cell
lines, in lectin studies, 61–62
Large cell undifferentiated colorectal
carcinoma, 54, 56
Laser surgery, 129–134
complications with, 133
mechanism of, 129–130
methods using, 130–131
reduction of tumor volume with, 134
results of treatment with, 131–132
variables in treatment with, 131
see also specific types of lasers
Lausanne System for staging, 261
Lectins
biochemical studies of colorectal carcinoma
metastases with, 63–67
blood-borne lung colonization with, 59–61
liver metastases reactivity to, 65–66
murine B16 melanoma cell studies with,
58–61
murine RAW117 large cell lymphoma/
lymphosarcoma cell studies with, 61–62
specificity for particular types of cells
with, 63–64
structural features of carbohydrate chains
with, 61
Leiden classification system for hepatic
metastases, 170–171, 261
Liver metastases
adjuvant chemotherapy and, 12–13
computed tomography of, 227
cotton-top tamarin model of colorectal
cancer with, 31, 36, 37
extent of hepatic involvement with, 11–12,
256–258
lectin selectivity of, 65–66
local surgical treatment of, 117–125
lung metastases coexistent with, 17
multiplicity of, 6
natural history of, 3–19
nude mice study of spread of, 27–29
percentage of large bowel cancer patients
with, 6
peritoneovenous shunting for malignant
ascites in, 45

325

prevention of, 176–177
prognostic factors for, 7–9, 253–256
quality of life with infusion therapy for,
84–95
regional therapy for, 103–104
resection failure in, 267–279
resection surgery for, 159–177
size of metastasis in, 86
stage and grade of primary lesion in, 13
starch microspheres in hepatic arterial
chemotherapy (HAC) in, 142
survival rates after resection of, 7–9, 11–18
therapeutic failure in, 7–10
unresected, natural history of, 11–18
Liver resection, 159–177
adjuvant chemotherapy with, 160, 176
complications with, 166
data sheets used in, 171, 172–175
delaying resection in, 168
distribution of metastases in, 161
literature survey on, 165–170
number of metastases resected in, 161, 169
prognostic factors in, 161, 166,
167–168, 169
size of metastases in, 169
staging of hepatic metastases and, 170–171
survival rates in, 159, 161, 165–166
Local surgical treatment of hepatic
metastases, 117–125
implantable pumps compared with,
124, 125
patients in study of, 118
performance status in, 119, 122
results with, 119–121
surgical mortality rate in, 123
survival times for, 122–123
tumor recurrence data at time of death in,
120–121
unresectable liver metastases compared
with, 119, 121–122
LoVo human colon cell lines
5-fluorouracil (5-FU) and, 286
metastatic capacity study with, 28
LS174T cell line, in metastatic capacity
study, 28
Lung metastases
cotton-top tamarin model of, 36–37
lectin-reactive glycoprotein study of, 59–61
liver lesions coexistent with, 17
resection failure and, 276
Lymph node involvement
adjuvant radiation therapy and, 146, 153
computed tomography of, 227
cotton-top tamarin model of colorectal
cancer metastases and, 35

natural history of hepatic metastases and, 9
peritoneovenous shunting for malignant
ascites and, 43–45
Lymphoma, in lectin-reactive glycoprotein
studies, 61–62
Lymphosarcoma, in lectin-reactive
glycoprotein studies, 61–62

Macrophage activation, with radiolabeled
antibodies, 202
Magnetic resonance imaging (MRI), 185, 232
Mammary tumors, and metastatic cell
colonization, 45–46
Melanoma cells
lectin-reactive glycoprotein studies of,
58–61
nude mice study of metastatic capacity
in, 25
Methyl chloroethyl cyclohexyl nitrosourea
(CCNU)
adjuvant radiation therapy combined
with, 151
combination chemotherapy using, 102–103
response criteria for, 216–217
Mitomycin, with starch microspheres in
hepatic arterial chemotherapy (HAC),
143
Mitoxantrone, dose response effects of,
194, 195
Murine mammary tumors, and metastatic
cell colonization, 45–46

Natural history of liver metastasis, 3–19
adjuvant chemotherapy in, 12–13
extent of hepatic involvement in, 11–12
lung metastases coexisting with liver lesions
in, 17
multiplicity of metastases in, 6
need for data about, 4
present state of study of, 5–7
prognostic determinants in, 7–9
stage and grade of primary lesion in, 13
surgical treatment compared with
unresected metastases in, 18–19
survival rates in, 7–9, 11–18
therapeutic failure and, 7–10
unresected metastases in, 10–18
Neodymium YAG (Nd:YAG) laser, 129
complications with, 133
mechanism of, 130
methods using, 130–131
results with, 131–132
variables in treatment with, 131

Neurobehavioral approach to quality of
life issues, 75–81
application of findings with, 77–79
basis for use of, 75–76
mortality determinants in, 79
organic brain syndrome (OBS) in, 76–79
patient evaluation in, 76
sociologic phenomena in, 79–80
therapeutic success and, 75
Nude mice studies
human colon cancer malignant capacity
in, 27–29
metastatic spread of human tumor cell
in, 24–27

Organic brain syndrome (OBS)
establishing, 78
head and neck cancer and, 76–78
Ovarian cystadenocarcinoma, 43

Pancreas metastasis, 37
Paracentesis for malignant ascites, 41–42
PC3 cell line, in metastatic capacity study,
25, 26, 27
Peritoneovenous shunting
applicability of findings with, 48–49
cellular immune response in, 49
clinicopathologic studies of metastatic
spread with, 41–51
complications with, 49–51
diversity of metastatic tumors in, 43
indications for, 42
introduction of, 42
organ inhibitory effects in, 47–48
sites of metastatic cell colonization
in, 43–48
vascular and lymphatic drainage in, 43–45
Polyps, in laser treatment, 130–133
Prostate carcinoma, in metastatic capacity
study, 25

Quality of life
applicability of findings on, 77–79
asymptomatic patients and treatment issues
in, 90–91
brain function in, 78
chemotherapy use and, 91–92, 94
clinical trial use of, 84
cost issues and, 87–88, 93
doctor-patient interaction and, 90
head and neck cancer studies in, 76–77
hepatic metastases management and, 83–97

infusion therapies and, 83–97
medical reimbursement system and, 94–95
need for no-treatment control group and,
92–93
neurobehavioral approach to, 75–81
patient desire for treatment and, 86–87
patient evaluation in, 76
patient role in treatment selection in, 89–90
public interest in, 80–81
quantitation of data in, 97
sociologic phenomena in, 79–80
treatment disruption of patient lifestyle
in, 87

Radiation enteritis, 156
Radiation therapy, see Adjuvant radiation
therapy
Radiolabeled antibodies
characteristics of, 198–199
clinical trials with, 203–205
concentration of antigen in, 199–200
concentration of tumor of, 200
considerations in therapeutic use of, 197
factors in evaluation of, 198
gastrointestinal malignancies with, 197–206
immune recognition of, 202
isotope characteristics of, 202–203
labeling index of, 201–202
molecular state of, 201
steps to implement applications of,
205–206
Radionuclide imaging, 179, 230
RAW117 large cell lymphoma/lymphosarcoma
cell lines, in lectin studies, 61–62
Recurrent metastases
adjuvant radiation therapy in, 153
diagnostic technique accuracy for, 225–232
local surgical treatment and, 120–121, 124
resection failure and, 279
serial marker data on, 236–237
Regional infusion chemotherapy, 101–114
advantages and disadvantages of, 95–96
anatomic anomalies and, 104–110
best route for, 103–104
implantable, 104
operative technique in, 106–107
quality of life issues in use of, 83–97
results of therapy with, 107–108
systemic chemotherapy compared with,
110–114
toxicity of chemotherapy in, 109–110, 114
tumor response to, 108–109
Renal adenocarcinoma, in metastatic capacity
study, 25

327

Resection
clinical evaluation and management in,
268-269
clinical patterns of failure after, 267-279
patient referral pattern in, 268
survival curves in, 275-276
Response criteria, 211-223
biologic principles of, 214-216
categories of, 212
clinical trials with, 212
data analysis alternatives in, 216-220
growth models with, 215-216
need for revisions to, 222-223
problems with current state of, 213-214
sample size reduction with, 221-222

Sandwich technique in adjuvant radiation
therapy, 151
Senile dementia, Alzheimer's type, 77
Serial tumor markers, 235-250
carcinoembryonic antigen (CEA) as,
239-240
clinical study of, 237-240
five-year suvival rates and, 243-247
recurrence risk prediction with, 236-237
second-look surgery with, 240-243
white blood cell (WBC) counts as, 239
769 cell line, in metastatic capacity study, 25,
26, 27
786-Q cell line, in metastatic capacity study,
25, 26, 27
Signet ring cell colorectal carcinoma, 54
SK-23 cell line, in metastatic capacity study,
25, 26, 27
Social worker, 90
Soft agar cloning technique, 187-195
bypass resistance mechanisms on, 193-194
collateral sensitivity with, 193
drug resistance studies with, 298-299
drug response effects with, 194
drug sensitivity testing with, 190-192
evaluable growth with, 188-189
factors affecting growth in, 189
methods for improving growth in, 189-190
Sonography, 180, 230
Staging
adjuvant radiation and, 146, 147, 150-151
liver metastasis survival rate and, 13
liver resection prognosis and, 170-171
metastatic colorectal carcinoma and, 53
recurrence of disease and, 225-227
soft agar cloning technique and, 189
Starch microspheres in hepatic arterial
chemotherapy (HAC), 140-142
Stomach cancer, with laser treatment, 134

Strip technique with adjuvant radiation
therapy, 155-156
Survival rates
adjuvant chemotherapy in liver metastases
and, 12-13
chemotherapy and, 94
classification schema in, 261
extent of hepatic involvement and, 11-12,
256-258
host factors and, 259
liver metastases resection and, 7-9, 11-18,
159, 161, 165-166
local surgical treatment of hepatic
metastases and, 117-125
lung metastases coexistent with liver lesions
and, 17
mean, 102
multifactorial analyses in, 259-260
performance status (PS) in, 259
primary tumor and, 254-256
serial tumor markers and, 243-247
stage and grade of primary tumor and, 13
surgical treatment compared with
unresected metastases in, 18-19

T-cell dependent antibody toxicity, 202
Tiazofurin, in soft agar sensitivity testing,
191
Treatment Trauma Scale, 97
Tumor markers
response criteria and, 223
serial, 235-250

Unresectable tumors
adjuvant chemotherapy in, 12-13
adjuvant radiation therapy in, 153
extent of hepatic involvement in, 11-12
local surgical treatment compared with,
119, 121-122
natural history of, 10-18
survival rates for, 11-18
treatment approaches to, 124

Villous adenomas, in laser therapy, 133

White blood cell (WBC) counts, as serial
marker, 239

YAG laser, see Neodymium YAG (Nd:YAG)
laser
Yttrium-90 starch microspheres in hepatic
arterial chemotherapy, 141-142

328